SUICIDE
Indian Perspectives

SUICIDE
Indian Perspectives

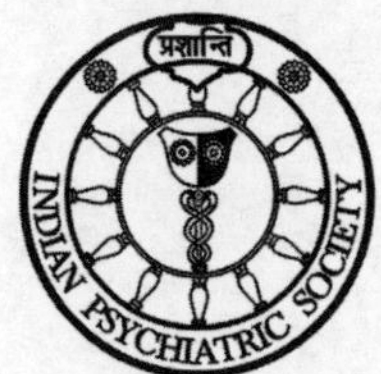

Indian Psychiatric Society Publication

Editors

Sujit Sarkhel MD DPM
Professor of Psychiatry
Institute of Psychiatry
Kolkata, West Bengal, India

Vinay Kumar MD
Consultant Psychiatrist
Manoved Mind Hospital
Patna, Bihar, India

Lakshmi Vijayakumar
MBBS DPM PhD FRCP (Edin) FRCPsych (Hon)
Founder SNEHA
Head Psychiatry
Voluntary Health Services
Chennai, Tamil Nadu, India

Shubhangi R Parkar
DPM MD (Mumbai) MSc PhD (Basel, Switzerland)
Dean
Vedantaa Institute of Medical Sciences
Dahanu, Palghar, Maharashtra, India

Foreword

Danuta Wasserman
President-Elect
World Psychiatric Association

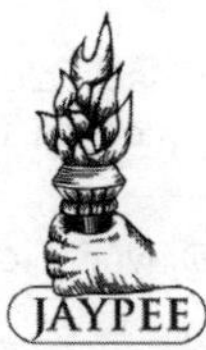

JAYPEE BROTHERS MEDICAL PUBLISHERS
The Health Sciences Publisher
New Delhi | London

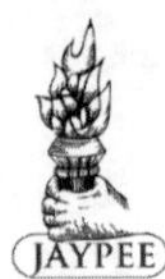 **Jaypee Brothers Medical Publishers (P) Ltd**

Headquarters

Jaypee Brothers Medical Publishers (P) Ltd
EMCA House, 23/23-B
Ansari Road, Daryaganj
New Delhi 110 002, India
Landline: +91-11-23272143, +91-11-23272703
+91-11-23282021, +91-11-23245672
Email: jaypee@jaypeebrothers.com

Corporate Office

Jaypee Brothers Medical Publishers (P) Ltd
4838/24, Ansari Road, Daryaganj
New Delhi 110 002, India
Phone: +91-11-43574357
Fax: +91-11-43574314
Email: jaypee@jaypeebrothers.com

Overseas Office

JP Medical Ltd
83 Victoria Street, London
SW1H 0HW (UK)
Phone: +44 20 3170 8910
Fax: +44 (0)20 3008 6180
Email: info@jpmedpub.com

Website: www.jaypeebrothers.com
Website: www.jaypeedigital.com

Suicide: Indian Perspectives

First Edition: **2023**

ISBN: 978-93-5465-763-4

Printed at: Sterling Graphics Pvt. Ltd. India

Contributors

Abdul Faheem MD
Additional Professor and Senior Resident
Department of Psychiatry
Jawaharlal Institute of
Postgraduate Medical Education and Research
Puducherry, India

Amrit Pattojoshi MD DPM
Professor, Department of Psychiatry
Hi-Tech Medical College
Bhubaneshwar, Odisha, India

Anish V Cherian PhD
Associate Professor
Department of Psychiatric Social Work
National Institute of Mental Health and
Neurosciences (NIMHANS)
Bengaluru, Karnataka, India

Anuradha Patil MD
Assistant Professor, MGM Medical College
Aurangabad, Maharashtra, India

Anuranjan Vishwakarma MD
Senior Resident, Department of Psychiatry
All India Institute of Medical Sciences
New Delhi, India

Bevinahalli Nanjegowda Raveesh
MBBS MD PGDMLE
Professor, Department of Psychiatry
Mysore Medical College and Research Institute
(MMCRI)
Mysore, Karnataka, India
Former Director
Dharwad Institute of Mental Health and
Neurosciences (DIMHANS)
Dharwad, Karnataka, India

Chandrima Naskar MD
Senior Resident
Department of Psychiatry
Post Graduate Institute of Medical Educational
and Research
Chandigarh, India

Chhitij Srivastava
MD DNB MRCPsych CCT (Child and Adolescent Psychiatry)
Associate Professor
Department of Psychiatry
Moti Lal Nehru Medical College, Prayagraj
Center of Behavioral and Cognitive Sciences,
University of Prayagraj
Prayagraj, Uttar Pradesh, India
Institute of Psychiatry, King's College
London, United Kingdom

Debasish Basu MD DNB
Professor and Head
Department of Psychiatry
Post Graduate Institute of Medical Sciences and
Research (PGIMER)
Chandigarh, India

Farheen Fatma MD
Senior Resident
Department of Psychiatry
All India Institute of Medical Sciences
Patna, Bihar, India

Guru S Gowda MBBS MD DNB PGDMLE MNAMS
Assistant Professor
Department of Psychiatry
National Institute of Mental Health and
Neurosciences (NIMHANS)
Bengaluru, Karnataka, India

Jayant Mahadevan MBBS MD DM
Assistant Professor
Department of Psychiatry
National Institute of Mental Health and
Neurosciences (NIMHANS)
Bengaluru, Karnataka, India

Koushik Sinha Deb MD
Additional Professor
Department of Psychiatry
All India Institute of Medical Sciences
New Delhi, India

KS Shubrata MD
Professor of Psychiatry
Subbaiah Institute of Medical Sciences
Shimoga, Karnataka, India

Lakshmi Vijayakumar
MBBS DPM PhD FRCP (Edin) FRCPsych (Hon)
Founder SNEHA
Head Psychiatry, Voluntary Health Services
Chennai, Tamil Nadu, India
Honorary Associate Professor
University of Melbourne, Australia
Honorary Adjunct Professor
University of Griffith, Australia
Member, WHO Network on Suicide Prevention
and Research

Manik C Bhise MD
Professor and Head
Department of Psychiatry
MGM Medical College
Aurangabad, Maharashtra, India

Naresh Nebhinani MD DNB
Additional Professor
Department of Psychiatry
All India Institute of Medical Science
Jodhpur, Rajasthan, India

Natarajan Varadharajan MD
Additional Professor and Senior Resident
Department of Psychiatry
Jawaharlal Institute of Postgraduate Medical
Education and Research
Puducherry, India

Nidhi Sharma MD DM (Addiction Psychiatry)
Assistant Professor, Department of Psychiatry
Indira Gandhi Medical College
Shimla, Himachal Pradesh, India

Nidhi Varghese MPhil
Clinical Psychologist, Department of Psychiatry
All India Institute of Medical Sciences
Patna, Bihar, India

Om Prakash Singh MD
Consultant Psychiatrist
West Bengal, Kolkata, India
Honorary Editor
Indian Journal of Psychiatry

Pallavi Rajhans MD
Visiting Consultant
Indian Institute of Technology
New Delhi, India

Pankaj Kumar MD
Additional Professor and Head
Department of Psychiatry
All India Institute of Medical Sciences
Patna, Bihar, India

Pratap Sharan MD PhD
Professor, Department of Psychiatry
All India Institute of Medical Sciences
New Delhi, India

Priya Sreedaran MD
Associate Professor, Department of Psychiatry
St John's Medical College Hospital
Bengaluru, Karnataka, India

Rajeev Ranjan MD
Assistant Professor
Department of Psychiatry
All India Institute of Medical Sciences
Patna, Bihar, India

Rakesh K Chadda MD FAMS FRCPsych DFAPA
Head, Department of Psychiatry
All India Institute of Medical Sciences
New Delhi, India
Chief
National Drug Dependence Treatment Center
(NDDTC)

Ravindra Neelakanthappa Munoli
MBBS MD
Associate Professor, Department of Psychiatry
Kasturba Medical College
Manipal Academy of Higher Education
Manipal, Karnataka, India

Rija Rappai MPhil MSW
Assistant Professor, Department of Social Work
WMO Arts and Science College
Wayanad, Kerala, India

Roshan V Khanande MD
Associate Professor, Department of Psychiatry
Central Institute of Psychiatry
Ranchi, Jharkhand, India

Sai Krishna Tikka MD DPM
Associate Professor, Department of Psychiatry
All India Institute of Medical Sciences
Hyderabad, Telangana, India

Seshadri Sekhar Chatterjee MD DNB
Registrar, PCP, CQMHAODS, Queensland Health
Associate Lecturer (Adjunct)
Department of Psychiatry
University of Queensland
Rockhampton, Queensland, Australia

Shobit Garg MD DPM
Professor and Head, Department of Psychiatry
Sri Guru Ram Rai Institute of Medical Sciences
Dehradun, Uttarakhand, India

Shubh Mohan Singh MD
Professor, Department of Psychiatry
Post Graduate Institute of Medical Educational
and Research
Chandigarh, India

Shubhangi R Parkar
DPM MD (Mumbai) MSc PhD (Basel, Switzerland)
Dean
Vedantaa Institute of Medical Sciences
Dahanu, Palghar, Maharashtra, India

Sujit Sarkhel MD DPM
Professor of Psychiatry, Institute of Psychiatry
Kolkata, West Bengal, India

Surendra Paliwal MD
Associate Professor, Department of Psychiatry
Central Institute of Psychiatry
Ranchi, Jharkhand, India

Swati Choudhary MD
Senior Resident, Department of Psychiatry
All India Institute of Medical Science
Jodhpur, Rajasthan, India

Tanu Gupta PhD
Clinical Psychologist, Department of Psychiatry
All India Institute of Medical Science
Jodhpur, Rajasthan, India

Varun S Mehta MD DNB MRCPsych
Associate Professor, Department of Psychiatry
Central Institute of Psychiatry
Ranchi, Jharkhand, India

Venkata Senthil Kumar Reddi MBBS MD
Professor, Department of Psychiatry
National Institute of Mental Health and
Neurosciences (NIMHANS)
Bengaluru, Karnataka, India

Vikas Menon MD DNB
Additional Professor and Senior Resident
Department of Psychiatry
Jawaharlal Institute of Postgraduate Medical
Education and Research
Puducherry, India

Vikas Sharma MD
Assistant Professor, Rheumatology Cell
Department of Medicine
Indira Gandhi Medical College
Shimla, Himachal Pradesh, India

Vinay Kumar MD
Consultant Psychiatrist
Manoved Mind Hospital
Patna, Bihar, India

Vivek Agarwal MD
Professor and Head
Department of Psychiatry
King George's Medical University
Lucknow, Uttar Pradesh, India

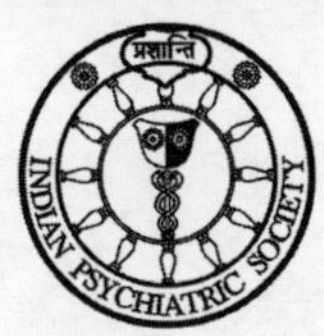

Indian Psychiatric Society

Dear Friends

I deem it a privilege to write a few lines for the textbook *"Suicide: Indian Perspective"* to be released in the annual conference of Indian Psychiatric Society 2023 to be held in Bhubaneswar, Odisha, India.

It is a timely attempt that the publication on an unnecessary death—suicide and to bring an Indian perspective is more laudable. The knowledge of the latest developments in suicidology is not only important but also challenging to the Psychiatrist and any additional information through publications will be very handy to learn. Many changes have occurred in the way suicide is studied over the years thanks to new scientific understanding. A thorough knowledge of the underpinnings of fatal self-harm is mandatory for any practitioner and more so for a practicing psychiatrist. I am happy to note that a book on suicide in India authored by experts in the field, and I congratulate them for their efforts in an area alien to the public. The discussion about suicide is still a taboo even in advanced and educated sections of the society in India.

The recent upsurge in the incidence of suicide in the last three to four years is a concern for medical and social scientists alike. While lot of advance is made in understanding the science of suicide, a lot is still to be explored both in assessment and prevention. A standardized tool to assess the risk of suicide applicable to all sections of the population is desirable but difficult to find in view of diverse socio-cultural variations in addition to economic inequality. I am sure more attention to suicidal behavior and suicidal attempts give some directions in the prevention of these unfortunate deaths.

I congratulate all who contributed to bring out the book on current burning issue, especially in youth. I am certain that more information would lessen the stigma and taboo that are prevailing in the society. I wish Dr. Sujit Sarkhel and his team all the very best!

Long Live IPS!

NN Raju	**Vinay Kumar**	**Arabinda Brahma**
President	Vice-President	Honorary General Secretary

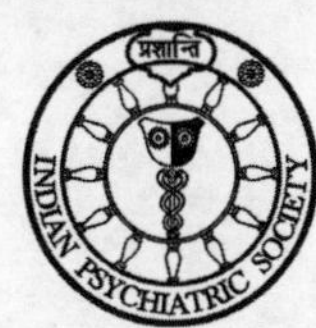

Publication Committee

It is a matter of great pleasure to write a message for a book on *"Suicide: Indian Perspectives"* which is a unique book; addressing the psychiatric issues related to suicide in India extensively.

It is heartening to see Indian Psychiatric Society (IPS) coming up with lots of books in Psychiatry; it is not just textbooks but books on many specialty topics and niche areas. The in-depth knowledge of pressing issues like suicide with special emphasis to Indian context is of paramount importance not just for students but also all mental health professionals and the additional information through publications will be very handy to learn.

Psychiatrists now have to handle varied illness related to all specialties unlike in the past when they were confined to treating mainly mental illness in mental hospitals. I feel glad to highlight that the book on *"Suicide: Indian Perspectives"* covers all aspects of suicide from an Indian context.

The authors, Dr Sujit Sarkhel, Dr Vinay Kumar, Dr Shubhangi R Parkar and Dr Lakshmi Vijaykumar have put their hard work to make this book a reality. The publication committee congratulates all of them for editing this book which will be released in ANCIPS 2023.

I on behalf of the publication committee thank the IPS office bearers for their continued support and cooperation. I also thank Jaypee Publications for their efforts.

I am sure this book will be a hugely popular and will be a significant contribution in the field Suicide.

Long Live IPS!

Anil Kakunje
Chairperson

Dipayan Sarkar
Convener

Mrugesh Vaishnav
Advisor

Foreword

I am happy to know that the Indian Psychiatric Society (IPS) has brought out a textbook on suicide covering various aspects of the phenomenon with special emphasis on the Indian perspective. I have been working in this area for several decades and have found that there needs to be a perspective of low- and middle-income countries (LAMIC) in this matter. This is important because there are many variations in socio-demographic as well as other associated factors in relation to suicide between the western world and the LAMIC countries. Since India and China form the major chunk of the population of LAMIC countries, the current textbook highlighting Indian perspectives fills an important gap in this area. The editorial team consisting of Dr Lakshmi Vijayakumar, Dr Vinay Kumar, Dr Sujit Sarkhel and Dr Subhangi R Parkar is a mix of young and the experienced with interest in the area of suicidology. I have personally known and worked with Dr Lakshmi Vijayakumar, and she is an accomplished researcher in the field of suicidology, especially in the Asian context.

The chapters of the textbook cover all the facets of the intriguing phenomenon called suicide. The emphasis has been to create a document with special attention to the available Indian data. A total of 20 chapters cover psychological, biological and socio-cultural theories, medical disorders, psychiatric disorders, personality disorders and substance use disorders associated with suicide. The chapters also cover suicide in various age and demographic groups- the young, the old, the women and the farmers. There are two important chapters on risk assessment and nomenclature which are essential elements on any textbook on suicide. The chapter covering the role of media in general and Indian media in particular has covered an area which has generated much controversy over the last few decades. Non-suicidal self-injury is an important concept related to suicide and has been adequately dealt with. Similarly, "survivors of suicide" is a very important area which is frequently neglected in the standard texts. Finally, very important chapters on epidemiology and gaps in data, legal aspects, suicide helplines and suicide prevention strategies highlight the core aspects of the Indian scenario.

Overall, this book serves as a very important document in the field of suicidology, especially in the Indian context. Whether it is psychiatrists, clinical psychologists, psychiatric social workers, psychiatric nurses, medical doctors of various specialties and researchers and students in the field of social sciences- the IPS publication *"Suicide: Indian Perspectives"* will be a useful resource to all. In the light of that, suicide is an unnecessary death and can be prevented.

Danuta Wasserman MD PhD
Professor of Psychiatry and Suicidology
Head and Founder of National Center for
Suicide Research and Prevention of Mental Ill-Health (NASP)
Karolinska Institutet, Stockholm, Sweden
Director for WHO Collaborating Center for
Research, Methods Development and Training in Suicide Prevention
President-Elect for the World Psychiatric Association (WPA)

Preface

While the entire human civilization across the centuries has evolved and strived for betterment, every individual has primarily been driven by the instinct of survival and self-preservation. Suicide is a condition which stands in direct contradistinction to this basic instinct of self-preservation—the opposing force of self-destruction drives the affected individual to his end brought about through his own efforts. This enigmatic phenomenon has influenced people across all walks of life—writers, poets, artists, filmmakers, anthropologists and makers of health policy across the world. Suicide is a core psychiatric emergency, but the multiple factors that come into play leading to an act of suicide have made it a public health problem.

India lost more than 1.6 lakh individuals to suicide in 2021 and the figure reported is the highest in the last 50 years. The greatest shock is that about 65% of these individuals were under 65 years of age. Thus, suicide leads to a huge loss of young, productive lives which could have gone a long way in nation building. While India has been trying to come to terms with the increasing curve of suicidal deaths, there is a lack of a comprehensive document on suicide which highlights the Indian perspectives. Dr Vinay Kumar, one of the editors of the book who was also the General Secretary of the Indian Psychiatric Society (IPS), conceived of the idea which was readily approved by the Publication Committee and the Office Bearers of IPS. Subsequently, in a National CME of the Suicide Prevention Specialty Section of the IPS held at Kolkata, Dr Vinay Kumar, Dr Lakshmi Vijaykumar, Dr Subhangi R Parkar and Dr Sujit Sarkhel met together and finalized the broad outlines of the chapters which went through several rounds of refinement. The aim was to create an authentic updated document on suicide with emphasis on Indian facts, figures and perspectives which would remain a source of reference for mental health and allied professionals as well as experts in public health policies. The authors were chosen with utmost care from among the experts working in the field of suicide.

We have tried our best to cover all aspects of suicide. Chapters have delved into the psycho-social theories of suicide to its neurobiological underpinnings, medical disorders leading to suicide to various psychiatric disorders associated with suicide. A separate chapter on nomenclature tries to provide clarity amongst confusing and overlapping terms related to suicide. Suicide in the youth, suicide in women and suicide in farmers have been dealt with separately because of their special importance. The role of media in suicide contagion as well as suicide prevention has been talked about all over the world. The chapter on media and suicide talks about the role of Indian media in influencing suicide. A chapter on risk assessment has been kept to fill the gap of lack of risk assessment across emergency settings in the country.

A chapter deals with available suicide helpline services in the country. Awareness of the laws in relation to the act of suicide is essential to deal with suicidal patients and their family members. Hence, this has been made a separate chapter. The perspective of suicide survivors has been effectively dealt with in a separate chapter. Finally, the concluding chapter deals with strategies and policies of the government directed at suicide prevention. Overall, the book has the potential to be used as a textbook as well as a reference for all health professionals, students of humanities, public health and research.

We thank President, Professor NN Raju; Honorary General Secretary, Dr Arabinda Brahma; Treasurer, Dr Aleem Siddiqui; and Honorary Editor, Professor Om Prakash Singh for their support and encouragement in compiling this book. We thank all the authors for their contributions and for accepting our suggestions. We also thank Shri Jitendar P Vij (Group Chairman), Mr Ankit Vij (Managing Director), Mr MS Mani (Group President), Ms Chetna Malhotra (Senior Director–Professional Publishing, Marketing and Business Development), and Nikita Chauhan (Senior Development Editor), M/s Jaypee Brothers Medical Publishers (P) Ltd, New Delhi, India for all their support and help. We hope that all health professionals in general and mental health professionals in particular will find this book useful.

Sujit Sarkhel
Lakshmi Vijayakumar

Vinay Kumar
Shubhangi R Parkar

Contents

Introduction and Overview

Sujit Sarkhel, Ravindra Neelakanthappa Munoli

■ INTRODUCTION

Suicide is a global public health problem which also happens to be a common psychiatric emergency. The entire globe is facing a rising trend in suicidal acts and India is no exception. The last data released by the National Crime Records Bureau showed the highest rate of suicide in the country in the last 50 years. With such a situation in front of us, an authentic document on the Indian perspectives of suicide is the need of the hour. Our book intends to fill a long void in the field of suicide studies in India. The book covers all the aspects of suicide with special emphasis on the Indian scenario.

The chapter "Changing Theories of Suicide" describes how various theories have been proposed over the years to explain a multifactorial phenomenon such as suicide. Starting from Durkheim's theories to present-day "ideation-to-action" theories, the chapter describes all.

The chapter on nomenclature tries to look at the varied and confusing nomenclature which have been used to describe various forms of suicidal behavior and have often created confusion among clinicians and researchers. The authors try to provide clarity regarding the terminology as much as possible.

The chapter on sociocultural aspects of suicide takes a journey through the varying sociocultural influences of our country and how this has affected suicide—starting from the times of self-immolation to the present days of rise of technology and loss of coherence of the family.

The chapter on neurobiology goes through various neurobiological and genetic underpinnings of suicide. The chapter on epidemiology looks at the available modes of gathering suicide data in India and what are its pitfalls. Nonsuicidal self-injury is related to suicidal behavior and is often neglected in emergency setups. The chapter deals with the concept, etiology, assessment, and management.

The next three chapters deal with various psychiatric comorbidities in individuals with suicidal behavior—psychiatric disorders, substance-use disorder, and personality disorders. The next chapter deals with various medical conditions, especially the chronic ones, which are associated with suicidal behavior. The chapter "Suicide in Indian Women" deals with the varying gender picture in our country in terms of stressful effects of marriage which can be a stressful factor for suicide rather than a protective factor. The chapter "Suicide in the Young" deals with youth suicide in India and what are the factors related to it.

The chapter on farmer's suicide reviews the existing Indian literature on farmer's suicide and discusses possible steps that could be taken to ameliorate this crisis. The role of media in influencing suicide has been widely debated worldwide, and India is no exception. The chapter discusses the available media guidelines in our country and how they could be implemented. The next chapter documents the stages through which suicide survivors must pass and what could be done to incorporate "postvention" programs in general health care. The next chapter deals with the current status of various available suicide helplines in India.

The chapter on suicide risk assessment makes a detailed description of the steps to be followed in formulating a risk for suicides. The chapter highlights the need for a thorough clinical interview rather than depending on rating scales with doubtful efficacy. The chapter on legal and ethical aspects of suicide deals with various Indian laws in relation to suicide including the existence of Section 309 IPC which still poses a hurdle in the complete decriminalization of suicide.

Finally, the chapter on suicide prevention strategies provides an overview of the national-level policies and what is the road ahead for framing and implementation of policies for achieving the goal of consistent reduction in the number and rate of suicides.

Theories of Suicide

Pallavi Rajhans, Pratap Sharan

ABSTRACT

Suicide is a global phenomenon. With an age-standardized rate of 9.0 per 100,000 globally, completed suicide occurs more often in men than women. Suicide rates are not evenly distributed and tend to vary with sociocultural, economic, and environmental factors. Suicide has a heterogeneous etiology with multiple risks, and protective factors interact with each other in its determination. A better understanding of suicide and its underlying mechanisms will help with the goal of prevention and timely intervention. Early theories on suicide looking at various determinants of suicide considered suicidal ideation and behavior as a single outcome category and hence mainly explained the determination of suicidal ideation. Risk factors for suicide do not follow a unitary model and they are different for ideators and attempters. Newer theories explain the process of development of suicidal ideation and its transition to suicidal attempt.

Keywords: Suicide theories; Psychosocial theories.

■ INTRODUCTION

Worldwide, suicide is an area of global public health concern. With an age-standardized rate of 9.0 per 100,000 globally, suicide is among the leading causes of death. Around 703,000 lives were lost due to suicide in 2019.[1,2] India has a high suicide rate with two age peaks, one in the 15–24 years age group and the other around 65 years of age.[3] Besides the emotional and physical consequences of suicide, the economic impact is also significant. It causes direct and indirect financial losses. In the United States, in the year 2019, suicide and nonfatal self-harm cost around $490 billion.[4] This included the medical, work loss, and quality of life costs. Suicide also impacts the lives of family members, friends, and colleagues of the affected person and the community at large.

Suicide is often viewed from different perspectives including psychiatric, philosophical, sociological anthropological, ethical, and religious. The healthcare strategy of suicide prevention includes identification of risk factors, diagnosis, treatment, and rehabilitation. For effective prevention and management, it is important to improve our understanding of the etiology and course of suicide. In the field of suicidology, various theories and models have been proposed to understand suicide. These include the traditional sociological–economic theories and psychological theories. More recently, ideation-to-action theories including Joiner's interpersonal-psychological theory of suicide (IPTS), three-step theory of suicide (3ST), fluid vulnerability theory (FVT), and integrated motivational volitional theory (IMVT) have been proposed.

■ RISK FACTORS FOR SUICIDE

Multiple factors seem to interact in a complex manner in the determination of suicidal behavior.[2] The risk factors for suicide (e.g., age, gender, ethnicity, and culture) also show varying strengths and patterns of association. The risk factors can be broadly divided into population-level and individual-level risk factors.[5] At the individual level, risk factors can be divided into precipitating and predisposing factors. Genetic, personality, and psychological factors can act as mediating factors for predisposing and precipitating factors.

Durkheim stressed upon the role of various social factors (population level) in the determination of suicide rates.[6] According to him, social changes which disrupt the traditional social structure are risk factors for suicide. Homogeneous societies on the contrary, which share common values and high levels of cohesion, were believed to have lower suicide rates.[5] Natural disasters, economic crisis, death of celebrity, and inappropriate media reporting are also population-level risk factors. Greater stress might be present in those who are unskilled, making them more vulnerable to suicide. Also, the suicide rates are higher in those who can access lethal measures such as medical professionals, farmers, and police officials. The strength of association of these individual factors with suicide is variable and not all are strongly and equally associated with suicide.[2]

Sociodemographic correlates, psycho-social and biological factors, and family history of suicide can act as individual-level predisposing risk factors for suicide. Rates are higher in males, older individuals, those living alone, divorced/ widowed, and those belonging to sexual or gender minority.[7]

Exposure to physical, emotional, or sexual abuse in childhood, parental neglect, or other early life adversity can act as a risk factor for suicide. Early life adversity can lead to long-term changes in the brain by bringing about epigenetic changes in gene pathways and epigenetic modification of certain genes which have a role in neuroprotection, neuronal growth, and plasticity.[5] Physical illness, adverse and traumatic life experiences in adulthood, and interpersonal stressors can all act as risk factors for suicide. Once considered as totally harmless, latent toxoplasmosis may also be a risk factor for suicidal behavior. Immunological responses caused by this brain-tropic parasite infection has been proposed as a possible underlying mechanism for suicide-related outcome.[8]

Psychopathology is an important predictor of suicide and suicidal behavior. Mental disorders are present in over 90% of the individuals who die by suicide in global studies.[9] Neuropsychiatric disorders have a strong association with suicide in life-course models. The life-course models suggest that different risk factors act at different life stages and suicide results due to the cumulative risk in one's lifetime. An increased risk of suicide may be associated with specific neuropsychiatric illnesses. These include mood disorders, substance-use disorders, schizophrenia-spectrum disorders, traumatic brain injury, and epilepsy. The odds of completed suicide increases by a factor of >3, when the abovementioned disorders are present.[2] In the developing nations, post-traumatic stress disorder, substance dependence, and conduct disorder are more predictive of suicide attempts.[10] Depression is a strong predictor for the development of suicidal ideation. Ideas of hopelessness or pessimistic views about future are also a risk factor for suicidal ideation. Recent research shows mixed results for hopelessness and depression regarding prediction of suicide attempts and death due to suicide.[11]

Personality factors such as impulsivity and perfectionism seem to be associated with suicide risk. Association between self-reported impulsivity and suicidal ideation, attempts and death has been reported and the association may be more salient in the younger individuals. Perfectionism, especially socially prescribed perfectionism, is associated with suicidal ideation and attempts.[11] Low extroversion and high neuroticism in combination may act as a risk factor for suicidal ideation and behavior. The role of impulsivity is debated to be critical, as conceptually it seems to be the link between thoughts and actions, but recent evidence suggests that even impulsivity is a modest predictor of suicide attempts.[7]

Certain cognitive factors can act as risk factors for suicide. A tendency to ruminate and keep brooding, being cognitively inflexible, having poor problem-solving and coping skills, having a sense of burdensomeness, having few reasons of living, a tendency to suppress one's thoughts, autobiographical memory biases, and attentional biases may be associated with suicidality.[11] A key step toward prevention of suicide is to identify the risk factors. But the accuracy with which these factors predict suicide is a matter of debate, and the studies need to be seen in the light of various methodological limitations.[12]

■ THEORIES OF SUICIDE

Any activity which moves a man to an earlier physical death and over which he has at least some volitional control is defined as self-destructive.[13] The three theories of self-destruction include the death instinct theory, mental illness theory, and adaptational failure theory.[13] Sigmund Freud conceptualized death instinct as the key driving force to return to a state of inertia that is present in all living beings. The second theory suggests that self-destruction takes place in those who have a mental illness. The theory of adaptational failure suggests that the task of man is to adjust or adapt to his situation, needs, goals, and capabilities. A failure to do so may lead to adaptational failure and self-destruction.

Sociological Theories of Suicide

Emile Durkheim propounded the first comprehensive suicide theory. He stressed the key role that society played in determining suicide rates.[6] His empirical study in 1897 and consequent theory had two basic principles. The first was that the social relationship structure of a group or class of people determines the suicide rates. The second principle stated that the level of moral regulation and integration determined the social relationship. The dimensions of regulation and integration were not clearly defined. Sociologists interpret regulation as the extent to which the attitudes and behavior of people are controlled by the collective's moral order and integration is conceptualized in terms of social relationships.[6] Durkheim proposed two continua of suicide and four different types depending on the level of imbalance between the two key social forces, i.e., regulation and integration. The four types of suicide described by Durkheim were:

1. Egoistic (less integration)
2. Altruistic (more integration)
3. Anomic (less regulation)
4. Fatalistic (more regulation).

Egoistic suicide: When an individual develops a sense of poor integration in his community, he develops a sense of nonbelonging. He becomes more vulnerable to die by suicide due to the lack of perceived social support.

Altruistic suicide: Conceptually, this is the exact reverse of egoistic suicide. When the extent of integration of an individual in his society is extreme, they may die by suicide or kill themselves on society's behalf.

Anomic suicide: When the level of moral regulation is low, anomic suicide occurs. Less regulation causes economic and social disruption that leads to individual disappointment.

Fatalistic suicide: When societies are rigid and oppressive, disappointed individuals in the society prefer to die rather than to live in such society; thus, fatalistic suicide results.

Among the two major social dimensions of Durkheim, integration had a more salient place in suicidology.[14] Social integration and cohesion were seen as protective factors and so was moral clarity. Social groups in which individuals relate to their society are believed to have high social capital and lower suicide rates. Social groups which lack moral regulation or clarity like those affected by collective or individual crises were believed to be more susceptible to suicide among its members.

Conceptualizing an individual death within the broad societal framework was one of the greatest strengths of this theory.[15] The concept helps in explaining population-level phenomena such as increased suicide rates after celebrity suicides and decreased rates at times of coming together.[15,16] Whether at an individual level or at a collective level, integration is protective against suicide.[17] On the contrary, some studies suggest that one should be cautious while linking social capital with population health as the incidence of suicide may actually be high in societies with greater social integration.[18] The societal variations may explain differences in suicide rates across culture and nations.[19]

A major limitation of Durkheim's theory is its inability to account for the ecological fallacy. The mechanism through which broad societal dimensions such as regulation and integration affect individual behavior, which is a microlevel parameter, is unclear. Questions such as how societal changes translate into individuals' decision to die remained unanswered.

Psychological Theories of Suicide

General Theories

The theories of self-destruction originated from Freud's emphasis on the death instinct. Most of the contemporary models of suicide originate from the concept of stress diathesis and focus on the cognitive aspects.[11]

Hopelessness theory: In the 1970s, Aaron Beck developed the pessimism scale, also known as hopelessness scale. In 1985, he proposed that hopelessness is the main mechanism for the development of suicidal ideation.[20] Abramson and colleagues in 1989 hypothesized that suicidality might be a central symptom of hopelessness in depression.[21] Hopelessness described as bleak pessimistic and negative views of future was believed to activate the cognitive system, which subsequently activated the affective, behavioral, conscious control, and motivational systems. These disturbed systems are believed to create a toxic environment in which suicidal ideation and behavior can develop.[22] The mediating effect of hopelessness on suicide was backed by findings of studies conducted on patients in outpatient and inpatient settings.[23,24]

Stress-diathesis model of suicide: This model states that when individuals with preexisting vulnerability to suicidality experience stress, they develop suicidal ideation.[25] Aggression and impulsivity may then lead to suicide attempts. Schotte and Clum came up with the stress/problem-solving model of suicidal behavior while studying a college population. They proposed that when people are exposed to highly stressful situations, those with poor problem-solving skills are at a higher risk of hopelessness, depression, and suicidal behavior.[26] The clinical stress-diathesis model of suicide by Mann and colleagues suggests that psychiatric disorders act as stressors rather than as sole etiological agents for suicide. They interact with preexisting diathesis (e.g., impulsivity) to lead to suicide.[11] This model was based on the findings of a clinical study which compared patients with a history of suicide attempts with those without a past history of attempts. Those attempters had very few reasons for living and scored higher in domains of subjective depression and suicidal ideation. They also had higher lifetime rates of impulsivity, aggression, substance use, abuse in childhood, family history of suicide acts, and comorbid borderline personality disorder. The study suggested that stress (psychiatric disorder) as well as diathesis (e.g., being more impulsive) determines the suicidal act. Borderline personality, impulsivity, and aggression are partly determined by genetic factors or early life adversity. So, a genetic or familial component could possibly be responsible for the association between aggression/impulsivity and suicidal behavior (independent of the transmission of depressive or psychotic disorders). The role of serotonin neurotransmission was also proposed based on links between low serotonin activity and suicidal behavior.[26]

A suicide model needs to consider proximal and distal factors and their interaction. Suicidal behavior cannot be explained solely by stress model as everyone experiencing extreme stress do not exhibit suicidal behavior.[27] When one encounters stress, it is the diathesis or one's vulnerability which predisposes to suicidal behavior. Cognitive vulnerability traits (e.g., impaired decision-making) can also be a part of diathesis to suicidal behavior as they can lead to problems in affective relationships (e.g., with family members or partners) of people who attempt suicide.[28]

Cubic model of suicide: This model has three primary dimensions: the degree of stress, psychache, and perturbation. The three dimensions are rated from low to high (1–5) for an individual. When a person has a score of 5 in all dimensions, which represents a 5–5–5 cube, he is believed to be experiencing extreme psychache and has an increased risk of dying by suicide.[15] Shneidman states that psychache (psychological or emotional pain) is the main factor that motivates one to attempt suicide.[7] Suicide is attempted when the pain exceeds a person's threshold for tolerating emotional and psychological pain (intense feelings of fear, loneliness, anxiety, or guilt). The impulsive act of suicide that takes place in the wake of psychache is expected to be fatal by the attempter.[29] In a study conducted on 41 students who were suicidal ideators, psychache uniquely predicted changes in suicidal ideation over time.[30] The role of psychache in predicting suicidal ideation was also established in longitudinal follow-up studies in general and high-risk undergraduate students.[31,32]

Escape theory: This theory of suicide was put forward by Baumeister in 1990. According to him, three constructs, i.e., cognitive, personality, and social, play a role in suicide.[15] According to Baumeister, the motivation for attempting suicide comes from a desire to escape painful self-awareness. He proposed a six-step chain of events to explain suicide.

1. Recent setbacks or unreasonable expectations
2. Negatively attributing the setbacks to oneself leading to self-blame and poor esteem
3. Self-awareness and comparing oneself with relevant standards leading to a state of aversion
4. Negative affective state
5. Cognitive deconstruction where an individual avoids/rejects constructive thoughts to escape the negative affective state
6. Irrational thoughts, passivity, apathy, and disinhibition (disinhibition appears to be the critical component).

Although all these six factors could be independent risk factors for suicide, there is limited research evidence for putting them in a causal chain.[33-35] However, when the escape theory as a whole was applied for understanding the suicidal behavior of undergraduate university students, the findings were in line with Baumeister's predictions.[36]

Emotion dysregulation theory: This theory was developed in the context of borderline personality disorder. According to Linehan's theory, intense negative affective states or emotional dysregulation occurs in individuals in critical/invalidating environments. Individuals look for ways (including suicidal behavior) to distract themselves from these negative emotional states.[15,37] The dialectical behavior therapy for borderline personality disorder is based on this theory.[38,39] However, a major limitation of the theory is that emotional dysregulation is common to several psychiatric illnesses but not all

patients suffering from these illnesses are ideators or attemptors.[40]

Ideation-to-action Theories

The earlier psychological theories have been found to be predictive of suicidal ideation rather than suicidal attempt. The development of suicidal ideation and its progression from desire to attempt are distinct phenomena. "Ideation-to-action" theories have been proposed to explain the transition from desire to attempt. Such theories include Joiner's IPTS, 3ST, FVT, and IMVT.[41]

Interpersonal-psychological theory of suicide: This theory was put forward by Joiner. According to ITPS, the perception of self in relation to others results in suicidal thinking.[42] Perceived burdensomeness and thwarted belongingness are the two main negative cognition at the interpersonal level. The feeling of being a burden on others is described as perceived burdensomeness and feeling "as if you don't belong here" is described as thwarted belongingness. When hopelessness sets in and the person feels that the state is not going to change, suicidal ideation starts developing. Thwarted belongingness and perceived burdensomeness can individually lead to passive desire for suicide. But suicidal desire is not enough for a suicide attempt, so the concept of acquired capability was introduced in this theory. When one gets habituated to pain and develops fearlessness of death, the transition from ideation to act occurs.[29,42] The habituation occurs because one develops tolerance to the physical pain of self-harm because of repeated previous encounters with painful experiences (e.g., childhood abuse, NSSI, previous suicide attempt, etc.).[21] A meta-analysis conducted on cross-national research available on interpersonal theory of suicide supports the theory.[43]

Integrated motivational-volitional theory: The key components of earlier theories were integrated and mapped into a process, progressing from ideation to attempt in the integrated motivational-volitional model (IMVM).[41,44] This theory was articulated in 2011 by O'Conner, and it suggests that suicidal behavior progresses through motivational and volitional phases.[44] Rather than considering suicide to be a consequence of psychiatric disorder, this theory identifies suicide as a behavior. Life situations such as feeling humiliated/ defeated, in the presence of moderators such as poor coping and problem-solving skills, make one feel trapped. An inability to move out of the humiliating/stressful situations and a sense of feeling trapped or defeated are the important driving forces for suicide in the IMVM. During the volitional phase, moderators such as impulsivity, knowledge about or access to lethal means, or increased capacity to act come into play and the intentions are carried out. The IMVM differs from IPTS as it does not feature burdensomeness or belongingness as paths to suicidal ideation and is not restricted to only acquired capabilities for self-harm in the volitional phase.[11] As this theory is relatively new, limited testing is available. A preliminary self-report survey on healthy adults found the proposed paths in IMVM to be significant.[45]

Three-step theory of suicide: The 3ST was developed by Klonsky and May in 2015.[46] The three main constructs of the three-step theory include pain and hopelessness, suicide capacity, and connectedness. Pain from any source [physical, psychological (e.g., psychache, perceived burdensomeness, thwarted belongingness), social] is postulated to decrease the desire to live (based on principles of conditioning: one avoids behaviors that are punished). However,

usually, individuals in pain often hope for things to get better with time and work for getting things better. So, pain by itself usually does not lead to suicidal ideation. Suicidal ideation occurs when one loses hope of things improving in future. According to the model, the combination of pain and hopelessness leads to the development of suicidal ideation.

The second step in the model is the loss of connectedness. Connectedness in 3ST includes connections with people, a role, an area of interest, or anything that adds purpose to one's life. The theory suggests that when one has feelings of pain and hopelessness but remains invested in these connections, suicidal ideation would be moderate and not lethal (e.g., passive desire, "it would be better if I were dead"). If the connectedness becomes weaker than the pain and suffering, stronger suicidal ideations emerge, and one considers taking one's own life. Thus, connectedness is given special importance in the 3ST. However, connectedness does not negate the role of factors such as depression, mental disorders, adverse life events, and personality traits in the development of suicidal ideation, but these are believed to contribute to pain and hopelessness.

The third and final step in the 3ST is progression from ideation to attempt. In this last step, Klonsky and May discuss the conditions that lead to conversion of strong suicidal ideas to attempt. They believe that the life instinct is quite strong; hence, many individuals with strong suicidal ideation do not attempt suicide. It is only when one overcomes the fear of self-harm that a suicide attempt takes place. The researchers agree with Joiner on this point and expand it further.

According to the 3ST, three variables contribute to the capacity for attempting suicide. These are dispositional variables, e.g., pain sensitivity (low pain sensitivity is likely to be associated with suicide attempt); acquired variables (e.g., habituation to injury, pain, etc.); and practical variables (the ones which make suicide easy, e.g., knowledge about or expertise in the use of lethal means, access to lethal means, etc.).[7,41,46] A few studies conducted on university students provide support to this theory.[46,47]

Fluid vulnerability theory: Rudd in 2006 first articulated this theory.[48] It was an extension of Beck's psychopathology theory which followed a cognitive behavioral framework. However, rather than specific thoughts such as hopelessness, FVT talks about much broader suicidal belief systems. According to this theory, emotional regulation issues and cognitive inflexibility (the two main components of this theory) make one vulnerable to suicidal behavior. To prevent suicides, both these components need to be addressed.

Due to its stress on the suicidogenic thoughts, this theory exhibits similarities to the IPTS, IMVT, and 3ST. However, FVT's stress upon the dynamic nature of suicide risk differentiates it from the other "ideation-to-action" theories. The FVT conceptualizes suicide risk along two dimensions: *baseline* (chronic or stable properties of suicide risk, e.g., genetics, trauma, demographics, and previous suicidal behavior) and *acute* (dynamic properties of suicide risk that are reactive to external forces). The baseline dimension corresponds to the homeostatic point of equilibrium for an individual's low-risk state. The acute dimension, on the other hand, is influenced by risk factors that fluctuate in response to environmental features and/or internal experiences (e.g., sadness, hopelessness, substance use), and corresponds to within-person differences in risk. The risk of suicide resolves when multiple domains are targeted effectively and adequately. The assumptions of this theory follow nonlinear change process and finds support from the recent literature.[49]

■ CONCLUSION

Suicide is a global problem with a heterogeneous etiology. Various theories have been put forward to explain/understand suicidal thoughts and behavior, e.g., the sociological theory by Durkheim or hopelessness theory by Beck. Some authors have suggested that biological vulnerability and environmental triggers work in combination to lead to suicidal behavior. Newer "ideation-to-action" theories attempt to account for what motivates individuals to move from suicide ideation to suicide attempts. It will be useful to assess the validity and utility of these theories to help fill the knowledge gap on suicidality and address issues in the adequate and timely management of a global crisis.

■ REFERENCES

1. World Health Organization (2021). Suicide. [online] Available from: https://www.who.int/news-room/fact-sheets/detail/suicide. [Last accessed January, 2023].
2. Fazel S, Runeson B. Suicide. N Engl J Med. 2020;382(3):266-74.
3. Mythri SV, Ebenezer JA. Suicide in India: Distinct epidemiological patterns and implications. Indian J Psychol Med. 2016;38(6):493-8.
4. Peterson C, Miller G, Barnett S, Florence C. Economic Cost of injury - United States, 2019. MMWR Morb Mortal Wkly Rep. 2021;70(48):1655-9.
5. Turecki G, Brent D. Suicide and suicidal behaviour. Lancet. 2016;387(10024):1227-39.
6. Mueller A, Abrutyn S, Pescosolido B, Diefendorf S. The Social Roots of Suicide: Theorizing how the External Social World Matters to Suicide and Suicide Prevention. Front Psychol. 2021;12:621569.

7. Klonsky ED, May AM, Saffer BY. Suicide, suicide attempts, and suicidal ideation. Annu Rev Clin Psychol. 2016;12(1):307-30.

8. Flegr J. How and why Toxoplasma makes us crazy. Trends Parasitol. 2013;29(4): 156-63.

9. Bertolote JM, Fleischmann A. Suicide and psychiatric diagnosis: a worldwide perspective. World Psychiatry. 2002; 1(3):181-5.

10. Nock M, Hwang I, Sampson N, Kessler R, Angermeyer M, Beautrais A, et al. Cross-national analysis of the associations among mental disorders and suicidal behavior: findings from the WHO World Mental Health Surveys. PLoS Med. 2009;6(8):e1000123.

11. O'Connor R, Nock M. The psychology of suicidal behaviour. Lancet Psychiatry. 2014;1(1):73-85.

12. Franklin JC, Ribeiro JD, Fox K, Bentley KR, Kleiman EM, Huang X, et al. Risk factors for suicidal thoughts and behaviors: A meta-analysis of 50 years of research. Psychol Bull. 2017;143(2):187-232.

13. Tabachnick N, Poze P, Fielder E. Theories of self-destruction. Am J Psychoanal. 1972;32(1):53-61.

14. Berkman LF, Glass T, Brissette I, Seeman TE. From social integration to health: Durkheim in the new millennium. Soc Sci Med. 2000;51(6):843-57.

15. Stanley I, Hom M, Rogers M, Hagan C, Joiner T. Understanding suicide among older adults: a review of psychological and sociological theories of suicide. Aging Ment Health. 2015;20(2):113-22.

16. Menon V, Kar S, Marthoenis M, Arafat S, Sharma G, Kaliamoorthy C, et al. Is there any link between celebrity suicide and further suicidal behaviour in India? Int J Soc Psychiatry. 2020;67(5):453-60.

17. Wray M, Colen C, Pescosolido B. The sociology of suicide. Annu Rev Sociol. 2011;37(1):505-28.

18. Kushner H, Sterk C. The limits of social capital: Durkheim, suicide, and social cohesion. Am J Public Health. 2005;95(7):1139-43.

19. Shah A, Bhat R, McKenzie S, Koen C. Elderly suicide rates: cross-national comparisons and association with sex and elderly age-bands. Med Sci Law. 2007;47(3): 244-52.

20. Beck A. Hopelessness as a predictor of eventual suicide. Ann NY Acad Sci. 1986;487:90-6.

21. Joiner T, Rudd MD (Eds). Suicide Science: Expanding the Boundaries. New York: Springer Science & Business Media; 2007.

22. Beck A, Brown G, Berchick R, Stewart B, Steer R. Relationship between hopelessness and ultimate suicide: a replication with psychiatric outpatients. FOCUS. 2006;4(2):291-6.

23. Beck AT, Brown G, Berchick RJ, Stewart BL, Steer RA. Relationship between hopelessness and ultimate suicide: a replication with psychiatric outpatients. Am J Psychiatry. 1990;147(2):190-5.

24. Kazdin A, French N, Unis A, Esveldt-Dawson K, Sherick R. Hopelessness, depression, and suicidal intent among psychiatrically disturbed inpatient children. J Consult Clin Psychol. 1983;51(4):504-10.

25. Rubinstein D. A stress-diathesis theory of suicide. Suicide Life Threat Behav. 1986;16(2):182-97.

26. van Heeringen K. Stress-diathesis model of suicidal behavior. In: Dwivedi Y (Ed). The Neurobiological Basis of Suicide. Boca Raton, FL: CRC Press/Taylor & Francis; 2012. 2012;51:113.

27. Hawton K, van Heeringen K. Suicide. Lancet. 2009;373(9672):1372-81.

28. Jollant F, Guillaume S, Jaussent I, Castelnau D, Malafosse A, Courtet P. Impaired decision-making in suicide attempters may increase the risk of problems in affective relationships. J Affect Disord. 2007;99(1-3):59-62.

29. Cramer R, Kapusta N. A social-ecological framework of theory, assessment, and prevention of suicide. Front Psychol. 2017;8:1756.

30. Troister T, Holden R. A two-year prospective study of psychache and its relationship to suicidality among high-risk undergraduates. J Clin Psychol. 2012;68(9):1019-27.

31. Troister T, Davis M, Lowndes A, Holden R. A five-month longitudinal study of psychache and suicide ideation: Replication in general

and high-risk university students. Suicide Life Threat Behav. 2013;43(6):611-20.

32. Montemarano V, Troister T, Lambert C, Holden R. A four-year longitudinal study examining psychache and suicide ideation in elevated-risk undergraduates: A test of Shneidman's model of suicidal behavior. J Clin Psychol. 2018;74(10):1820-32.

33. Anestis M, Soberay K, Gutierrez P, Hernández T, Joiner T. Reconsidering the link between impulsivity and suicidal behavior. Pers Soc Psychol Rev. 2014;18(4):366-86.

34. Chatard A, Selimbegović L. When self-destructive thoughts flash through the mind: Failure to meet standards affects the accessibility of suicide-related thoughts. J Pers Soc Psychol. 2011;100(4):587-605.

35. Hirsch J, Duberstein P, Conner K, Heisel M, Beckman A, Franus N, et al. Future orientation and suicide ideation and attempts in depressed adults ages 50 and over. Am J Geriatr Psychiatry. 2006;14(9):752-7.

36. Tang J, Wu S, Miao D. Experimental test of escape theory: accessibility to implicit suicidal mind. Suicide Life Threat Behav. 2013;43(4):347-55.

37. Linehan M, Comtois K, Murray A, Brown M, Gallop R, Heard H, et al. Two-year randomized controlled trial and follow-up of dialectical behavior therapy vs therapy by experts for suicidal behaviors and borderline personality disorder. Arch Gen Psychiatry. 2006;63(7):757.

38. Lynch T, Trost W, Salsman N, Linehan M. Dialectical behavior therapy for borderline personality disorder. Annu Rev Clin Psychol. 2007;3(1):181-205.

39. Linehan M, Korslund K, Harned M, Gallop R, Lungu A, Neacsiu A, et al. Dialectical behavior therapy for high suicide risk in individuals with borderline personality disorder. JAMA Psychiatry. 2015;72(5):475.

40. Gross J, Muñoz R. Emotion regulation and mental health. Clin Psychol: Sci Pract. 1995;2(2):151-64.

41. Klonsky E, Saffer B, Bryan C. Ideation-to-action theories of suicide: a conceptual and empirical update. Curr Opin Psychol. 2018;22:38-43.

42. Van Orden K, Witte T, Cukrowicz K, Braithwaite S, Selby E, Joiner T. The interpersonal theory of suicide. Psychol Rev. 2010;117(2):575-600.

43. Chu C, Buchman-Schmitt J, Stanley I, Hom M, Tucker R, Hagan C, et al. The interpersonal theory of suicide: A systematic review and meta-analysis of a decade of cross-national research. Psychol Bull. 2017;143(12):1313-45.

44. Tucker R, O'Connor R, Wingate L. An Investigation of the Relationship Between Rumination Styles, Hope, and Suicide Ideation Through the Lens of the Integrated Motivational-Volitional Model of Suicidal Behavior. Arch Suicide Res. 2016;20(4):553-66.

45. Dhingra K, Boduszek D, O'Connor R. A structural test of the Integrated Motivational-Volitional model of suicidal behaviour. Psych Research. 2016;239:169-78.

46. Klonsky E, May A. The Three-Step Theory (3ST): A New Theory of Suicide Rooted in the "Ideation-to-Action" Framework. Int J Cognit Ther. 2015;8(2):114-29.

47. Dhingra K, Klonsky E, Tapola V. An empirical test of the Three-Step Theory of Suicide in U.K. university students. Suicide Life Threat Behav. 2018;49(2):478-87.

48. Rudd M. Fluid Vulnerability Theory: A Cognitive Approach to Understanding the Process of Acute and Chronic Suicide Risk. In: Ellis TE (Ed). Cognition and Suicide: Theory, Research, and Therapy. Washington DC: American Psych Assoc; 2006. pp. 355-68.

49. Bryan C, Rudd M. Nonlinear change processes during psychotherapy characterize patients who have made multiple suicide attempts. Suicide Life Threat Behav. 2017;48(4):386-400.

Suicide Nomenclature

Vikas Menon, Natarajan Varadharajan, Abdul Faheem

ABSTRACT

Consistent terminology, definitions, and classification of suicidal behavior are critical to promote theoretical understanding, research, and suicide prevention activities. However, for many decades now, the absence of a universally accepted nomenclature and classification system has hindered research in suicide and affected comparability of findings. In this chapter, we briefly trace the evolution and conceptualization of the range of suicidal behaviors. Various classifications and components of suicide are described. The key components of suicide are the agency of the act, outcome, intent, and awareness of the act. Probably, the most important advancement in classifying a behavior as suicidal versus nonsuicidal is the presence of some degree of intent to die ("nonzero" intent). Contemporary definitions of a range of suicide-related behaviors and communications are presented to aid understanding. We describe the underpinnings and relevance of considering the range of suicidal behaviors on a spectrum from presuicidal syndrome to suicide. This is essential to identify factors that may predict transition through various stages of the "suicide process" and identify opportunities for suicide prevention. Finally, we discuss the strengths and limitations of the current suicide nomenclature with special relevance to the Indian context.

Keywords: Suicide; Attempted suicide; Suicide ideation; Non-suicidal self-injury; Classification.

INTRODUCTION

Worldwide, it is estimated that close to 800,000 people die annually by suicide. Asia accounts for >60% of global suicides and the South-East Asian region, comprising 11 low- and middle-income countries including India, has the dubious distinction of one of the highest regional suicide rates amounting to 17.7 per 100,000 population.[1,2] Suicide is viewed as a preventable issue and, therefore, many countries have invested hugely in suicide prevention strategies to bring down their suicide burden.

Prevention of suicide hinges on accurate understanding, identification, assessment, and prediction of risk. For many decades now, lack of conceptual clarity, universally accepted definitions of suicide and suicide-related phenomena, and standardized classification of suicidal behaviors have hindered research in the domain of suicidology. There is a distinct need to develop a nomenclature system of suicide that is anchored in theoretical and conceptual understanding to facilitate uptake; lack of this can hinder suicide prevention, clinical care, as well as research activities.

This chapter initially provides an overview of our understanding of suicidal behavior from a theoretical perspective. Next, we examine classification, comparative nosology, and components of suicidal behavior. Subsequently, we present the major definitions of a range of suicide-related phenomena (behavior and communication).

Finally, we end with a discussion on the importance of conceptualizing suicide behavior on a continuum and the strengths and limitations of the current suicide nomenclature. In so doing, we present the relevant Indian evidence and contextualize the findings against global perspectives.

HISTORY, EVOLUTION, AND CONCEPTUALIZATION OF SUICIDAL BEHAVIOR

Origin of the Word Suicide

The concept of suicide dates back to 1303–1213 BCE, where there are descriptions of two brothers who died by suicide during Egyptian Pharaoh Ramses II (although the word-suicide was not explicitly mentioned).[3] The first mention of the word "suicide" can be traced to Sir Thomas Browne's Religio Medici (1643) and its roots from the modern Latin word "suicidium" where "sui" refers to "of oneself", and "cidium" refers to "killing".[4,5]

Sociological Perspective of Suicide

Ever since Esquirol described suicide, in *Dictionnaire des sciences médicales (1821)*,[6] as "a disease or a symptom of disease", there has been a paradigm shift in how suicide was viewed from a criminal perspective to a sociological perspective.[7] The major contribution toward the sociological study of suicide is through Emile Durkheim's "Suicide—A study of sociology" (1897); in this treatise, he emphasized the role of society in determining suicide. Individuals were governed by the society and its rules, which provided an identity and moral regulation with the society. Failure of integration or moral regulation results in suicide. Based on the imbalance between the two, he proposed four types of suicide: altruistic, egoistic, fatalistic, and anomic suicide.[8]

Psychoanalytic Theory of Suicide

In 1917, Freud published the "Mourning and melancholia" paper, where he formulated the dynamics of melancholic depression and suicide. He proposed that suicide results from anger turned inward against an introjected and ambivalently cathected love object. He also stated that there would be no suicide without an earlier repressed desire to kill somebody else. In "Man against Himself," Karl Menninger built further on Freud's ideas and explained suicide in terms of balance between death instinct (Thanatos) and life instincts. Suicide occurs when the balance is obliterated, and it is the extreme manifestation of the death instinct, which he divided into three components: wish to kill, wish to be killed, and wish to die. Hendin put forward that suicide can be best understood by observing both its affective and cognitive components. Hopelessness, anger, rage, shame, despair, and guilt are some affective states that are essential when intolerable combined with the meaning given for suicide (including both conscious and unconscious affect and perception) results in suicide. He identified six reasons behind suicidal attempts on psychodynamic grounds, namely death as:

1. Retaliatory abandonment
2. Retroflexed murder
3. Reunion with a loved one
4. Rebirth of the self after death
5. Self-punishment
6. Seeing oneself as already dead.

These psychoanalytic concepts, along with the sociological perspective, serve as the foundation for understanding the idea of suicide better.[9-11]

Psychological Orientation toward Death

In an attempt to describe suicide attempts from the perspective of psychological orientation toward death, many new terms such as deliberate self-harm, parasuicide, and pseudo-suicide were coined. The main motive of all of them was to produce changes which the subject desired via actual or expected consequences of his actions.[12] Deliberate self-harm was derived from deliberate self-injury/self-poisoning suggested by Kessel,[13] highlighting the nature of the act ignoring the intent. Kreitman and his colleagues introduced "parasuicide", which is the behavioral analog of suicide, ignoring the psychological orientation toward death that would bridge the continuum between attempted suicide and suicide.[14] Parasuicide was operationally defined in the World Health Organization/Europe (WHO/EURO) multicenter study on suicidal behavior as follows: *"an act with nonfatal outcome, in which an individual deliberately initiates a non-habitual behavior that, without intervention from others, will cause self-harm, or deliberately ingests a substance in excess of the prescribed or generally recognized therapeutic dosage, and which is aimed at realizing changes which the subject desired via the actual or expected physical consequences".*[15]

Operational Approaches for Determination of Suicide

Edwin Schneidman described suicide as a "conscious act of self-induced annihilation best understood as a multidimensional malaise in a needful individual who defines an issue for which the suicide is perceived as the best solution." Motto suggested that apart from intent elicited from direct inquiry, the final decision rests on subjective and intuitive judgment, and he denoted suicide as "self-inflicted, self-intentioned death".[16] Rosenberg et al. (1988) formulated the Operational Criteria for Determination of Suicide which was tailored explicitly for legal purposes; here, suicide is defined as *"death arising from an act inflicted upon oneself with the intent to kill oneself"*[17] which has three components: death by harm, acts against self, and intent.[12]

CLASSIFICATION AND COMPONENTS OF SUICIDAL BEHAVIOR

Nomenclature versus Classification

Despite various suicide-related nomenclatures and classificatory systems being proposed internationally,[15] none of them have a universal appeal which further reiterates the complexities of the phenomenon of suicide.[18,19] To better understand the phenomenon, one should know the distinction between nomenclature and classification. **Box 1** describes their basic definitions. Nomenclature deals with naming and defining terms explicitly, whereas

---

BOX 1: Definitions of nomenclature and classification as per O'Carroll et al. (1996)[20] and Silverman et al (2006).[21]

Nomenclature
"A set of commonly understood, widely acceptable comprehensive terms, that define the basic clinical phenomena of suicide and suicide-related behaviors and is based on a logical and minimum set of necessary component elements that has utility"

Classification
"Implies comprehensiveness, a systematic arrangement of items in groups or categories with ordered, nested subcategories; scientific validity; exhaustiveness; accuracy sufficient for research or clinical practice; and an unambiguous set of rules for assigning items to a single place in the classification scheme"

classification deals with the systematic arrangement of those terms in a scientifically meaningful way.

National Institute of Mental Health Summit (1970)

In 1973, the National Institute of Mental Health (NIMH) task force group chaired by Dr Aaron T Beck developed a classification of suicidal behavior to address inconsistencies in suicide-related behaviors. The suicidal phenomena were classified as completed suicides, suicide attempts, or suicide ideation (definitions in **Box 2**) based on the dimensions of intent (seriousness or degree or sincerity of the subject in his/her actual or contemplated action, in terms of ending his/her life), the lethality of the act (the risk of harm to self-resulting from a suicide attempt), mitigating circumstances, method, and certainty by the rater regarding individual's suicidality.[22]

This classification is quite broad. For example, repetitive self-harm behaviors without intent to die, typically seen in conditions such as borderline personality disorders, are grouped under suicide attempts. The above classification makes no distinction between various subtle forms of suicidal behaviors.

Components of Suicide

The WHO/EURO multicenter study on suicidal behavior[23] identified three essential elements that are considered prerequisites to define a suicide, namely the agency of the act, intent of the act, conscious awareness, and outcome of the behavior. It defined suicide as described in **Box 3**, which would serve as a common language between researchers and enable international comparisons. This culminated in different definitions proposed by Shneidman, Durkheim, and Rosenberg, as described above.[24]

These essential components are described briefly:[15]

- *Agency of the act:* The individual indulges in the act by himself and carries it out deliberately. Here, the emphasis is not on the performance of the behavior but the responsibility of the outcome, i.e., it includes even indirect/passive methods adopted for suicide. For example, a person stands on the railway track with the intent to die from the speeding train. Here, it is a passive suicide method because some degree of inaction rests with the person, and responsibility for the outcome lies with him (who initiates the act). Irrespective of the method adopted to achieve death, if the responsibility of the outcome lies with the person, it is considered self-initiated.
- *Outcome of the act:* The outcome of the act is always death (fatal, in other words). Although done with the intention of death, outcomes other than this are by definition not classified as suicide.

BOX 2: Classification of suicide as per NIMH conference.[22]

Completed suicide: "Willful, self-inflicted, life-threatening act which has resulted in death"

Suicide attempt: "Willful, self-inflicted, life-threatening act resulting in physical injury but not in death"

Suicide ideas: "Includes such suicidal ideation and acts that indicate a loss of desire to live but which have not yet resulted in physical injury"

BOX 3: Essential components of the definition of suicide.

"Suicide is an *act with a fatal outcome* which the deceased, *knowing or expecting a fatal outcome had initiated and carried out* with the *purpose of provoking the changes he desired*"

—*WHO/EURO Multicenter Study on Suicidal Behavior, 1986*[23]

- *Intent and awareness of the act:* It is the most defining and characteristic element of the definition of suicide. Intent also implies conscious awareness of the lethal consequences of the act.

CONTEMPORARY CLASSIFICATION SYSTEMS

Position of International Classification of Diseases-10 and Diagnostic and Statistical Manual of Mental Disorders-IV on Suicide

In International Classification of Diseases-10 (ICD-10), both suicide and parasuicide are included in the general category of self-harm, and there is no differentiation between the two. Likewise, in Diagnostic and Statistical Manual of Mental Disorders-IV (DSM-IV), there is no separate category for suicide and related behaviors.[25,26]

DSM-5 Position

Section-III of DSM-5 has included "conditions for further study" in which it has proposed criteria for entities such as "suicidal behavior disorder" and "nonsuicidal self-injury." These criteria were devised through expert consensus by the DSM Taskforce. It was mainly intended for research purposes to enhance communication between researchers and to facilitate greater understanding so that its inclusion in subsequent editions can be considered. The criteria proposed for suicidal behavior disorder and nonsuicidal self-injury behavior are given in **Boxes 4 and 5.**[27]

The basic premise of difference between these two conditions is the act's intent. For more detailed notes on suicide intent and how it can be inferred, see Section on Additional Notes on Suicide Intent.

The Comparative Nosology of Suicidal Behavior

In contrast to ICD-10, DSM-5 offers a clear delineation between suicide, suicide attempt, and other repetitive self-harm behaviors such as nonsuicidal self-injurious behavior (NS-SIB) for better understanding. However, these are not officially coded.

The Position of ICD-11

In the ICD-11 which has recently come into effect, suicide and related terminologies are listed outside the chapter on mental, behavioral, or neurodevelopmental disorders and in different chapters such as "symptoms, signs and clinical findings, not elsewhere classified" (Chapter 21) or "morbidity and mortality due to external causes (Chapter 23)."

BOX 4: Proposed criteria in DSM-5 for suicidal behavior disorder.[27]

Suicidal behavior disorder:
- Within the last 24 months, the individual has made a suicide attempt

Note: A suicide attempt is a self-initiated sequence of behaviors by an individual who, at the time of initiation, expected that the set of actions would lead to his or her own death. The "time of initiation" is the time when a behavior took place that involved applying the method
- The act does not meet criteria for nonsuicidal self-injury—that is, it does not involve self-injury directed to the surface of the body undertaken to induce relief from a negative feeling/cognitive state or to achieve a positive mood state
- The diagnosis is not applied to suicidal ideation or to preparatory acts
- The act was not initiated during a state of delirium or confusion
- The act was not undertaken solely for a political or religious objective

(DSM-5: Diagnostic and statistical manual of mental disorders-5)

> **BOX 5:** Proposed criteria in DSM-5 for nonsuicidal self-injury.[27]
>
> *Nonsuicidal self-injury:*
> - In the last year, the individual has, on 5 or more days, engaged in intentional self-inflicted damage to the surface of his or her body of a sort likely to induce bleeding, bruising, or pain (e.g., cutting, burning, stabbing, hitting, excessive rubbing), with the expectation that the injury will lead to only minor or moderate physical harm (i.e., there is no suicidal intent)
>
> *Note:* The absence of suicidal intent has either been stated by the individual or can be inferred by the individual's repeated engagement in a behavior that the individual knows, or has learned, is not likely to result in death
> - The individual engages in the self-injurious behavior with one or more of the following expectations:
>   - To obtain relief from a negative feeling or cognitive state
>   - To resolve an interpersonal difficulty
>   - To induce a positive feeling state
>
> *Note:* The desired relief or response is experienced during or shortly after the self-injury, and the individual may display patterns of behavior suggesting a dependence on repeatedly engaging in it.
> - *The intentional self-injury is associated with at least one of the following:*
>   - Interpersonal difficulties or negative feelings or thoughts, such as depression, anxiety, tension, anger, generalized distress, or self-criticism, occurring in the period immediately prior to the self-injurious act
>   - Prior to engaging in the act, a period of preoccupation with the intended behavior that is difficult to control
>   - Thinking about self-injury that occurs frequently, even when it is not acted upon
> - The behavior is not socially sanctioned (e.g., body piercing, tattooing, part of a religious, or cultural ritual) and is not restricted to picking a scab or nail biting
> - The behavior or its consequences cause clinically significant distress or interference in interpersonal, academic, or other important areas of functioning
> - The behavior does not occur exclusively during psychotic episodes, delirium, substance intoxication, or substance withdrawal. In individuals with a neurodevelopmental disorder, the behavior is not part of a pattern of repetitive stereotypies. The behavior is not better explained by another mental disorder or medical condition [e.g., psychotic disorder, autism spectrum disorder, intellectual disability, Lesch–Nyhan syndrome, stereotypic movement disorder with self-injury, trichotillomania (hair-pulling disorder), excoriation (skin-picking) disorder
>
> (DSM-5: Diagnostic and statistical manual of mental disorders-5)

The former includes nonsuicidal self-injury, suicide attempt, and suicidal behavior, whereas the latter comprises intentional self-harm classified by the method employed. Unlike the ICD-10, nonsuicidal self-injury (parasuicide in ICD-10) and attempted suicide are differentiated based on intent despite being included in the broad category of "symptoms, signs or clinical findings, not elsewhere classified". Further, extension codes are created for supplementary use to identify greater details in individual categories. In the extension codes, under dimensions of external causes, various aspects of intentional self-harm events such as proximal risk factors, previous nonintentional self-harm attempts, and intent to die aspects of self-harm are included. However, these extension codes are not intended for usage in primary classification.[28]

CURRENT CLASSIFICATION AND DEFINITIONS OF SUICIDAL BEHAVIOR

Classification of Suicidal Behavior

An operational classification of suicidal behavior is necessary to inform risk assessment and further interventions aimed at mitigating suicide risk. Accumulating research over the last five decades points to a total of 19 different, yet overlapping, descriptive classifications of suicide. These are described in a recent systematic review by Goodfellow and colleagues,[29] who grouped them under three categories: comprehensive classification systems where the focus is on covering the wide spectrum of suicidal behaviors and acts, restrictive classification systems that focus on a particular subgroup of suicidal behaviors (such as nonfatal suicidal behavior), and suicidal behaviors that require to be added to existing classifications. They are briefly discussed here.

Comprehensive Classification Systems (n = 10)

Ten different comprehensive classification systems have been proposed so far, of which the most popular, perhaps, are the classification by O'Caroll and colleagues,[20] where they delineated nine defined categories of suicide related thoughts and behaviors, and subsequently, the one by Silverman and colleagues,[21] where they built on available evidence and proposed a new classification comprising 11 categories, with the significant addition of a category named suicide related communication. Precise operational definitions of suicide categories that would facilitate communication and research were the central feature of most comprehensive classification systems.

Restrictive Classification Systems (n = 6)

This category included six classifications of which Litman's classification of suicide,[30] based on degree of suicide intent, and Rosenberg and colleagues Operational Criteria for Determination of Suicide (OCDS),[17] which

described method to assess intent, focused on fatal suicidal behavior. Other models such as those by Lester (1990)[31] and Brown et al.[32] classified nonfatal suicidal behavior, based on evidence of intent and knowledge (foreseeability of self-harm due to act).

Suicidal Behaviors that Require to be Added to Existing Classifications (n = 3)

More than two decades ago, Barber and colleagues[33] introduced the term aborted suicide attempt and provided a set of rules as well as a scale to correctly identify the behavior; this was subsequently incorporated into the Columbia Classification Algorithm of Suicide Assessment (C-CASA) by Posner and colleagues,[34] as a category to help predict suicide. The DSM-5 has included two new suicide-specific diagnostic categories—*suicide behavioral disorder and nonsuicidal self-injury*, under the section "Conditions for further study" and has proposed a set of diagnostic criteria for both these entities.

Contemporary Definitions of Suicide-related Behavior and Communication

The field of suicide research is plagued by use of inconsistent, or worse still, lack of proper definitions of suicide. A scoping review of suicide studies in South Asia, including India, found that four out of five published studies failed to explicitly define suicide;[35] similar findings were noted in reviews of studies related to NSSIBs in India.[19] Even most clinical trials focusing on attempted suicide failed to clearly define a suicide attempt.[36] These results underscore the need to develop and adopt uniform definitions so that findings can be compared across studies.

The aim in this section is to provide a snapshot of different contemporary and popular definitions of suicide-related behaviors and suicide-related communications available in literature; the latter was proposed as a superset category by Silverman and colleagues[21] to impart greater clarity to terms such as suicide threat and suicide plan, which are deeply enshrined in popular communication and, thus, difficult to eliminate.

Definition of Suicide-related Behaviors

Suicide ideation: The definitions of suicide ideation are given in **Table 1**.

Definition of suicide attempt: The definitions of suicide attempt are given in **Table 2**.

Definition of suicide: The definitions of suicide are given in **Table 3**.

Definition of self-harm: The definitions of self-harm are given in **Table 4**.

Definition of Suicide-related Communication

Suicide threat: The definitions of suicide threat are given in **Table 5**.

TABLE 1: Definitions of suicide ideation.

Author(s)	Proposed definition
O'Caroll et al. (1996)[20]	"Any self-reported thoughts of engaging in suicide-related behavior"
American Psychiatric Association (2006)[37]	"Thoughts of serving as the agent of one's own death"
Posner et al. (2007)[34]	"Passive thoughts about wanting to be dead or active thoughts about killing oneself, not accompanied by preparatory behavior"
Crosby et al. (2011)[38]	"Thoughts of engaging in suicide-related behavior"
Diagnostic and Statistical Manual of Mental Disorders (DSM)-5 (2013)[27]	"Thoughts about self-harm, with deliberate consideration or planning of possible techniques of causing one's own death"

TABLE 2: Definitions of suicide attempt.

Author(s)	Proposed definition
O'Caroll et al. (1996)[20]	"A potentially self-injurious behavior with a nonfatal outcome, for which there is evidence (either explicit or implicit) that the person intended at some (nonzero) level to kill himself/herself. A suicide attempt may or may not result in injuries"
American Psychiatric Association (2006)[37]	"Self-injurious behavior with a nonfatal outcome accompanied by evidence (either explicit or implicit) that the person intended to die"
Posner et al. (2007)[34]	"A potentially self-injurious behavior, associated with at least some intent to die, as a result of the act. Evidence that the individual intended to kill himself/herself, at least to some degree, can be explicit or inferred from the behavior or circumstance. A suicide attempt may or may not result in actual injury"
Silverman et al. (2007)[21]	"A self-inflicted, potentially injurious behavior with a nonfatal outcome for which there is evidence (either explicit or implicit) of intent to die"
Diagnostic and Statistical Manual of Mental Disorders (DSM)-5 (2013)[27]	"A self-initiated sequence of behaviors by an individual who, at the time of initiation, expected that the set of actions would lead to his or her own death"

TABLE 3: Definitions of suicide.

Author(s)	Proposed definition
Rosenberg et al. (1998) (Operational Criteria for Definition of Suicide)[17]	"Death from injury, poisoning, or suffocation where there is evidence (either explicit or implicit) that the injury was self-inflicted and that the decedent intended to kill himself/herself"
American Psychiatric Association (2006)[37]	"Self-inflicted death with evidence (either explicit or implicit) that the person intended to die"
De Leo et al. 2006[15]	"Act with fatal outcome, which the deceased, knowing or expecting a potentially fatal outcome, has initiated and carried out with the purpose of bringing about wanted changes"
Posner et al. (2007)[34]	"A self-injurious behavior that resulted in fatality and was associated with at least some intent to die as a result of the act"
Silverman et al. (2007)[21]	"Self-inflicted death with evidence (either explicit or implicit) of intent to die"

TABLE 4: Definitions of self-harm.

Author(s)	Equivalent term and proposed definition
O'Caroll et al. (1996)[20]	*Instrumental suicide-related behavior:* "Potentially self-injurious behavior for which there is evidence (either implicit or explicit) that (a) the person did not intend to kill himself/herself (i.e., had zero intent to die), and (b) the person wished to use the appearance of intending to kill himself/herself in order to attain some other end (e.g., to seek help, to punish others, and to receive attention)"
American Psychiatric Association (2006)[37]	*Deliberate self-harm:* "Willful self-inflicting of painful, destructive, or injurious acts without intent to die"
Posner et al. (2007)[34]	*Self-injurious behavior:* "Self-injurious behavior associated with no intent to die. The behavior is intended purely for other reasons, either to relieve distress (often referred to as "self-mutilation", e.g., superficial cuts or scratches, hitting/banging, or burns) or to effect change in others or the environment"
Silverman et al. (2007)[21]	*Self-harm:* Self-harm is defined as a "self-inflicted, potentially injurious behavior for which there is evidence (either implicit or explicit) that the person did not intend to kill himself/herself" (i.e., had no intent to die)
Diagnostic and Statistical Manual of Mental Disorders (DSM)-5 (2013)[27]	Nonsuicidal self-injurious behavior (see Section on Nonsuicidal Self-injurious Behavior)

TABLE 5: Definitions of suicide threat.

Author(s)	Proposed definition
O'Caroll et al. (1996)[20]	"Any interpersonal action, verbal or nonverbal, stopping short of a directly self-harmful act, that a reasonable person would interpret as communicating or suggesting that a suicidal act or other suicide-related behavior might occur in the near future"
Silverman et al. (2007)[21]	"Any interpersonal action, verbal or nonverbal, without a direct self-injurious component, that a reasonable person would interpret as communicating or suggesting that suicidal behavior might occur in the near future"

TABLE 6: Definition of suicide plan.

Author(s)	Proposed definition
Silverman et al. (2007)[21]	"Proposed method of carrying out a design that will lead to a potentially self-injurious outcome; a systematic formulation of a program of action that has the potential for resulting in self-injury"

Suicide plan: The definition of suicide plan is given in **Table 6**.

Suicide gesture: The term suicide gesture was historically used to refer to behaviors "where the intended purpose was to alter one's life circumstances (interpersonal or intrapersonal) in a manner that was without suicidal intent, but involved self-inflicted behaviors (whether or not it resulted in injuries)".[21] However, due to the pejorative connotations that this term acquired with time, the same authors[21] have suggested that this behavior be relabeled as self-harm.

Other terms—aborted and interrupted suicide attempt/preparatory acts or behaviors: The term aborted suicide attempt was introduced by Barber and colleagues[33] to refer to an "event in which an individual is one step away from attempting suicide but does not complete the act and thus incurs no physical injury". The authors proposed three essential characteristics of an aborted attempt as the intent to kill oneself, change of mind just before the actual act, and absence of injury. Interrupted suicide attempts "occur when individuals initiate action to end their lives but are stopped by *someone or something* external to the individual before actually carrying out the act".[39] A related term is preparatory act or behavior toward suicide which refers to any preparatory behavior or act that heralds an imminent suicide attempt; examples include preparatory acts such as making/revising a will, giving away personal belongings or securing a method such as buying pesticide or firearms.[40]

Self-injurious Behavior

The first major aspect in assessing any case of suicidal behavior is the intent to die, which may be answered either affirmatively, negatively, or in uncertain terms.[15,41] This is referred to as suicide intent, in other words, the seriousness of the wish to die. If suicide intent is present to any degree, then it is called suicide attempt and, if intent is absent, it is called self-harm. A major precondition to establish suicidal or nonsuicidal behavior is the presence of deliberate or intentional self-injurious behavior; it follows that any self-harm or potential for self-harm accrued as a result of the behavior is a deliberate consequence of the behavior.[40] The Centers for Disease Control and Prevention (CDC) has used the term self-directed violence which has the same meaning and is often used interchangeably with self-injurious behavior.[38] In this context, it must be noted that the lethality of the act is immaterial in determining the classification of self-injurious behavior; as an example, someone who pulls the trigger of a loaded gun directed at his/her head but the gun fails to fire for some reason will still be classified as having performed a self-injurious behavior. In other words, any behavior carried out with the goals of inflicting harm on oneself is termed self-injurious behavior; depending on intent, the behavior may be classified as suicidal or non-NSSIB. Intent is absent.[40]

Nonsuicidal Self-injurious Behavior

The term NSSIB, as mentioned in the previous section, refers to self-injurious behavior where the end goal is to inflict harm to oneself, but there is no intent to die; common examples of NSSIB include nonlethal cuts or lacerations and head banging. NSSIB acts are typically stereotyped and occur repetitively; in contrast, suicide attempt is a discrete single or intermittent behavior.[42] This distinction, however, should not lull a clinician into a false sense of confidence when performing a suicide risk assessment because a history of NSSIB confers increased risk of subsequent suicide attempt; more than half of individuals with NSSIB have a history of at least one lifetime suicide attempt.[43]

The clinical value of distinguishing NSSIB from a suicide attempt appears to lie in directing appropriate clinical interventions and risk mitigation measures. In this regard, it is important to note that NSSIB has been found to serve the following purposes:[44]

- Affect regulation—to release emotional tension and re-establish a sense of control
- Distraction from (emotional) pain
- Sense of self-punishment—for relief from a sense of shame or remorse
- To provide a concrete evidence, in the form of a scar or wound, that permits individual to self-validate the emotional distress
- Mitigation of feelings of emotional numbing or depersonalization
- Discharge of anger and negative emotions—self-directed anger seems more acceptable and less disruptive than anger at others.

Clear definitions of NSSIB would facilitate research, understanding, and validation of the distinction between this entity and suicide attempt.

Additional Notes on Suicide Intent

Assessment of suicide intent, perhaps the single most important step in assessment of self-injurious behavior, is a field replete with misunderstandings and misconceptions. Intent can be assessed based on statements made by the person, information gathered from family and friends, or from circumstantial evidence; in other words, suicide intent may be stated or inferred.[45] Intent may not always correlate with medical lethality (defined as objective danger to life associated with a suicide method or action); as an example, if someone consumes three tablets of acetaminophen with some intent to die, then it should be labeled as suicide attempt; in other words, use of nonlethal methods should not automatically imply a lack of intent.[40] Circumstantial evidence may be used to infer intent or lack thereof; if an individual cuts the hand or leg, it is not usually indicative of suicide intent. Finally, an awareness and subjective understanding of the potential consequences of the act are necessary; this may be unclear in cases of psychosis. For instance, if a person jumps from a height due to a delusional belief that he/she can fly, then the presence of intent cannot be inferred in such cases and should be stated as such.[46]

SUICIDAL BEHAVIOR AS A SPECTRUM

Presuicidal Syndrome

The term denotes the psychological state preceding suicide. It was first described in 1949 by Ringel based on analysis of suicide notes and had three principal components:

1. *Constriction*, which may be situational or dynamic or combined, may be of human relations or values
2. *Inhibited aggression,* which becomes autoaggression
3. *Suicidal fantasies*—preoccupation with suicide ranging from passive death wishes to the specific plan for committing suicide.[47]

Suicidal Logic

This was a cognitive model proposed by Shneidman[48] to explain the progression from suicidal ideation to the act of suicide. According to this model, a person experiences unbearable psychological pain coupled with negative lived experiences and a state of mental perturbation. The person feels the need to end the prolonged psychological distress, but due to the negative effects of prior experiences, the individual moves to a rigid/dichotomous reasoning; the result of this is an inability to see any solution other than suicide, to their suffering. Thus, suicide ideation may culminate in suicide.

Continuum from Suicidal Ideation to Completed Suicide

Suicidal behaviors may lie on a continuum from suicidal ideation to attempted suicide and completed suicide.[49] It is the severity of the clinical situation that would determine the outcome of suicidal behavior while the strength of intention determines the position of an individual on the suicidal spectrum. Based on the outcome of the act, suicide can be divided into those who had a serious suicide attempt (medical outcome), those who made a violent attempt (based on the method used), and those who did not fit into either of these categories. Those with violent or serious attempts share characteristics with the population who complete suicide, such as a higher proportion of males, a history of previous attempts, a family history of suicidal behavior, and advanced age.[50]

Studies comparing single attempters and repeat suicide attempters have found that the latter group had higher rates of mood/anxiety disorder and substance use disorder especially alcohol, prior history of exposure to early trauma, greater hopelessness and trait impulsivity, and increased rates of family history of suicide compared to the former group.[51,52] More research into characteristics of different sub-groups among suicide attempters is necessary to ascertain their validity; in this regard, a large retrospective study from India found that age at onset could be a useful marker to delineate early and late-onset subgroup among suicide attempters.[53] Such studies could have potential implications in terms of customization of suicide prevention strategies.

IMPORTANCE OF DISTINGUISHING SUICIDAL IDEATION VERSUS SUICIDAL BEHAVIORS

Individuals harboring suicidal ideas must be differentiated from ones with other suicidal behavior so that an accurate assessment of suicide risk can be made and appropriate follow-up action initiated. The suicide risk after expression of suicidal ideation in the 1st year of follow-up was higher in psychiatric patients than in nonpsychiatric participants.[54] It is estimated that around 60% of individuals' transition from suicidal ideation to actual attempt within a year of the onset of ideation.[55] Simultaneously, it is also important to note that not all suicide ideators may go on to attempt suicide.[56] Therefore, it becomes crucial to identify risk factors that may predict the transition from suicidal ideation to further suicidal behavior.[57] The clinical utility of identifying suicidal ideation may lie in identifying a sub-group of people at risk for future attempts and broadening the scope of risk assessment weighted traditionally toward the use of past suicide attempts as a predictor for future suicidal behavior.[58,59]

More research is required to clearly understand the causes of suicide ideation, attempts, and death. Especially, short-term longitudinal studies assessing various factors at various micro timelines such as minutes, hours, days, years would help us to understand better and identify action points to prevent evolution from suicide ideation to action.[60] This is important because research on attempted suicide, in Indian settings, has shown that the median time of the suicidal process, defined as "progression from the emergence of ideas of harming self to the actual behavior of carrying out the suicidal act which may become a completed suicide or an attempted suicide depending on the subject's survival",[61] is 30 minutes;[62] thus, only a small, but definite, window of opportunity is available for risk mitigation interventions.

STRENGTHS AND LIMITATIONS OF CURRENT SUICIDE NOMENCLATURE

Strengths

The existing nomenclature provides an overview of different suicidal behaviors. It recognizes the need for and tries to bring in some uniformity in interpreting a range of key suicide-related behaviors. It also helps to understand the fundamental differences between suicidal behaviors.[29] The Silverman et al.[21] nomenclature is widely accepted and may be considered for defining suicide-related behaviors in clinical activities and research.

Limitations

Prior Indian investigators, using a record-based design, have found poor inter-rater reliability for currently accepted definitions of suicide-related ideation and behavior.[63] Further, current suicide nomenclature does not include certain culture-specific practices, specific to the Indian setting, such as "sati",[64] wherein a widow immolates herself on the funeral pyre of her deceased husband, and "Thalaikoothal", an end of life practice specific to southern districts of Tamil Nadu wherein a close relative hastens the death of the elderly in households.[65]

In developing countries such as India, massive underreporting of suicides exists because of the social stigma attached to the behavior and because attempted suicide, until recently, was a punishable offense under Section 309 of the Indian Penal Code.[66] These cultural and legal factors pose additional unique challenges in correctly identifying and classifying suicidal behaviors in India.[67]

CONCLUSION

The last couple of decades have seen significant efforts to develop a standardized suicide nomenclature. Several influential publications propose intent to die as the cornerstone of classifying self-injurious behaviors. However, because our knowledge of the basis of suicidal behavior is constantly evolving, we must be prepared to refine existing definitions in light of new information accrued from time to time. The inclusion of new suicide-related categories in DSM-5 is an important initial step that shows a commitment to move toward a uniform system of classifying suicidal behaviors. Nevertheless, much work remains to be done to develop a universally agreed-upon set of terms and definitions that will have wide uptake and augment suicide intervention, prevention, and research activities.

REFERENCES

1. Beautrais AL. Suicide in Asia. Crisis. 2006; 27(2):55-7.
2. Vijayakumar L, Daly C, Arafat Y, Arensman E. Suicide prevention in the Southeast Asia region. Crisis. 2020;41(Suppl 1):S21-9.
3. Tondo L. Brief history of suicide in Western cultures. In: Nemeroff CB, Ruiz P, Koslow SH (Eds). A Concise Guide to Understanding Suicide: Epidemiology, Pathophysiology and Prevention. Cambridge: Cambridge University Press; 2014. pp. 3-12.

4. Barraclough B, Shepherd D. A necessary neologism: the origin and uses of suicide. Suicide Life Threat Behav. 1994;24(2):113-26.

5. Rosen G. History in the study of suicide. Psychol Med. 1971;1(4):267-85.

6. Biblioteket H. (1838). Des maladies mentales. Considérées sous les rapports médical, hygiénique et médico-légal. Tome Premier - Second & Atlas. Paris, J.-B. Baillière, libraire de l'Acadèmie Royale de Medecine, 1838. [Internet]. The Historical Library of Karolinska Institutet and the Swedish Society of Medicine. [online] Available from: http://hagstromerlibrary.ki.se/books/1560. [Last accessed July, 2022].

7. Solano P, Pizzorno E, Pompili M, Serafini G, Amore M. Conceptualizations of suicide through time and socio-economic factors: a historical mini-review. Ir J Psychol Med. 2018;35(1):75-86.

8. Mueller AS, Abrutyn S, Pescosolido B, Diefendorf S. The social roots of suicide: theorizing how the external social world matters to suicide and suicide prevention? Front Psychol. 2021;12:621569.

9. Hendin H. Psychodynamic motivational factors in suicide. Psych Quar. 1951;25(1):672-8.

10. Ronningstam E, Weinberg I, Maltsberger J (2009). Psychoanalytic theories of suicide. [online] Available from: https://oxfordmedicine.com/view/10.1093/med/9780198570059.001.0001/med-9780198570059-chapter-24. [Last accessed July, 2022].

11. Hendin H. The psychodynamics of suicide. J Nerv Ment Dis. 1963;136:236-44.

12. Giner L, Guija JA, Root CW, Baca-Garcia E. Nomenclature and definition of suicidal behavior. In: Courtet P (Ed). Understanding Suicide. Cham: Springer International Publishing; 2016. pp. 3-17.

13. Kessel N, Grossman G. Suicide in alcoholics. Br Med J. 1961;2(5268):1671-2.

14. Kreitman N, Philip AE, Greer S, Bagley CR. Parasuicide. Br J Psychiatry. 1969;115(523):746-7.

15. De Leo D, Burgis S, Bertolote JM, Kerkhof AJFM, Bille-Brahe U. Definitions of suicidal behavior: lessons learned from the WHO/EURO multicentre Study. Crisis. 2006;27(1):4-15.

16. Motto JA. An integrated approach to estimating suicide risk. Suicide Life Threat Behav. 1991;21(1):74-89.

17. Rosenberg ML, Davidson LE, Smith JC, Berman AL, Buzbee H, Gantner G, et al. Operational criteria for the determination of suicide. J Forensic Sci. 1988;33(6):1445-56.

18. Silverman MM, De Leo D. Why there is a need for an international nomenclature and classification system for suicide? Crisis. 2016;37(2):83-7.

19. Gandhi A, Luyckx K, Maitra S, Claes L. Non-suicidal self-injury and other self-directed violent behaviors in India: a review of definitions and research. Asian J Psychiatr. 2016;22:196-201.

20. O'Carroll PW, Berman AL, Maris RW, Moscicki EK, Tanney BL, Silverman MM. Beyond the tower of Babel: a nomenclature for suicidology. Suicide Life Threat Behav. 1996;26(3):237-52.

21. Silverman MM, Berman AL, Sanddal ND, O'carroll PW, Joiner TE. Rebuilding the tower of Babel: a revised nomenclature for the study of suicide and suicidal behaviors. Part 2: Suicide-related ideations, communications, and behaviors. Suicide Life Threat Behav. 2007;37(3):264-77.

22. Comstock BS. Suicide in the 1970s: a second look. Suicide Life Threat Behav. 1979;9(1):3-13.

23. Schmidtke A, Brahe UB, Leo DD, Kerkhof AJFM. (2004). The WHO/EURO Multicentre Study on Suicidal Behaviour: History and Aims of the Study. Suicidal Behaviour in Europe Results from: the WHO/EURO Multicentre Study on Suicidal Behaviour. [online] Available from https://psycnet.apa.org/record/2004-19472-002. [Last accesed July, 2022].

24. Bille-Brahe U, Schmidtke A, Kerkhof AJ, De Leo D, Lönnqvist J, Platt S, et al. Background and introduction to the WHO/EURO multicentre study on parasuicide. Crisis. 1995;16(2):72-8, 84.

25. World Health Organization. (1992). The ICD-10 classification of mental and behavioural disorders: clinical descriptions and diagnostic guidelines. [online] Available from: https://apps.who.int/iris/handle/10665/37958. [Last accessed July, 2022].

26. Bell CC. DSM-IV: Diagnostic and Statistical Manual of Mental Disorders. JAMA. 1994;272(10):828-9.

27. American Psychiatric Association. Diagnostic and statistical manual of mental disorders: DSM-5, 5th edition. Washington, D.C: American Psychiatric Association; 2013.

28. International Classification of Diseases. ICD-11 for Mortality and Morbidity Statistics. [online] Available from: https://icd.who.int/browse11/l-m/en. [Last accessed July, 2022].

29. Goodfellow B, Kõlves K, de Leo D. Contemporary nomenclatures of suicidal behaviors: a systematic literature review. Suicide Life Threat Behav. 2018;48(3):353-66.

30. Litman RE. Psychological-psychiatric aspects in certifying modes of death. J Forensic Sci. 1968;13(1):46-54.

31. Lester D. A classification of acts of attempted suicide. Percept Mot Skills. 1990;70(3_suppl):1245-6.

32. Brown G, Jeglic E, Henriques G, Beck A. Cognitive therapy, cognition, and suicidal behavior. In: TE Ellis (Ed.). Cognition and Suicide: Theory, Research, and Therapy. Washington, DC: American Psychological Association; 2006. pp. 63-74.

33. Barber ME, Marzuk PM, Leon AC, Portera L. Aborted suicide attempts: a new classification of suicidal behavior. AJP. 1998;155(3):385-9.

34. Posner K, Oquendo MA, Gould M, Stanley B, Davies M. Columbia Classification Algorithm of Suicide Assessment (C-CASA): Classification of Suicidal Events in the FDA's Pediatric Suicidal Risk Analysis of Antidepressants. Am J Psychiatry. 2007;164(7):1035-43.

35. Jordans MJ, Kaufman A, Brenman NF, Adhikari RP, Luitel NP, Tol WA, et al. Suicide in South Asia: a scoping review. BMC Psychiatry. 2014;14(1):358.

36. Mitra S, Kodancha PG. Defining suicide in clinical trials—how do we fare? Indian J Psychol Med. 2022;44(1):85-7.

37. Jacobs DG, Baldessarini CRJ, Conwell Y, Fawcett JA, Horton L, Meltzer H, et al. Practice Guideline for the Assessment and Treatment of Patients With Suicidal Behaviors. In: APA Practice Guidelines for the Treatment of Psychiatric Disorders: Comprehensive Guidelines and Guideline Watches. Arlington, VA: American Psychiatric Association; 2006.

38. Crosby AE, Ortega L, Melanson C. Self-directed violence surveillance; uniform definitions and recommended data elements. (Version 1.0). Atlanta, GA: Centers for Disease Control and Prevention; 2011. p. 90.

39. Burke TA, Hamilton JL, Ammerman BA, Stange JP, Alloy LB. Suicide risk characteristics among aborted, interrupted, and actual suicide attempters. Psychiatry Res. 2016;242:357-64.

40. Nock MK, Posner K, Brodsky B, Yershova K, Buchanan J, Mann J. The classification of suicidal behavior. In: Nock MK (Ed). The Oxford Handbook of Suicide and Self-Injury. Jericho: Oxford University Press; 2014.

41. De Leo D, Burgis S, Bertolote J, Kerkhof A, Bille-Brahe U. Definitions of suicidal behavior. In: DeLeo D, Bille-Brahe U, Kerkhof ADM, Schmidtke A (Eds). Suicidal Behavior: Theories and Research Findings. Washington, DC: Hogrefe & Huber; 2004. pp. 17-39.

42. Favazza AR. The coming of age of self-mutilation. J Nerv Ment Dis. 1998;186(5):259-68.

43. Brent DA, Oquendo M, Birmaher B, Greenhill L, Kolko D, Stanley B, et al. Familial pathways to early-onset suicide attempt: risk for suicidal behavior in offspring of mood-disordered suicide attempters. Arch Gen Psychiatry. 2002;59(9):801-7.

44. Gunderson J, Hoffman P. Understanding and treating borderline personality disorder: A guide for professionals and families. Washington, DC: American Psychiatric Publishing; 2005.

45. O'Carroll PW. A consideration of the validity and reliability of suicide mortality data. Suicide Life Threat Behav. 1989;19(1):1-16.

46. Beck A, Greenberg R. The nosology of suicidal phenomena: past and future perspectives. Bull Suicidol. 1971;8:10-7.

47. Ringel E. The presuicidal syndrome. Suicide Life Threat Behav. 1976;6(3):131-49.

48. Shneidman E. Suicidology: contemporary developments. New York: Grune & Stratton; 1976.

49. Sveticic J, De Leo D. The hypothesis of a continuum in suicidality: a discussion on its validity and practical implications. Ment Illn. 2012;4(2):e15.

50. Giner L, Jaussent I, Olié E, Béziat S, Guillaume S, Baca-Garcia E, et al. Violent and serious suicide attempters: one step closer to suicide? J Clin Psychiatry. 2014;75(3):e191-7.

51. Park CHK, Lee JW, Lee SY, Moon J, Jeon DW, Shim SH, et al. Suicide risk factors across suicidal ideators, single suicide attempters, and multiple suicide attempters. J Psychiatr Res. 2020;131:1-8.

52. Menon V, Kattimani S, Sarkar S, Mathan K. How do repeat suicide attempters differ from first timers? An exploratory record based analysis. J Neurosci Rural Pract. 2016;7(1):91-6.

53. Menon V, Kattimani S, Sarkar S, Sathyanarayanan G, Subramanian K, Velusamy SK. Age at onset of first suicide attempt: Exploring the utility of a potential candidate variable to subgroup attempters. Asian J Psychiatr. 2018;37:40-5.

54. Hubers AAM, Moaddine S, Peersmann SHM, Stijnen T, van Duijn E, van der Mast RC, et al. Suicidal ideation and subsequent completed suicide in both psychiatric and nonpsychiatric populations: a meta-analysis. Epidemiol Psychiatr Sci. 2018;27(2):186-98.

55. Nock MK, Borges G, Bromet EJ, Alonso J, Angermeyer M, Beautrais A, et al. Cross-national prevalence and risk factors for suicidal ideation, plans and attempts. Br J Psychiatry. 2008;192(2):98-105.

56. ten Have M, de Graaf R, van Dorsselaer S, Verdurmen J, van 't Land H, Vollebergh W, et al. Incidence and course of suicidal ideation and suicide attempts in the general population. Can J Psychiatry. 2009;54(12):824-33.

57. Kessler RC, Berglund P, Demler O, Jin R, Merikangas KR, Walters EE. Lifetime prevalence and age-of-onset distributions of DSM-IV disorders in the National Comorbidity Survey Replication. Arch Gen Psychiatry. 2005;62(6):593-602.

58. Kessler RC, Borges G, Walters EE. Prevalence of and risk factors for lifetime suicide attempts in the National Comorbidity Survey. Arch Gen Psychiatry. 1999;56(7):617-26.

59. Rudd MD, Joiner T, Rajab MH. Relationships among suicide ideators, attempters, and multiple attempters in a young-adult sample. J Abnorm Psychol. 1996;105(4):541-50.

60. Klonsky ED, Saffer BY, Bryan CJ. Ideation-to-action theories of suicide: a conceptual and empirical update. Curr Opin Psychol. 2018;22:38-43.

61. Wassermann D. A stress-vulnerability model and the development of the suicidal process. In: Wasserman D (Ed). In: Suicide – An Unnecessary Death. London: Dunitz; 2001. pp. 13-27.

62. Kattimani S, Sarkar S, Menon V, Muthuramalingam A, Nancy P. Duration of suicide process among suicide attempters and characteristics of those providing window of opportunity for intervention. J Neurosci Rural Pract. 2016;7(4):566-70.

63. Kattimani S, Bharadwaj B, Sarkar S, Mukherjee A. Interrater reliability of the Silverman et al. nomenclature for suicide-related ideations, behaviors, and communications. Crisis. 2015;36(1):61-4.

64. Bhugra D. Sati: a type of nonpsychiatric suicide. Crisis. 2005;26(2):73-7.

65. Ramalingam S, Ganesan S. End-of-life practices in rural South India: Sociocultural determinants. Indian J Palliat Care. 2019;25(2):224-7.

66. Vadlamani LN, Gowda M. Practical implications of Mental Healthcare Act 2017: Suicide and suicide attempt. Indian J Psychiatry. 2019;61(10):750.

67. Radhakrishnan R, Andrade C. Suicide: an Indian perspective. Indian J Psychiatry. 2012;54(4):304-19.

Sociocultural Aspects of Suicide

Koushik Sinha Deb, Anuranjan Vishwakarma, Rakesh K Chadda

ABSTRACT

The recently published suicide statistics of India [National Crime Records Bureau (NCRB), 2021] reported 12 suicidal deaths per 100,000 population for the year 2021. The "Global Burden of Diseases Study" and the "Million Death Study", often considered as landmark research on suicide in India, report even higher rates and greater demographic clustering. Wide variations in suicides (sometimes over 10 times) across geographic locations, gender, marital state, and occupation have also been reported. An in-depth exploration of the sociocultural and geopolitical determinants, which shape the lives of Indian people, becomes necessary to understand these suicide research findings.

This chapter begins by exploring the complex past civilizations, rituals, and religious connotations of suicide. Acceptance of suicide by the elderly and death by immolation in females are India-specific patterns, starkly in contrast with the West, and comprehensible only by understanding our past. The changing Indian family systems, urbanization of the villages, and the inescapable loss of pride in farming represent some of the economic and commercial determinants driving suicide rates. Migration, exploitation, discrimination, social disconnect, apathy, and anomie of the city life are consequences of a rapidly changing social landscape. The rapid expansion of technology, internet, and social media has further disrupted customs, morals, and values of individuals, families, and communities, contributing to newer stressors and traumas.

India and many similar developing countries are in state of unstable cultural flux due to rapid changes in all spheres of life. Developing an understanding of these agents of change is necessary, not only to comprehend the patterns of suicide, but also for devising appropriate strategies of prevention.

Keywords: Suicide; Social theories; Cultural theories.

INTRODUCTION

Suicide or the act of voluntarily and actively ending one's life is counter-biological, counter-evolutionary, and counter-adaptive.[1] Yet, suicide forms one of the most common causes of death in the young adults, second only to accidents. The World Health Organization, which has been monitoring and advocating against suicide since 1950, suggests that 78% of the suicides occur in the low- and middle-income countries.[2] India and China together account for more than half of the suicides across the world, and India records the highest suicide rates among all other South-East-Asian countries.[3] Despite India's overall rate being similar to many other nations, the female suicide rate of the country is one of the highest globally.[4] India's (possibly under-reported)[5] suicide statistics of 2022, published by the National Crime Records Bureau (NCRB), reported a national rate of 12 suicidal death per 100,000 population, the highest rate ever reported by the Bureau since its inception in 1967.[6] Almost 50% of all these deaths occurred in just five of India's 28 states and 8 union territories and 64.2% of the victims earned <1 lakh rupees per year.[7] The marked variability of the rates, in terms of gender, geography, and wage, suggests factors beyond the individual at play, the evaluation of which forms the focus for this chapter. The role of mental and substance use disorders as a precipitator of suicide cannot be underestimated and this write up, by no means, intends to underplay the pivotal role of mental morbidity in suicide.[2] The chapter instead intends to look beyond the obvious and aims to sensitize the reader about the sociocultural fabric that operates behind the proximate cause of depression and self-harm.

CIVILIZATION, CULTURE, RELIGION, AND SOCIETY

India is the land of ancient civilizations. The Indus valley (proto-Dravidian) civilization of the North and the Dravidian civilization of the South flourished around two to three millennia before the birth of Christ (2500 BCE) and envisioned philosophical doctrines on life, death, rebirth, and morality which were followed by its people.[8] Subsequent waves of conquests, expansions, and influences over the next two millennia have brought in ideas from the Persian, Greek, Arabic, Mughal, and British (Christian) culture into the region, which shaped the traditional Indian society. Postmodern influences of globalization and westernization of values, urban migration and emigration, and a gradual shift from collectivism to individualism have created an immensely complex, rich, multi-layered, intertwined, and amalgamated culture of the subcontinent. These traditional and modern pressures on individuals constitute the unseen threads that knit the tapestry of life

stories of people, and understanding them is vital to understanding the conclusion.

The Vedic Hindu philosophy believed in the doctrine of reincarnation and rebirth, with "Moksha" or "Mukti' providing liberation from this eternal circle. Unlike the strict proscription on suicide in the Islamic and Christian religion, the stance of the Vedas on suicide has been nuanced, resulting often in theological and religious debates.[9] The four Vedas, forming the oldest of Hindu scriptures of "Shruti" (what is heard), do not directly expound on suicide. The Vedas value life, with "ahimsa" being a virtue and "hatya" being a sin. Death, according to Vedas, comes naturally after living a full and pious life.[9] The Upanishads (written expositions of the Vedas), denounce suicides, stating that "he who takes his self, reaches after death the sunless region covered by impenetrable darkness".[10] Similar proscriptions are also found in the social-rules texts of Hinduism ("Shastras"). For example, "Arthashastra", written by Kautilya (advisor to Emperor Chandragupta Maurya), condemned men and women who committed suicide in the throes of sinful passions, and instituted a procedure for determination of death by commissioners.[11]

Acceptance and allowance of suicides are first noted in the text of "Dharma-shastra", the Hindu text on ethics. Death by starvation while on pilgrimage to Kailash (the place of Lord Shiva) at the end of fulfilling ones life's responsibilities forms the tradition of "Maha-Prasthana". Death by drowning in the Ganges at Kashi (Varanasi), jumping from a cliff at Amarkantak, and drowning at or jumping from a sacred tree at Prayag (confluence of the three holy rivers of Ganga, Yamuna, and Saraswathi) was suggested as a form of attaining Moksha. In the great Hindu epic, Ramayana, after the departure of Sita,

Lakshman, unable to bear the sorrow, kills himself by drowning in the river. Ram, Bharat, and Shatrughan follow suit by drowning in the Sarayu river, along with thousand inhabitants of their city Ajodhya.[11] The other religious epic of Mahabharata provides numerous examples of accepting death for the righteous reason and for the greater good (e.g., Dadhichi offering his life for creation of weapons from his bones) but denounces taking one's own life for shame or before time.[12]

Over time, the Vedic philosophies mutated into societal rules and the British India saw a large number of religious suicides to end personal suffering. Hunter, in 1872,[13] recorded religious suicides in Puri, Orissa at the "Ratha-Yatra" festival of Lord Jagannath, where devotees took their lives by throwing themselves under the wheel of the chariot which was pulled by thousands of devotees.[14,15] The custom of "Sati"[16] and "Jauhar"[14] fascinated the British rulers and numerous recorded descriptions of these events were documented.[17] Raja Rammohan Roy, between 1818 and 1829, wrote several articles detailing the various Hindu religious doctrines and their interpretations, successfully arguing against the custom of "sati". The established dogma of "sati" as ordained by the ruling pandits did not bear any Vedic validation, according to Roy.[18] A crusade that started in 1814 after observing the burning of his brother's widow ultimately succeeded after 15 years, when Governor-General of India, Lord William Bentinck, declared sati illegal and made it punishable as a criminal offence through Regulation XVII of December 4th, 1829.

Other Indian religions have a far uniform proscription against taking one's own life. Jainism, founded by Mahavira (600 BC), is characterized by extreme respect for life.[10] The tradition of "sallekhana" or fasting

unto death in Jainism represents a religious ritual intended to end the cycle of death and rebirth, and has the connotation of enlightenment, rather than suicide from suffering.[20] Buddhism similarly believes in the eternal cycle of life and suicide, therefore, does not alter or shorten any suffering. Islam, practiced by around 15% of the population of India, has the strongest moral and religious opposition to suicide, as life needs to follow the principles of "Allah".[21]

Indian family systems arising out of such cultures are also, therefore, understandably complex. The traditional Indian family would be classified as collectivistic, with group interests taking priority over individual aspirations.[22] The patrilineal and patriarchal structure of the traditional family provides security and safety of all, and shields members in times of hardships. Conversely, the subservient role of women in such families and the demands of the family on young adults to adhere to role obligations form an environment of conflict and oppression, making such collectivism far from the ideal harmonious social unit.[11,23] The society of India, imbued in its tradition, has undergone rapid changes postindependence, due to forces of urbanization and economics. Work, opportunity, and education have taken families to far away cities, with alien language, food, culture, moral, and social values, making everyday life a struggle for adaptation. Modern nuclear families of the city face newer conflicts, as members differentially imbibe diverse aspects of the urban culture. Intergenerational gaps in moral and ethical values increase exponentially, creating culture clash and further fragmentation of the family.[24]

URBAN AND RURAL DIVIDE

Urbanization has been cited as a major driver of social change and disruptor of stability, and has long been the focus of sociological studies of suicide. The most influential work comes from the French sociologist Émile Durkheim, whose 1897 book Suicide: A Study in Sociology (French: Le Suicide: Étude de sociologie) formed the basis of our understanding of suicide over the next decades.[25] Durkheim posited that the society exerts coercive influence on individuals through its rules and obligations which he labeled as "social facts". These social facts are not merely in the mind of the individual but external and real, similar to the natural facts of the world we live in. Integration of the individual into the society follows a continuum, with too little integration causing "egoism" or the feeling of being untethered to the society one stays in, and too complete integration resulting in "altruism", where the self is completely subservient to the society. The rigidity of societal control creates the second continuum, at one end of which lies complete social abandon

resulting in "anomie", while the other end being absolute control resulting in "fatalism". Sudden changes and upheavals in the social structure results in the social facts become skewed toward any extreme ends of these continuums, affecting the person living in the society. Durkheim rejected the psychological causation of suicide, and considered mental morbidity to be a result of the same societal forces, rather than in independent causative agent. Durkheim believed that social facts alone can predict the pattern of suicide and provided case studies and examples of the same **(Table 1)**.[26]

India with its 1.4 billion peoples ranks as the second most populous country in the world. Postindependence, India has seen a rapid growth in urbanization, with currently 35% of its population living in the cities.[28] Such accelerated urbanization exerts enormous pressure on city infrastructure, sanitation, transport, and public amenities, resulting in overcrowding and unsafe living. The migration to cities for better living standards transmutes into homelessness and slum dwelling. Indeed, 17.4% of Indians (one in every five family) currently live in slums, with the major metropolises of Mumbai (41.3%), Kolkata (29.6%), and Chennai (28.5%) far outpacing the national average.[29] The problems of urban India are further complicated by pressing public health issues. Urban India is home to 35 of the 50 most polluted cities of the world, with the national capital Delhi and the British capital Kolkata ranking as the top two most polluted cities world over. Delhi empties more than 3,500 million liters of municipal sewage in the Yamuna river, resulting in a 3,000-fold rise of fecal bacterial count and often covering the main water source of the city with toxic foam. Tuberculosis, pneumonia, and diarrheal diseases, as well as noncommunicable

TABLE 1: Émile Durkheim's types of suicides.[27]

Type	Durkheim's example	Indian example
Egoistic suicide: Lasting feeling of not being integrated into the community with excessive individualization	Individuals not sufficiently bound to social groups, example unmarried man	Urban youths, students living away from family for studies or work
Altruistic suicide: Suicide occurs when the individual is too integrated into society	Individuals' belief for good of their society—suicide bombers, soldiers	Self-immolation as a form of protest against reservation. Freedom fighters and the custom of Jouhar
Anomic suicide: Occurs when the regulation of the society is disrupted	In contrast to egoistic suicides, where the individual feels untethered, here the society is untethered, and fails to provide guidance	Urbanization and globalization resulting in ambiguous ethical and moral rules of the metropolis
Fatalistic suicide: Occurs due to overly regulated regime, where the individuals choose suicide over the oppressive control of the society	Suicide upon enslavement or suicide in prison inmates. Durkheim considered them to be of theoretical value with very few real-world example	Suicide of women in abusive authoritarian families. Farmers suicide, when in debt trap and no means of support and recovery

disorders such as heart diseases, cancer, and chronic lung disease have been consistently shown to be two to three times more common in the cities as compared to the villages.[30] In addition to the sociological factors, industrialization has significantly increased the friction of city life, by increasing health demands, which the existing infrastructure is often woefully inadequate in coping with.

Search adversities of the city life have prompted many theoreticians, including Durkheim, and postulate the link between urbanization and suicide. Loss of traditional support mechanisms resulting in anomic and egoistic suicide has been demonstrated in the urban France by both Durkheim and others.[31] Indeed, early studies conducted in postindependent India reflects a similar trend, with significantly higher number of suicides reported in cities as compared to the rural areas. Studies by Banerjee and Nandi et al. in West Bengal,[32] Venkoba Rao in Madurai,[33] and Phal et al. in Panaji (Goa)[34] found urban suicide rates to be as much as 10 times than the national average. Studies from the northern states of India by Verma et al. (1972)[35] and Mishra et al.[36] show a similar trend, although the rates of suicides are overall lesser than the south. A change in pattern emerged around the late 1990s, when authors started reporting increasing rates of rural suicides, and in contradiction to existing sociological theories.[37] High rates and high lethality suicides by poisoning were reported by Gautami et al. in 2001 from the Telangana region of Andhra Pradesh.[38] Indeed, analysis of Indian literature by Mayer et al. in 2016 suggested a paradoxical increase in rural suicides in Indian states with higher urbanization and human development.[39] Suicide in the villages surpassed city rates in the urban states of the South and West India, while the agrarian North continued to report comparatively low rural suicide rates.[40] Similar shift in trends in suicide rates over time, from urban to semiurban and rural areas, has also been reported by the European countries of Sweden, Greece, UK, and Scotland and studies from the US show higher suicide rates in the more sparsely populated areas.[41] Chinese data show suicide rates to be not only higher in rural areas but also to be more in females than in males.[42] The rates are perhaps most disparate in Japan, where suicide rates in the elderly are reported to be as high as 240/10,000 in rural areas compared to 40/100,000 in the cities.[43]

Scholars have argued that the flux of change to be the primary driver of anomie than modernization per se. Urban cities in the early days of their formation are expected to have higher suicide rates, but with time and with stabilization, the city culture will see a decrease in the rates. As urban societies develop newer means of support and integration for their dwellers, through clubs, associations, and societies, the pressures of anomie and egoism will abate. Urbanization, in contrast, might exert a disrupting influence in the way of life in its surrounding villages. These villages then experience the disruption of their traditional ethical, societal, and economic values, resulting in strife and struggle. The dissonance between the traditional and the modern ways of living results in the same societal forces affecting life, which the cities of the old once faced.[34]

■ GENDER AND FAMILY

Globally and in India, the rates of completed suicide have always been higher in males as compared to females.[44] Despite most cultures around the world being patriarchal, increased suicide in males has been such a consistent finding that Durkheim considered suicides "to be an essentially male phenomena".[27] The traditional male role of being the breadwinner

for the family exposes them to more societal demands and conflicts. Females, on the other hand, remain better integrated with family and society, decreasing anomic and egoistic forces. Even though suicide rates of countries have fluctuated over time, the proportion rated for each gender has remained remarkably stable. Only China, in recent times, has reported a higher suicide rate in rural females.[42] There have been some speculations on the possibility of increased suicide rates in females, with change in the traditional role and with the entry of women into the workforce. Modernization and gender equality may paradoxically increase the vulnerability of women to societal conflicts. However, globally this trend has not been observed, even in developed countries, where workforce parity has been achieved.[45]

Indian national data do suggest completed suicide rates to be higher in males. However, researchers have questioned on the veracity of the suicide data, as most attempted suicides are never reported, suicide being a criminal offence in the penal code.[46] Individual studies have reported that as many as 50% of "accidental" burn injuries in females may represent unreported self-harm attempt.[47] An analysis of the published data suggests female suicide rates in India to be significantly higher compared to global average even after correcting for national variances, making suicide rates almost equal between sexes. The Global Burden of Diseases study (GBD) of 2016 reported a male-to-female ratio of suicides at 1.34 in India, compared to the rates of 4.0 in Europe and 3.6 in the US.[48] A 2022 review by Ramesh et al.[46] suggests that the suicide rates in Indian females significantly outpace almost every other country in the world. India hosts 17.8% of the global population, yet accounts for 36.6% of the global suicide

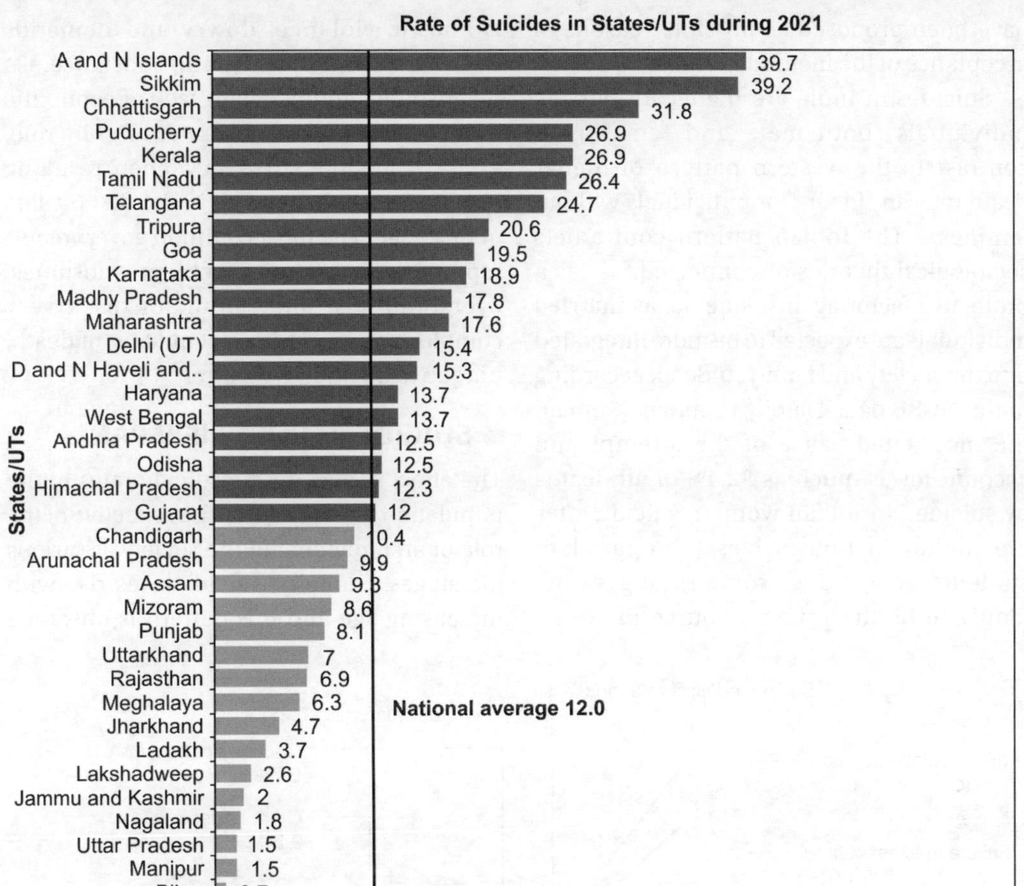

Fig. 1: Suicide rates across states of India. (UTs: union territories)

Courtesy: Data from National Crime Records Bureau, Ministry of Home Affairs. (2021). Accidental Deaths and Suicides in India-2021. [online] Available from: https://ncrb.gov.in/en/ADSI-2021. [Last accessed January, 2023]

deaths in women compared to 24.3% among men. Hanging remains the most common method of suicide in Indian females, in contrast to the global pattern of poisoning being the most common method in women. The western data and assumption, that men generally resort to more violent means of suicide, do not also apply to India, as hanging (followed by poisoning) remains the most common means used to end one's life. This change in pattern is partly explained by the stricter gun control laws in India and to the wider availability of pesticides for agriculture. Indeed, in the agricultural regions of India, pesticide consumption outpaces hanging as the method of suicide. Another distinctive pattern of Indian suicides in females involves the use of self-immolation as a means of suicide, a method that is rarely used by women in the west, due to possible concerns of disfigurement in death. Cultural memories of sati, Jauhar, and purification by fire of Sita have been proposed as possible reasons of acceptance of the method in India.[49]

Suicides in India are higher in married individuals (both male and female), in contrast to the western pattern of higher death rates in "loners" or individuals without families.[50] The Indian pattern contradicts sociological theories of connectedness as a protective factor against suicide, as married individuals are expected to be more integrated into the society and family. Indeed, according to the NCRB data, "family problems" remain the most cited cause of the attempt and account for as much as 32.4% of all deaths by suicide.[6] In Indian women, suicide rates are higher in housewives (compared to students or working women), suggesting family to be the primary source of stress.

Domestic violence, dowry and demands by the husband's family, and substance use by husband, coupled with lack of economic independence and subservient family role, exert tremendous stress on women, resulting in increased suicide rates in the first 5 years of marriage. The most common government-reported cause "family problem" subsumes, oversimplifies, and dehumanizes a very complex and layered social inducer of death, unique to the Indian culture.[51]

■ SUICIDE ACROSS LIFESPAN

The effect of age, on the suicide rates of the population, is intricate, and is reflective of the role of an individual in the society at various life stages. Globally, suicide rates rise with increasing age and this pattern is observed

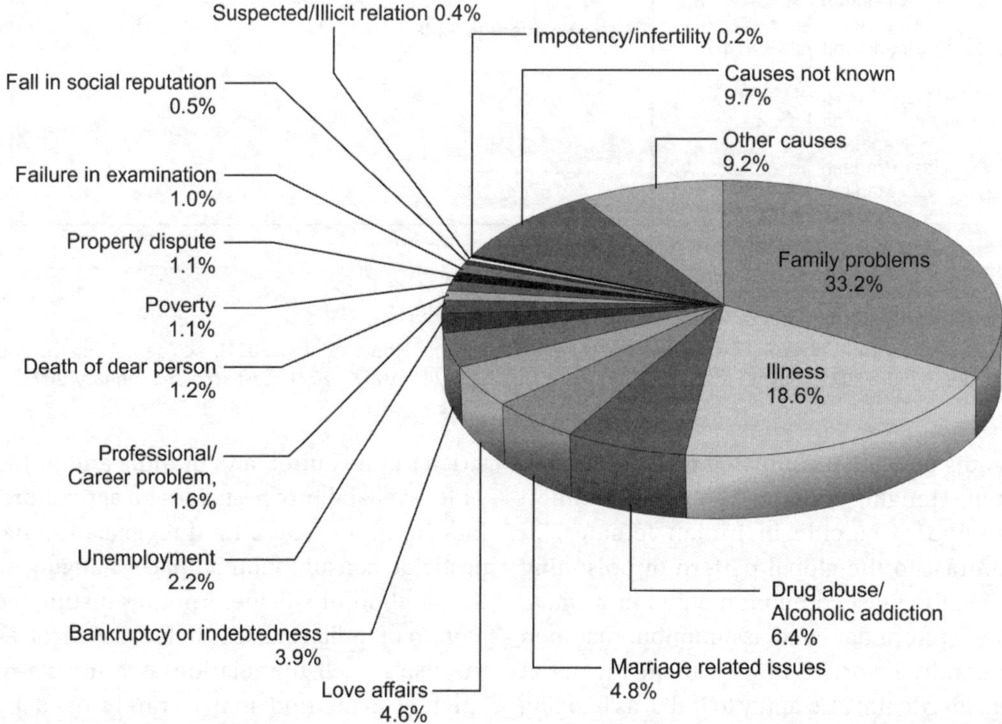

Fig. 2: Causes of suicide in India.

Courtesy: Data from National Crime Records Bureau, Ministry of Home Affairs. (2021). Accidental Deaths and Suicides in India-2021. [online] Available from: https://ncrb.gov.in/en/ADSI-2021. [Last accessed January, 2023]

more clearly in the male suicides. Suicide rates in females show additional peaks in early adulthood, between the ages of 15 and 25 years and again in the later life after 60 years. To explain the variability in rates with age, Lester, back in 1982, proposed that for females, suicide age distribution was tied to the level of the economic development of the country.[52] For low-income nations, young adult women were at the greatest risk of suicide whereas in the wealthiest nations, female suicide rates peaked after the middle ages. Girard, in 1993, similarly suggested upward or downward sloping patterns of suicide (in both sexes), dependent on the human development state of the country.[53] In underdeveloped countries, where family and societal ties dictate the way of life, most suicides are expected to occur in the young adulthood, the phase of maximum struggle. Whereas in industrialized nations, an upward sloping pattern is observed, as most suicides shift to middle or old age. In addition, Girard postulated a bimodal pattern of suicides in nations going through the intermediate stages of industrialization, reflecting a transition from traditional to modern stresses of living. Other researches have also highlighted the vulnerability of young Indian for suicide in the current sociocultural milieu. Women below the age of 30 face the intense expectation of forming successful marriages, integrating with in-laws and bearing a male child. Despite modernization and rise in education, women still have a subservient role in India's patriarchal culture. The sense of powerlessness in young females, "trapped between the conservative past and the promise of a liberated future", acts as a significant precipitator for suicide in this age group.

State-wise gender-based suicide data have been published by the National Crime Records Bureau (NCRB) since 2001. Analysis of the last two decades of data indeed reflects an early peak in suicide rates in the economically weak states of Bihar and Uttar Pradesh, while in the economically prosperous Maharashtra Gujarat, as well as in Kerala with its high development index suicides in both male and females peak at a later age. Globally and in India, the rise of suicide in young adults has become a cause of concern. By proportion, young adults (15–29 years) account for 34.5% of all suicides in India. In the states of Kerala, West Bengal,

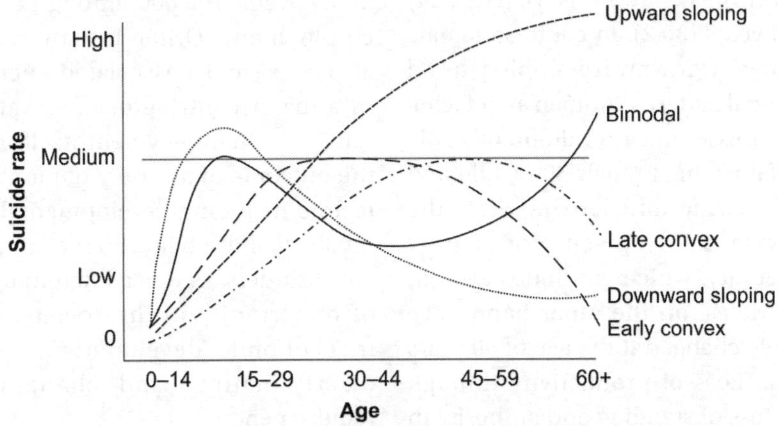

Fig. 3: Suicide patterns across age groups in various types of societies.
Source: Adapted from Mayer P.[34]

and in Pondicherry, death by suicide exceeds that by accidents, the most common cause of death in this age group.[49] >60% of completed suicides occur in women <25 years of age and one study reported that in even adolescent females (10–19 years), 50–75% of the deaths were due to suicide. The study reported very high rates of suicide in rural south India with 148 suicides per 100,000 in girls and a rate of 58/100,000 in boys.[11] Suicide attempts are considered to occur at rates 20 times that completed suicides. Studies from general hospital settings report suicidal ideations to be the most common in the 16–25 age groups. Other studies report female gender, history of sexual abuse and physical abuse, premarital sex, and lack of education to be significant predictors of suicide, particularly in rural women.

At the other end of the age spectrum, suicide rates increase past the age of 65 years, more so in men than in women. The 2012 "Million Death Study" by Patel et al.[4] reported a much higher suicide rate in Indian men (26.3/100,000) and women (17.5/100,000) as compared to the NCRB data. More relevantly, age trends from the survey showed male suicides to be bimodal in India, with peaks at 30–44 years (27.4) and post 70 years (30.2). In contrast, female suicides show a downward sloping trend similar to global patterns. Women after facing difficult life stresses in early adulthood settle better into family life in their 30s. Child and grandchild rearing and looking after the family provide the deep sense of identity and role stability, which continues even in later ages. Males, on the other hand, face significant life changes at the age of 60 years and beyond. Loss of productivity through retirement, loss of standing and authority in family, and the handing over of patriarchal title to the next generation result in significant narcissistic hurt. Social isolation, declining physical health (more in males as compared to females), functional disability, and a feeling of invalidity or becoming a burden to the family result in anomic and egoistic suicides in elderly males. One worrisome regional phenomenon regarding geriatric death in India revolves around the custom of "Thalaikoothal" or senicide through voluntary/involuntary euthanasia. Practiced primarily in the state of Tamil Nadu, the ritualistic process involves feeding the person tender coconut water exclusively, resulting in kidney failure and death. The practice finds covert social acceptance as a form of mercy killing of the debilitated elderly, although its abuse has raised alarm among social activist and states in recent times.[54]

■ OCCUPATION AND ECONOMICS

The effect of social stability and productivity on suicide is also visible in the variable rates of suicide associated with various occupations. Consistently, suicides are found to be significantly higher among the unemployed, and in the Indian states of Karnataka, Andhra Pradesh, Punjab, and Haryana, male suicide rates are reported to be over 200/100,000 among those without employment. Other Indian studies have also consistently associated unemployment as a major contributor to elevated suicide rates.[55-57] Unemployment itself, however, is the outcome of a variety of biopsychosocial factors including developmental disorders, intellectual disability, mental and substance use disorders, as well as stemming from lack of opportunity in the society, stagnation in economic development, caste-based discrimination, and changing skillset requirement.

The 2021 NCRB data records higher suicide rates in those working as daily wage earners (25.6%), rather than the unemployed (8.4%). A 10-year trend analysis shows a sharp increase in deaths among the daily workers in recent years (12% in 2014), making daily laborers the most common occupational group associated with suicidal death in 2021. Inter-state migration, lack of social security, urban exploitation, fluctuation in job market, COVID-19 pandemic, etc. have all been forwarded as reasons for this rise. The vulnerability of this group stems from their untethered life, uncertain tomorrow, and despondent future, with a slow drift between the choices of unemployment and exploitation.[7]

Beyond the city workers, India still remains an agrarian society and occupationally, >55% of its population remains involved in farming. In recent decades, a sharp rise in suicides among people involved in the agricultural sector has been a cause of national and international media concern. According to Durkheim and Morselli,[58] farmers living a more traditional way of life are more integrated into the society and, therefore, "classes addicted to agriculture, pastoral life [and] forestry [have] very low suicide rates".[59] Global literature, however, has repeatedly signaled increasing death rates over the past few decades in persons involved with agriculture. Although trends of rise in death in farmers correlate with rising suicide rates in rural areas, where the population resides, agricultural failure and economic burden have remained consistent themes in studies from US, Brazil, Australia, and Europe.[60]

A series of insightful articles has reported on the complex interplay between the changing social, economic, and political forces which have pushed India farmers to the brink of despondency.[61-64] The NCRB data suggests around 6,000 deaths in farmers every year, accounting for 7.8% of all suicides in the country. Suicide rates among Indian farmers are reported to be 47% higher than the national average, with the highest being at Maharashtra (60% higher), followed by Karnataka, Andhra Pradesh, Madhya Pradesh, Chhattisgarh, and Telangana.[65] The changing agricultural landscape precipitating these drastic outcomes needs to be viewed in light of the national policy changes over the last three decades. Post-1990s, economic reforms favored open market, globalization, and foreign investment. Entry of MNCs into the agriculture sector favored large landholders with the capacity to invest funds for hybrid (GMO) seeds, fertilizers, and pesticides. Unable to compete, many small farmers were forced to shift from food grains to commercial crops such as cotton and sugarcane. In the absence of government support, even a single season of drought or flood pushed many to irredeemable economic debt. Since 2018, a coalition of farmers and social activists has staged multiple protests demanding an increase in minimum market prices and agricultural loan waiver, culminating in the national protest of 2020 against the Agriculture Reform Bill.[66] Additionally, in the last two decades, the government policy focus has also shifted from agriculture to skilling population for industrial work. The national development policy of 2019 formally stated intention to "reduce the farming population of the country from 52 to 30% by 2022". This is reflected in the rapid increase in "nonfarm employment (NFE)" over the years, with 25–50% of village dwellers in various states remaining engaged in nonagricultural occupations.[64]

The other economic change contributing to the fall of agriculture stems from the gradual demise of large landowners from most parts of India. Land reforms in some states, selling off of land for debt and dowry payment in others, or property division between several children (itself a social result of failed national population control policies), have resulted in >85% of farmers holding <5 acres of land. Most of these smallholdings are family farmed, decreasing employment opportunities for the rural landless. Left with minimal prospect, many village folks become migrant in cities, with even less social security.[67] However, the most influential social change altering our villages, perhaps, stems from our loss of pride in tradition and farming. Gone are the days when "Jai Jawan Jai Kisan" was the national mantra, and when farmers of Punjab or Haryana would proudly declare tilling the land to be the sacred most of professions. Most farmers today would not do farming if they had alternatives, and almost all want their children to move to the cities. Across caste, migrants from rural India will accept jobs in the cities which they will not do in their own villages. For those with means, emigration to other countries serves the same purpose, as migration to cities. The states of Kerala, Punjab, and UP have significant rural NRI population residing in UAE, Canada, and UK, and emigration from other states of Maharashtra, West Bengal, and Haryana has been increasing rapidly in recent years.

It is improper to consider Indian villages as ideal, idyllic, unchanging traditional society. Dr BR Ambedkar, himself a Dalit from Maharashtra, had famously described villages as "cesspools of degradation, corruption, and worse", and the situation has little changed in the ensuing 75 years. A 2004 paper by Dipankar Gupta from the Centre of Social Studies, JNU discusses the sociocultural changes of Indian villages with great insight. According to Gupta, rather than modernization of the cities corrupting the village way of life, it is the stagnation in the villages that drives people to the city—"the

town is not coming to the country as much as the country is reaching out to the town, leaving behind a host of untidy rural debris. Nowhere else does one find the level of hopeless disenchantment as one does in the rural regions of India. In urban slums, there is squalor, there are filth and crime, but there are hope and the excitement that tomorrow might be quite different from today."[68]

At the other end of the spectrum, suicide rates are also significantly higher among professionals such as lawyers, doctors, and civil servants. Higher rates among persons engaged in the "science and the letter" have been reported world over,[69] but form a small part of the national proportion in developing countries such as India. However, the relative risk of suicide in these professions is two to eight times higher than in the general population, and the risk may be even higher in certain subpopulations, such as in psychiatrists, anesthetists, and dentists among other healthcare professionals.[70] The loss of skilled professionals at the highest economic strata is a reminder of the universality of mental health issues and marks a philosophical discontent with the modern way of living. Another consistent pattern in these suicides is the equality in gender distribution, or even a female preponderance, compared to the male predominance in the general population. Even among the theoretically "safe" group of educated, married, people, working in stable government jobs, a female preponderance in suicides in the states of Tamil Nadu, Kerala, Assam, Rajasthan, UP etc. have perplexed researchers and do suggest other social pressures at play.[11] Suicide among students has come under media focus in recent times, although the actual numbers remain quite less. In addition to the age- and gender-related stressors described before, academic

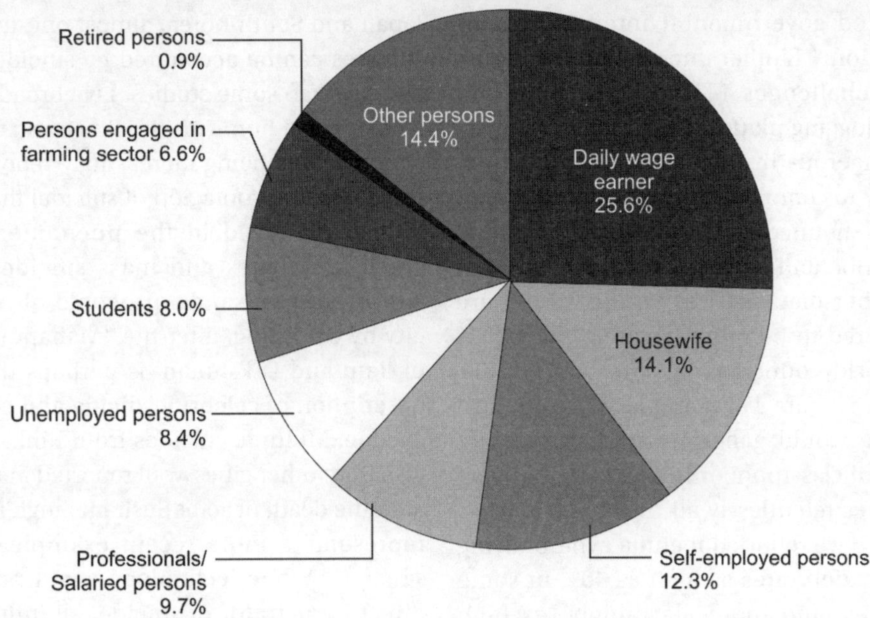

Fig. 4: Proportion of suicide by occupation.

Courtesy: Data from National Crime Records Bureau, Ministry of Home Affairs. (2021). Accidental Deaths and Suicides in India-2021. [online] Available from: https://ncrb.gov.in/en/ADSI-2021. [Last accessed January, 2023]

failure, bulling, ragging, physical and sexual abuse, and substance use form unique stressors of this age group.

■ THE CULTURE OF TECHNOLOGY

The intertwining of technology in modern culture has affected the life of all, but more so of our young. Digital and social media determine the value systems, peer group behavior, and social mores for most adolescents and young adults. Internet is, therefore, a resource, a support, a stressor, as well as an addiction in the modern life. The vast amount of unregulated information on suicide available on the free web itself has been a cause of concern for researchers. A 2008 study of Google search results reported easy availability of details on suicidal means and methods, and a neutral or prosuicide sentiment in 42% of the sites searched. Subsequent international advocacy and

social activism resulted in Google adding a "Suicide Prevention Result" (SPR) in 2010 on keyword search around the topic of suicide. SPR, started in 14 countries, provided contact details for the relevant suicide crisis support and Google's original blog post reported a 9% increase in calls to the US National Suicide Prevention Lifeline following its release.[71] Although recent articles have further analyzed Google's SPR, or the lack thereof, in non-English languages or when searches are made for celebrity suicide, the case exemplifies the promotive as well as the preventive power of Internet in relation to suicides.[72]

In schoolchildren, improper exposure to age-inappropriate content and contact to strangers posing as peer have resulted in an increase of digital sexual abuse.[73] Internet trends such as the "Blue Whale challenge" where participants were provided 50 tasks culminating in self harm and suicide prompted governmental intervention for prevention.[74] Similar microtrends, cropping up as challenges (TikTok challenge) in microblogging platforms from time to time, are dangerous in themselves. In addition, inability to complete them often causes peer group denouncement and shame, resulting in isolation and depression.[75] Cyberbullying and cyber-blackmail of young adults are considered to be more harming than their real-world counterparts, due to their all-pervasive nature. For example, while physical bullying would generally stop in the safe spaces of classroom or home, cyberbullying continues relentlessly all times and spaces. Studies have reported lifetime cyberbullying victimization rates as high as 40% in some countries, and more alarmingly, as high as 20% students admitted to perpetrating the same. Peer group pressure, ease, and anonymity, and the distant nonempathic nature of the victimization are suggested as reasons for the high-perpetration rate.[76]

In adolescents and young adults, advertent exposure of intimate life, revenge posting of pornographic materials, cyber harassment, and cyberstalking have all been often reported as the cause for suicide.[77] The advent of multiple dating Apps (Tinder), end-to-end encrypted video chat Apps (Snapchat), and live broadcast Apps (Tango), where strangers establish various levels of intimacy for tokens and gifts in private or in public broadcast, makes a very dangerous digital landscape for young adults. Finally, the traditional suicide pact, where two or more close acquaintances make a contract to commit suicide at the same time and by the same method, has undergone digitization in form of cybersuicide. Cybersuicides are more insidious, as victims make pacts with strangers in anonymous chat rooms, where recruiters of the dark web often crawl for victims.[78] In Japan and South Korea, almost one-thirds of suicides can be accounted by suicide pacts according to some studies. Live broadcast of suicides and homicide-suicide events, while shocking, are being increasingly reported in media. Media contagion of suicidal thoughts is also observed in the phenomenon of copycat suicides and mass suicides. The suicide of thousands of people of Ayodha city by drowning, after the "Mahaprasthan" of Ram and Lakshman, is perhaps the first description of celebrity suicide and copycat suicide. Multiple suicides from Kolkata and also from other cities, well reported in media, after the death of actor Sushant Singh Rajput, represents a more recent example of the same.[79,80] While technology might not be a direct perpetrator of suicide, all influences blend in our cultural fabric, creating a milieu against which the value of life and the worth of survival are judged by individuals.

■ CONCLUSION

India is a vast country with a myriad of cultures and with extensive social variations. Any discourse on the sociocultural factors affecting suicidal behavior invariably falls short in light of the complex geo-socioeconomic variations of our country. The factors affecting suicidal behavior in the urban centers of the country will be completely different from the trials and tribulations of the tribal population. National statistics, which provides us a context to understand the rates of suicide, cannot explain the reasons for geographical variations. The factors driving people to self-harm in the North-Eastern states, the Southern states, and in the heartland of the country are so diverse that they defy generalization of causes. The only thematic consistency, across all data and all discourse, suggests that India is indeed going through a silent epidemic of suicide of its young adults, both males and females, consequent to the rapidly changing sociocultural fabric of the nation. Subsequent to the COVID-19 pandemic of 2020–2022, the world is reeling from war, climate crisis, and the looming recession. The rapidly changing world brings us back to Durkheim's original description of a time of social upheaval, anomie, and fatalism, when suicides are expected to increase. More than by numbers, it is therefore important as mental health professionals to understand the cultural subtext of the life of our people. Only then we can even begin to design social interventions, which integrate people, stabilize their identity, and empower them with social capital to make their lives a joyous and worthy.

■ REFERENCES

1. Aubin HJ, Berlin I, Kornreich C. The evolutionary puzzle of suicide. Int J Environ Res Public Health. 2013;10(12):6873-86.
2. Bachmann S. Epidemiology of suicide and the psychiatric perspective. Int J Environ Res Public Health. 2018;15(7):1425.
3. World Health Organization. (2019). Suicide in the world: global health estimates. [online] Available from: https://apps.who.int/iris/handle/10665/326948. [Last accessed January, 2023]
4. Patel V, Ramasundarahettige C, Vijayakumar L, Thakur JS, Gajalakshmi V, Gururaj G, et al. Suicide mortality in India: a nationally representative survey. Lancet. 2012; 379(9834):2343-51.
5. Arya V, Page A, Armstrong G, Kumar GA, Dandona R. Estimating patterns in the under-reporting of suicide deaths in India: comparison of administrative data and Global Burden of Disease Study estimates, 2005–2015. J Epidemiol Community Health. 2021;75(6):550-5.
6. National Crime Records Bureau, Ministry of Home Affairs. (2021). Accidental Deaths and Suicides in India-2021. [online] Available from: https://ncrb.gov.in/en/ADSI-2021. [Last accessed January, 2023]
7. Singh OP. Startling suicide statistics in India: Time for urgent action. Indian J Psychiatry. 2022;64(5):431-2.
8. Balodhi JP. Indian mythological views on suicide. NIMHANS J. 1992;10(2):101-5.
9. Vijayakumar L. Hindu religion and suicide in India. In: Wasserman D, Wasserman C (Eds). Oxford Textbook of Suicidology and Suicide Prevention. London: Oxford University Press; 2009.
10. Vijayakumar L, John S. Is Hinduism ambivalent about suicide? Int J Soc Psychiatry. 2018;64(5):443-9.
11. Radhakrishnan R, Andrade C. Suicide: An Indian perspective. Indian J Psychiatry. 2012;54(4):304-19.
12. Somasundaram OS, Babu CK, Geethayan IA. Suicide behaviour in the ancient civilizations with special reference to the Tamils. Indian J Psychiatry. 1989;31(3):208-12.
13. Hunter WW. Orissa ; Or The Vicissitudes of an Indian Province Under Native and British Rule: In Two Volumes: Being the Second and Third Volumes of The Annals of Rural Bengal. London: Smith, Elder & Company; 1872.
14. Vijayakumar L. Altruistic Suicide in India. Arch Suicide Res. 2004;8(1):73-80.
15. Ghosh U. Chariots of the Gods: The Many Histories of Jagannath, "Juggernaut," and the Rathayatra in the Nineteenth Century. Hist Relig. 2018;58(1):64-88.
16. Shamsuddin M. A brief historical background of sati tradition in India. Din Ve Felsefe Araştırmaları. 2020;3(5):44-63.
17. Hunter WW. The Annals of Rural Bengal. London: Smith, Elder; 1868.
18. Siddharth M. A study on Raja Ram Mohan Roy and abolision of sati system in India. Int J Soc Sci Econ Res. 2018;3(12):7173-80.
19. Tagore S. Raja Rammohun Roy. New Delhi: Publications Division Ministry of Information & Broadcasting; 2017.
20. Somasundaram O, Tejus Murthy AG, Raghavan DV. Jainism - Its relevance to psychiatric practice; with special reference to the practice of Sallekhana. Indian J Psychiatry. 2016;58(4):471-4.
21. Ineichen B. The influence of religion on the suicide rate: Islam and Hinduism compared. Ment Health Relig Cult. 1998;1(1):31-6.

22. Chadda RK, Deb KS. Indian family systems, collectivistic society and psychotherapy. Indian J Psychiatry. 2013;55(Suppl 2):S299-309.

23. Vijayakumar L. Indian research on suicide. Indian J Psychiatry. 2010;52(Suppl1):S291-6.

24. Chandra PS, Shiva L, Nanjundaswamy MH. The impact of urbanization on mental health in India. Curr Opin Psychiatry. 2018;31(3):276-81.

25. Durkheim E. Suicide: A Study in Sociology, 2nd edition. London: Routledge; 2002.

26. Wray M, Colen C, Pescosolido B. The Sociology of Suicide. Sociol Suicide. 2011; 37:505-28.

27. Hassan R. One hundred years of Emile Durkheim's Suicide: A Study in Sociology. Aust N Z J Psychiatry. 1998;32(2):168-71.

28. Parida JK. Rural-urban migration, urbanization, and wage differentials in urban India. In: Internal migration, urbanization and poverty in Asia: Dynamics and interrelationships. Singapore: Springer; 2019. pp. 189-218.

29. Firdaus G. Urbanization, emerging slums and increasing health problems: a challenge before the nation: an empirical study with reference to state of Uttar Pradesh in India. J Environ Res Manag. 2012;3(9):146-52.

30. Neiderud CJ. How urbanization affects the epidemiology of emerging infectious diseases. Infect Ecol Epidemiol. 2015; 5:10.3402/iee.v5.27060.

31. Halbwachs M. The causes of suicide: translated by Harold Goldblatt. Oxfordshire: Routledge and Kegan Paul; 1978.

32. Banerjee G, Nandi DN, Nandi S, Sarkar S, Boral GC, Ghosh A. The vulnerability of Indian women to suicide a field-study. Indian J Psychiatry. 1990;32(4):305-8.

33. Rao VA, Chinnian RR. Attempted suicide and suicide among 'students' in Madurai. Indian J Psychiatry. 1972;14(4):389-97.

34. Mayer P. Suicide and society in India. Oxfordshire; Routledge; 2010.

35. Varma P. Suicide in India and abroad. Agra: Sahitya Bhawan; 1976.

36. Mishra S. Suicide mortality rates across states of India, 1975-2001: a statistical note. Econ Polit Wkly. 2006;41(6):1566-9.

37. Singh L, Bhangoo KS, Sharma R. (2019). Agrarian distress and farmer suicides in North India. [online] Available from: https://www.taylorfrancis.com/books/mono/10.4324/9780429270628/agrarian-distress-farmer-suicides-north-india-lakhwinder-singh-kesar-singh-bhangoo-rakesh-sharma. [Last accessed January, 2023]

38. Gautami S, Sudershan R, Bhat RV, Suhasini G, Bharati M, Gandhi K. Chemical poisoning in three Telengana districts of Andhra Pradesh. Forensic Sci Int. 2001;122(2–3):167-71.

39. Mayer P. Thinking clearly about suicide in India: Desperate Housewives, Despairing Farmers. Econ Polit Wkly. 2016;51(14):44-54.

40. Arya V, Page A, Dandona R, Vijayakumar L, Mayer P, Armstrong G. The geographic heterogeneity of suicide rates in India by religion, caste, tribe, and other backward classes. Crisis. 2019;40(5):370-4.

41. Hirsch JK. A review of the literature on rural suicide: Risk and protective factors, incidence, and prevention. Crisis J Crisis Interv Suicide Prev. 2006;27:189-99.

42. Phillips MR, Li X, Zhang Y. Suicide rates in China, 1995–99. The Lancet. 2002;359(9309):835-40.

43. Watanabe N, Hasegawa K, Yoshinaga Y. Suicide in later life in Japan: Urban and Rural differences. Int Psychogeriatr. 1995;7(2):253-61.

44. Steen DM, Mayer P. Modernization and the Male–Female Suicide Ratio in India 1967–1997: Divergence or Convergence? Suicide Life Threat Behav. 2004;34(2):147-59.

45. Chang Q, Yip PSF, Chen YY. Gender inequality and suicide gender ratios in the world. J Affect Disord. 2019;243:297-304.

46. Ramesh P, Taylor PJ, McPhillips R, Raman R, Robinson C. A scoping review of gender differences in suicide in India. Front Psychiatry. 2022;13:884657.

47. Batra AK. Burn mortality: recent trends and sociocultural determinants in rural India. Burns. 2003;29(3):270-5.

48. Dandona R, Kumar GA, Dhaliwal RS, Naghavi M, Vos T, Shukla DK, et al. Gender differentials and state variations in suicide deaths in India: the Global Burden of Disease Study 1990–2016. Lancet Public Health. 2018;3(10):e478-89.

49. Vijayakumar L. Suicide in women. Indian J Psychiatry 2015;57(Suppl 2):S233-238.

50. Snowdon J. Indian suicide data: What do they mean? Indian J Med Res. 2019;150(4):315.

51. Ponnudurai R. Suicide in India. Indian J Psychol Med. 1996;19(1):19-25.

52. Lester D, Reeve C. The suicide notes of young and old people. Psychol Rep. 1982;50(1):334.

53. Girard C. Age, gender, and suicide: A cross-national analysis. Am Sociol Rev. 1993;58(4):553-74.

54. Sunger V. Senicide as a modern problem in india: a Durkheimian perspective of thalaikoothal. Crossing Bord Stud Reflect Glob Soc Issues. 2020;2(1):1-5.

55. Kar N. Profile of risk factors associated with suicide attempts: A study from Orissa, India. Indian J Psychiatry. 2010;52(1):48.

56. Arya V, Page A, River J, Armstrong G, Mayer P. Trends and socio-economic determinants of suicide in India: 2001–2013. Soc Psychiatry Psychiatr Epidemiol. 2018;53(3):269-78.

57. Aggarwal S. Suicide in India. Br Med Bull. 2015;114(1):127-34.

58. Rozenblatt D. (2014). Madness and Method: Enrico Morselli and the Social Politics of Psychiatry, 1852-1929. [online] Available from: https://escholarship.org/content/qt9jv5016s/qt9jv5016s_noSplash_2a978211b680d66cf687bc7af57ce16c.pdf. [Last accessed January, 2023]

59. Capstick A. Urban and rural suicide. J Ment Sci. 1960;106(445):1327-36.

60. Barbosa Junior M, Sokulski CC, Salvador R, Pinheiro E, de Francisco AC, Trojan F. What kills the agricultural worker? A systematic review on suicide. Rural Remote Health. 2021;21(3):6067.

61. Behere PB, Chowdhury D, Behere AP, Yadav R. Psychosocial aspects of suicide in largest industry of farmers in Vidarbha Region of Maharashtra. Ind Psychiatry J. 2021;30 (Suppl 1):S10-4.

62. Chinnasamy P, Hsu MJ, Agoramoorthy G. Groundwater Storage Trends and Their Link to Farmer Suicides in Maharashtra State, India. Front Public Health. 2019;7:246.

63. Carleton TA. Crop-damaging temperatures increase suicide rates in India. Proc Natl Acad Sci U S A. 2017;114(33):8746-51.

64. Merriott D. Factors associated with the farmer suicide crisis in India. J Epidemiol Glob Health. 2016;6(4):217-27.

65. Sundar M. Suicide in farmers in India. Br J Psychiatry. 1999;175(6):585-6.

66. Kennedy J, King L. The political economy of farmers' suicides in India: indebted cash-crop farmers with marginal landholdings explain state-level variation in suicide rates. Glob Health. 2014;10(1):1-9.

67. Mohanty BB. 'We are like the living dead': farmer suicides in Maharashtra, western India. J Peasant Stud. 2005;32(2):243-76.

68. Gupta D. Whither the Indian village?: culture and agriculture in 'rural' India. Rev Dev Change. 2005;10(1):1-20.

69. Virga A. Suicide is not for the poor: Self-death in Veristi Authors, Luigi Capuana and Giovanni Verga. Suicide in Modern Literature. Berlin: Springer; 2021. pp. 95-108.

70. Ventriglio A, Watson C, Bhugra D. Suicide among doctors: A narrative review. Indian J Psychiatry. 2020;62(2):114.

71. Kirtley OJ, O'Connor RC. Suicide prevention is everyone's business: Challenges and opportunities for Google. Soc Sci Med. 2020;262:112691.

72. Arendt F, Haim M, Scherr S. Investigating Google's suicide-prevention efforts in celebrity suicides using agent-based testing: A cross-national study in four European countries. Soc Sci Med. 2020;262:112692.

73. Biddle L, Derges J, Mars B, Heron J, Donovan JL, Potokar J, et al. Suicide and the Internet: Changes in the accessibility of suicide-related information between 2007 and 2014. J Affect Disord. 2016;190:370-5.

74. Mukhra R, Baryah N, Krishan K, Kanchan T. 'Blue Whale Challenge': A Game or Crime? Sci Eng Ethics. 2019;25(1):285-91.

75. Khasawneh A, Madathil KC, Dixon E, Wiśniewski P, Zinzow H, Roth R. Examining the self-harm and suicide contagion effects

of the blue whale challenge on YouTube and Twitter: Qualitative Study. JMIR Ment Health. 2020;7(6):e15973.

76. Maurya C, Muhammad T, Dhillon P, Maurya P. The effects of cyberbullying victimization on depression and suicidal ideation among adolescents and young adults: a three year cohort study from India. BMC Psychiatry. 2022;22(1):599.

77. Gavrilovic Nilsson M, Tzani Pepelasi K, Ioannou M, Lester D. Understanding the link between Sextortion and Suicide. Int J Cyber Criminol. 2019;13(1):55-69.

78. Durkee T, Hadlaczky G, Westerlund M, Carli V. Internet Pathways in Suicidality: A Review of the Evidence. Int J Environ Res Public Health. 2011;8(10):3938-52.

79. Saini T, Arora V, Sharma S, Kumar D, Parmar V, Sharma S. A Study on Copycat Suicides and Werther Effect: Myth or Reality. Int J Ethics Trauma Vict. 2021;7(01):11-3.

80. Kar SK, Arafat SY, Ransing R, Menon V, Padhy SK, Sharma P, et al. Repeated celebrity suicide in India during COVID-19 crisis: An urgent call for attention. Asian J Psychiatry. 2020;53:102382.

Neurobiology of Suicide: An Overview

Jayant Mahadevan, Guru S Gowda, Venkata Senthil Kumar Reddi

ABSTRACT

Suicide and Suicidal behavior (SB) are acknowledged as a significant cause of morbidity and mortality, globally. Over the years, a large body of research has been conducted suicide and SB, in different contexts. The current understanding of the basis of suicide and SB suggests a complex etiology resulting from an interplay of biological, psychological, social, and environmental factors. The stress–diathesis models of suicide and SB elegantly explain this interaction between social and environmental factors (stress) and, biological and psychological factors (diathesis). The application of advanced research techniques and approaches, particularly, over the preceding one and half decades strongly indicate a biological basis to suicide and SB.

These approaches have included the identification of markers of genetic susceptibility, demonstration of epigenetic alterations triggered by environmental stimuli such as childhood adversity and chronic stress, identification of brain regions and neuronal circuitry changes and neurochemical abnormalities, that are associated with suicide and SB. This chapter provides a brief overview of findings from genetic, epigenetic, neurochemical, neuroendocrine, neuroimmune, cellular, neuroanatomical, and neuroimaging studies on suicide and SB, including studies on the same from India. Furthermore, it discusses the implications of these findings in the context of patient care and management.

Keywords: Suicide; Suicidal behavior; Neurobiology; Neurocircuits.

■ INTRODUCTION

Suicide and suicidal behavior (SB) are acknowledged as a significant cause of morbidity and mortality, globally. Over the years, extensive research has been conducted on epidemiology, risk factors, identification, and management of suicide and SB, in different contexts. However, findings from these studies have been unable to accurately delineate those at risk and this constitutes a major public health challenge.

Our current understanding of the basis of suicide and SB suggests a complex etiology resulting from an interplay of biological, psychological, social, and environmental factors. The stress–diathesis model of suicide elegantly explains this interaction between social and environmental factors (stress) and biological and psychological factors (diathesis). While proposed as early as 1980,[1] over subsequent years, it has attempted to link neurobiology with psychopathology based on emergent findings.[2]

The application of advanced research techniques and approaches, particularly, over the preceding one and half decades strongly indicates a biological basis to suicide and SB. These approaches have included the identification of markers of genetic susceptibility, demonstration of epigenetic alterations triggered by environmental stimuli such as childhood adversity and chronic stress, identification of brain regions, and neuronal circuitry changes and neurochemical abnormalities that are associated with suicide and SB.

This line of enquiry had its origin in data from large epidemiological, family, twin, and adoption studies, which suggested that suicide and SB were familial. Further, given the benefits of antidepressant medications in attenuating suicidality, the synaptic and cellular targets of pharmacological agents became a basis for exploring the biological basis of suicide and SB. Hence, monoamine neurotransmitters systems such as serotonin and noradrenaline, as well as other neuro-modulators and their downstream signaling pathways became the focus of the investigations exploring the biology of suicide and SB. These revealed abnormalities in serotonin, noradrenaline, and their metabolites, which were confirmed by subsequent research that evaluated neuromodulator receptor-linked signaling systems.

In addition to neurotransmitters, the role of the hypothalamic–pituitary–adrenal (HPA) axis has been extensively investigated, particularly given its involvement in the body's stress response. A chronic dysregulation of the HPA axis system has been noted across studies with several recent investigations also pointing to alterations in neuroimmune functioning in suicide and SB.

Finally, advancements in neuroimaging techniques, especially structural and functional brain imaging, have helped to demonstrate changes in brain regions and networks, such as the prefrontal cortex (PFC), insula, and default mode network (DMN), which are associated with suicide and SB.

This chapter provides a brief overview of findings from genetic, epigenetic, neuro-chemical, neuroendocrine, neuroimmune, cellular, neuroanatomical, and neuroimaging studies on suicide and SB, including studies on the same from India. Furthermore, it discusses the implications of these findings in the context of patient care and management.

■ GENETICS OF SUICIDE AND SB

Family, Twin and Adoption Studies

Family, twin and adoption (FTA) studies have consistently demonstrated that suicide and SB are familial with heritability estimated to be between 17 and 55%.[3,4] This raises two important questions, namely: Is familial transmission attributable to shared genes or shared environment? And, is familial transmission of suicide explainable solely based on family transmission of associated psychiatric syndromes?

Two recent family-based studies using Swedish National Registry data have attempted to answer the first question and disentangle the effects of genetics and environment in the intergenerational transmission of suicide and SB. The first found that genetic factors appear to be primary,[5] while the second reported contributions of both genes and environment, with the latter mediated by parental psychopathology.[6] Twin studies have also shown that there is an increased concordance for suicide in monozygotic (MZ) versus dizygotic twins (DZ), not explicable by differential grief responses (environmental influence).[7] Adoption studies using data from the Danish and Swedish National adoption registers found that the transgenerational transmission of suicide is likely genetic and not mediated by the early environmental influences.[8-10] These indicate that genetic factors play an important role in the etiology of suicide and SB.

Family-based studies have also concluded that the familial risk for suicide and SB seems to be independent of that of familial transmission of psychiatric disorders, which are also associated with the suicide and SB.[8,11,12] However, a recent large family study found that the association between lifetime suicide attempts in patients and first-degree relatives was not statistically significant after adjustment for comorbid conditions.[13] Thus, findings from family, twin and adoption studies are an area, which merit further exploration.

Candidate-gene Studies

Candidate-gene studies investigate the association between a phenotype and a pre-determined DNA marker that is decided based on prior knowledge of disease biology. Associations may either be as a consequence of the marker itself being the causal variant or because the marker is in linkage disequilibrium (LD) with a causal variant.

A number of candidate genes have been investigated for an association with suicide and SB. These include genes linked to serotonergic system (*5HTR1A, 5HTR1B, 5HTR2A, TPH1, TPH2,* and *SLC6A4*), dopaminergic system (*DRD2*), monoamine catabolism (*COMT* and *MAOA*), HPA axis (*CRHR, CRHR1, CRHR2, CRHBP,* and *FKBP*), and neurotrophic factors [*brain-derived neurotrophic factor (BDNF)*]. Meta-analyses support the association of variants such as *TPH1*-rs1800532, *SLC6A4*-5-HTTLPR, *COMT*-rs4680, and *BDNF*-rs6265 with suicide and SB.[14]

There are four studies from India that have investigated the genetic underpinnings of suicide and SB. They have all employed candidate gene-based approaches and predominantly focused on single nucleotide polymorphisms (SNPs) in monoamine genes. The first study aimed to study the differences in the clinical profiles between first-degree relatives and other relatives (second degree or further) of patients presenting with a suicidal attempt. This study also investigated allele frequency differences of variants in *BDNF* (Val66Met), *COMT* (Val158Met), *5-HTT* (STin2), and *5-HTTLPR* between the two groups as a secondary objective, but found no significant differences.[15] A second study evaluated the relationship between SNPs in *5-HTTLPR, 5HTR1A, 5-HTR2A* and symptom dimensions including suicidality in patients with major depressive disorder (MDD), but found no significant associations.[16] The third study investigated differences in *5-HTT* (STin2) and *5-HTTLPR* between patients with a suicidal attempt compared to controls and found a higher frequency of the S10 haplotype among cases and evidence of gene-environment interaction mediated by stressful life events.[17] The fourth study investigated sixteen SNPs reported to be previously associated with SB and found that seven SNPs (in six genes—*IL7, RHEB, CTNN3, KCNIP4, ARFGEF3,* and *NUGCC*) were significantly different between cases and controls using different genetic models. These were also found to be in interaction with known candidate genes using pathway analysis.[18]

Candidate gene studies have offered support for the role of neurotransmitters such as serotonin, norepinephrine (NE), and BDNF in the etiology of suicide and SB. However, similar to the case for other complex phenotypes, they have suffered from problems related to inadequate sample size and replicability of findings, which has led to the increasing popularity of genome-wide approaches discussed in the subsequent section.

Genome-wide Association Studies

Genome-wide association studies (GWAS) employ an atheoretical approach, using a large number of markers spread across the genome, which are then tested for association with the phenotype, after correction for multiple testing. This unbiased approach has greatly facilitated genetic discovery in a number of complex traits. However, adequate statistical power requires large sample sizes, which are not typically attainable through single studies. This has been addressed by the formation of consortia, such as the Psychiatric Genomics Consortium (PGC) and population level biobanks, such as the UK Biobank. Similar to other studies, they have used broad and varying definitions of what constitutes suicide and SB.

A recent large GWAS evaluated genetic associations of self-reported suicidal ideation (N = 36,599), self-harm with unknown suicidal intent (N = 2,498) or suicidal attempt (N = 2,666) and controls (N = 83,557) from UK Biobank. Only three loci were found to be genome-wide significant, and strongest genetic correlations were observed with MDD. Polygenic risk score (PRS) was tested in an independent sample and was associated with a higher risk of suicide. SNP-based heritability for the broadly defined construct described above was estimated at 7.6%.[19]

Another recent GWAS which used clinically ascertained cohorts of European Ancestry from the Psychiatric Genomics Consortium with and without a lifetime suicidal attempt and diagnosed with MDD ($N_{attempters}$ = 1,622, $N_{nonattempters}$ = 8,786), bipolar disorder (BD) ($N_{attempters}$ = 3,264, $N_{nonattempters}$ = 5,500) and schizophrenia ($N_{attempters}$ = 1,683, $N_{nonattempters}$ = 2,946) yielded three associated genome-wide significant loci. MDD PRS was found to be associated with risk of suicidal attempt in people with MDD, BD, and schizophrenia.

SNP-based heritability for suicidal attempt was not significantly different from zero.[20]

A large GWAS of completed suicide in individuals of European ancestry found that unlike the case for suicidal attempt or broadly defined SB, completed suicide had a significant SNP-based heritability of 25%.[21] This finding was replicated in another study from Japan, which found a SNP-based heritability ranging between 35 and 48%.[22] The first study was also able to use a suicide PRS for prediction in two independent cohorts. Additionally, completed suicide cases were observed to have elevated PRS for multiple psychiatric traits, including behavioral disinhibition, MDD, and schizophrenia.[21]

These findings suggest that there is a strong contribution of common genetic variation in completed suicide when compared to suicidal ideation and suicidal attempts. There are also strong overlaps with genetic risk for major psychiatric disorders and traits related to impulsivity, which reinforces epidemiological and clinical observations. Further, a genetic risk score for suicide has had moderate success in being able to predict the likelihood of completed suicide and SB, which is a positive step in identifying those vulnerable to suicide.

Whole Exome and Whole Genome Sequencing Studies

In addition to investigating the association of common variation with suicide and SB, the role of rare variation, both single nucleotide variants (SNVs) and copy number variants (CNVs), has now begun to be investigated. This is possible using next-generation sequencing techniques such as whole-exome and genome sequencing. Two whole-exome sequencing studies have concluded that rare SNVs may be linked to suicidal attempts in BD[23] and suicide in MDD.[23,24] Another recent study of rare protein coding SNVs that used samples from the Utah Suicide Genetic Risk Study (USGRS) (N = 2,676) also identified five rare protein-coding SNVs to be significantly associated with suicide.[25] However, these studies are still in their nascence due to small sample sizes.

EPIGENETICS OF SUICIDE AND SB

Genetic studies in the area of suicide and SB have yielded some interesting insights into possible genetic associations, correlations with psychopathology, and polygenic architecture.

However, the interaction between genetic and environmental factors that are consistently observed in epidemiologic studies also requires to be studied for a more complete understanding of neurobiology. Epigenetic changes are proposed as the mechanism for this interaction by influencing transcription, protein expression, and ultimately behavioral phenotypes. The three most frequently studied epigenetic mechanisms are DNA methylation, micro-RNA (mi-RNA) interference, and histone modifications. As is the case with genetic studies, these can be studied using both targeted (gene-based) and agnostic (epigenome-wide) approaches.

DNA Methylation Studies

Deoxyribonucleic acid methylation involves the transfer of a methyl group onto the C5 position of the cytosine to form 5-methylcytosine. These typically occur at sites where cytosine precedes guanine in the DNA sequence and are called CpG sites.[26]

Deoxyribonucleic acid methylation is the most commonly studied epigenetic mechanism in the context of suicide and SB. From a candidate gene perspective, genes linked to the HPA axis could mediate the interaction between childhood adversity or trauma and suicidality. Studies have investigated epigenetic changes in HPA axis genes such as *NRC31*, *SKA2*, *CRH*, *CRHBP*, *CRHR1*, and *CRHR2*, but results have been mixed.[27] A comprehensive study that investigated individual CpG sites in PFC samples of patients with MDD who died by suicide found evidence of *SKA2 3′* UTR (cg13989295) hypermethylation and reduced *SKA2* gene expression, which was associated with increased waking cortisol and suicidality.[28] The spindle and kinetochore-associated protein 2 (SKA2) is a part of the HPA axis and aids in chaperoning and transactivation of glucocorticoid receptor (GR).[29] Apart from HPA axis genes, there are a few studies which have investigated BDNF promoter methylation and found that hypermethylation is associated with reduced BDNF synthesis, suicide, and SB. Additionally, studies have also investigated methylation of serotonergic pathway genes including *5HT2A* and *TPH2* but results have been inconsistent.[27]

Epigenome-wide association studies (EWAS) have investigated differential methylation levels globally and at individual CpG sites between cases (suicidal ideation, attempts, or completed suicide) and controls, in peripheral blood and postmortem brain tissue. The results from EWAS investigating methylation levels globally have been mixed with both hypermethylation[30] and hypomethylation[31] seen in patients with completed suicide compared to nonpsychiatric controls. These studies have not yielded any specific gene level methylation differences, possibly due to the lack of statistical power to detect such differences.

Micro-RNA Expression Studies

Micro-RNAs are small noncoding RNAs that mediate post-transcriptional gene silencing by controlling the translation of mRNA into proteins. There are ~1,500 mi-RNAs identified in humans. While some mi-RNAs have specific targets, others can regulate the expression levels of several genes at the same time.[32]

A number of hypothesis-free mi-RNA studies have been conducted comparing expression levels in different brain regions between individuals with psychiatric illness who died by suicide and controls (both with psychiatric illness and healthy), but findings have been equivocal.[33]

However, a candidate gene approach which compared 10 mi-RNAs that influence expression of polyamine genes *SAT1* and *SMOX* found increased levels of four mi-RNAs in the prefrontal brain of suicide completers compared to psychologically healthy controls.[34] This provides support for the role of polyamines in the biology of suicide and will be discussed further in subsequent sections.

Overall, epigenetic studies show promise in unraveling the potential mechanisms of gene–environment interactions that confer an enhanced susceptibility to suicide and are an area, which will require further exploration.

NEUROTRANSMITTERS IN SUICIDE AND SB

As mentioned previously, neurotransmitters and their role in the biology of suicide and SB have been extensively investigated. These include studies of levels of neurotransmitters and their metabolites, in blood (serum and plasma), platelets, and body fluids such as urine, as well as receptor density and expression levels in specific areas of the brain. This section reviews research on neurotransmitters such as serotonin [5-hydroxytryptamine (5-HT)], NE, and others, with relevance to suicide biology.

Serotonin

Serotonin (5-HT) is found in the serotonergic nerve endings, other cells, and platelets. While synthesized from tryptophan by enzyme tryptophan hydroxylase (TH), it undergoes enzymatic degradation to 5-hydroxyindoleacetic acid (5-HIAA). Serotonin has been known to have role in mood, anxiety, sleep, cognition, memory, and aggression[35] and is the most studied neuromodulator in suicide.

Early studies measured the levels of 5-HT and its metabolite 5-HIAA in platelets, blood, and cerebrospinal fluid (CSF) in patients with suicidality both with and without psychiatric disorders (MDD, BD, schizophrenia, and personality disorders). These studies have consistently found lower levels of 5HT in blood and/or platelets of patients with SB, in comparison to investigations of 5HT or 5HIAA levels in postmortem brains.[36] Further, lower levels of CSF-5-HIAA but not 5HT correlated with severity of lifetime impulsive aggressive behavior, predicted future suicide attempts, and completed suicide.[37] A study from India also found decreased levels of CSF-5-HIAA in suicide attempters. It also noted an inverse association between urine and CSF-5-HIAA, and the intensity of suicidal ideation among attempters.[38] Another Indian study also found that CSF-5-HIAA levels were considerably lower in violent suicide attempters compared to nonviolent suicide attempters and normal controls.[39]

Subsequent research has focused on investigating the density of different subtypes of 5HT receptors (such as $5HT_{1A}$, $5HT_{2A}$, and $5HT_{2C}$) by measuring mRNA and protein expression levels in specific brain areas of individuals who died by suicide. Two studies found increased expression levels of $5HT_{2A}$ receptors in PFC and the hippocampus of suicide victims,[40,41] while one study found that they did not differ between suicide attempt victims with and without depression.[42] The higher $5HT_{2A}$ receptor levels in suicide victims could be linked to abnormalities of the HPA axis and higher cortisol levels. They may also indicate a higher genetic risk of suicide. Studies have also shown altered $5HT_{2C}$ pre-mRNA editing with low-functional activity $5HT_{2C}$ receptor expression noted in the PFC of suicide victims.[43] However, findings of $5HT_{1A}$ receptor studies remain inconsistent and inconclusive. Taken together, this suggests that serotonergic dysregulation seems to play a role in the pathophysiology of suicide and SB.

Dopamine

Dopamine is a monoamine neurotransmitter present in the brain's ventral tegmental region and substantia nigra. It binds to dopamine (D_1-D_5) receptors. The most common dopamine receptors in the human nervous system are D_1 and D_2. Dopamine is synthesized from L-Phenylalanine and Tyrosine and converted into neurotransmitters NE and epinephrine by dopamine β-hydroxylase. Dopamine is degraded through a set of enzymes such as monoamine oxidase (MAO), catechol-O-methyltransferase (COMT), and aldehyde dehydrogenase (ADH). It degraded into inactive metabolite such as dihydroxyphenylacetaldehyde (DOPAL) and homovanillic acid (HVA) through methylation.[44]

Studies that have looked at the HVA and DOPAL in the CSF and urine and found that patients with MDD who attempted suicide during a 5-year follow-up period had significantly lower urinary HVA urinary than those who did not.[45] Another study found that DOPAL concentrations in the caudate, putamen, and nucleus accumbens of antidepressant-naive suicides were significantly lower than controls

(who were on antidepressants).[46] However, a study from India found that CSF and urine HVA levels were not associated with the intensity of suicidal ideation among patients with MDD.[38]

Studies have also found reductions in dopamine transport and increase in D_2/D_3 receptors in the amygdala of patients with MDD, supporting the hypothesis of decreased mesolimbic dopaminergic transmission in MDD and suicide.[47] Later studies have supported these findings, as evidenced by an impaired growth hormone (GH) response to apomorphine (dopaminergic agonist) among individuals diagnosed with MDD and a past suicidal attempt, suggesting that the same could be a marker of suicide risk.[48] Studies on mRNA levels expression found no differences in the D_1 and D_2 receptor binding areas or the D_4 receptor binding area in the caudate nuclei of suicide victims. Taken together, dopamine appears to play a role in suicide biology, possibly through decreased dopaminergic activity in specific brain areas medicated through various mechanisms, resulting in inward self-directed aggression and increased neuroticism.[49,50]

Adrenaline and Noradrenaline

Norepinephrine, an excitatory neurotransmitter, is produced primarily by neurons in the locus coeruleus (LC). NE is synthesized from amino acid tyrosine by tyrosine hydroxylase, a rate-limiting enzyme. Through vesicular monoamine transporters (VMAT2), NE is released into the synaptic cleft via calcium-dependent exocytosis. NE tracts from the LC project to the entire brain with NE signaling occurring via α_1, α_2, β_1, and β_2 receptors. NE degraded into inactive metabolites such as 3-methoxy-4-hydroxyphenylglycol (MHPG) and 3-methoxy-4-hydroxymandelic acid (VMA).[51] NE is associated with stress response, attention, memory, the sleep–wake cycle, decision-making, and sympathetic response regulation. It is one of three catecholamine neurotransmitters in the brain that has been widely investigated in relation to suicide biology.[52]

Initial studies looking at levels of NE and its metabolite MHPG found lower levels in urine, plasma, and CSF of suicide attempters compared to nonattempters.[53] However, subsequent studies showed no clear link between CSF, plasma, or urine MHPG levels and SB in patients with MDD.[36,38]

Immunolabeling studies have observed increased expression of α_2-adrenergic receptors in the cortex and hippocampus of suicide victims compared with normal control subjects, indicating a chronic activation of the LC possibly related to chronic stress that may result in depletion of synaptic NE and compensatory changes in receptor concentrations. As these receptor changes could be the result of a change in noradrenergic innervation to the cerebral cortex, researchers investigated pigmented neurons in the LC and found a reduction in neuron numbers localized to the rostral two-thirds of the LC in suicidal victims compared to controls.[54] Additionally, the immunoreactivity of tyrosine hydroxylase in LC also exhibits diminished responsiveness or insignificant results.[55] This points to a NE deficit in the brain in suicide victims. However, studies of other adrenergic receptors and their subtypes are few and inconsistent.[36]

Glutamate and Gamma-aminobutyric Acid

Glutamate is an excitatory neurotransmitter that has been linked to suicide neurobiology. Few postmortem studies among suicide victims have shown reduced level of high-affinity glutamatergic receptors in post-mortem brain of suicidal victims.[56] Other findings including increased α-amino-3-hydroxy-5-methyl-4-isoxazolepropionic acid (AMPA) (glutamate receptor) activity in the caudate nucleus, as well as a change in zinc interaction at the N-methyl-D-aspartate (NMDA) receptor in the hippocampus, Lithium's antisuicidal action mediated via a glycogen synthase kinase-3 (GSK3) inhibitor, and effects of NMDA receptor antagonist, ketamine, in rapidly reducing suicidality support the idea of glutamatergic dysfunction in the biology of suicide.[50,57]

In contrast, GABA (gamma-aminobutyric acid) is an inhibitor neurotransmitter. Only a few studies have been done on the association between suicide and GABA dysfunction. Despite studies showing lower GABA levels in both CSF and the dorsolateral prefrontal and occipital cortex of depressed patients,[58] there is no difference in GABA, glycine, taurine, and aspartate levels, with the exception of a low glutamate level in the frontal cortex, between those who commit suicide and those who do not.[59] However, studies found lower mRNA expression of GABA-A receptor α_1, α_3, α_4, and δ subunits in the frontal cortex and subcortical regions. Additionally, upregulation of GABA-A receptor α_1 and β_3 subunits in the cerebral cortex of postmortem victims supports the notion of GABA role in suicide. This lends support to impaired inhibitory GABAergic function across specific brain regions in depression and suicide. The studies on GABA, glutamate receptor density, and GABA-A receptor subunit mRNA expression are limited. Given the same, the specific mechanisms through which glutamate and GABA dysfunction lends vulnerability to SB are yet to be unraveled.[50]

Other Neuromodulators

There have been a few studies on the links between suicide and SB and the opioid system, acetylcholine, and the endocannabinoid system, given their inherent roles in mood, cognitive functions such as attention and memory, as well as motivation.

With respect to the opioid system, two early studies found that younger individuals who completed suicide had a greater density of μ-opioid (mu-opioid) receptors in their frontal and temporal lobes.[60,61] However, a recent study did not find any difference in μ-opioid density or binding affinity in PFC and pre-postcentral gyri (PPCG) between suicide victims and controls.[62]

With respect to acetylcholine, there was no difference between the suicide victims and controls in terms of mAChR (muscarinic acetylcholine receptor) binding affinity or density in the frontal cortex.[63]

There have been no studies till date that have measured the levels of endocannabinoids such as arachidonoyl ethanolamide (anandamide) and 2-arachidonoylglycerol (2-AG) in suicide victims. However, studies have looked at the density and immunoreactivity of cannabinoid CB1 receptors in the dorsolateral PFC of suicide victims with alcohol addiction[64] and found higher receptor expression and immunoreactivity suggesting a possible role of the endocannabinoid system in the pathophysiology of suicide.

Hence, current research is insufficient to draw conclusions with respect to the role of opioid system, acetylcholine, and cannabinoid system dysfunction in suicide.[50,57]

■ STRESS AND IMMUNE SYSTEM

Acute and chronic stressors are both associated with the dysregulation of the HPA axis, polyamines, and neuroinflammation pathway. The consequent complex pathophysiological processes arising from stress have been linked to various psychiatric disorders, primarily mood disorders, and suicide. This section will provide an overview of the pathways mentioned above, as well as their implications for suicide biology.

Hypothalamic–Pituitary–Adrenal Axis

The HPA axis is primarily involved in the regulation of stress in the body. In response to stress, the paraventricular nucleus (PVN) of the hypothalamus releases corticotropin-releasing factor (CRF) and arginine vasopressin (AVP). This hormone stimulates the anterior pituitary gland, which secretes adrenocorticotropic hormone (ACTH). In turn, ACTH stimulates glucocorticoid (cortisol) synthesis in the adrenal gland, which acts on mineralocorticoid (type-I) and glucocorticoid (type-II) receptors. The functioning of the HPA axis is regulated through a negative feedback mechanism and also by many neurotransmitters via their inhibitory (e.g., GABA and endogenous opioids) and excitatory (e.g., NE and serotonin) effects on the PVN.[65]

The dexamethasone suppression test (DST), used to test HPA function, typically suppresses the release of cortisol. Failure to suppress the same (nonsuppression) indicates HPA dysfunction possibly from chronic stress. Studies have demonstrated that nonsuppression to DST was associated with a higher likelihood of suicidal ideation, self-inflicted harm, suicidal attempts, and high lethality suicidal attempts.[66,67] The Trier Social Stress Test (TSST) and Maastricht Acute Stress Test (MAST) showed that previous suicide attempts are associated with lower cortisol reactivity and blunted HPA axis activity.[68]

Conversely, research has identified increased CRF and vasopressin levels in certain brain regions such as the forebrain, raphe, and LC, as well as increased adrenal weight, total cortical thickness, and adrenal cortical hypertrophy among depressed individuals who died by suicide compared to healthy controls, suggesting HPA hyperactivity.[69,70] Subsequent research has showed a decrease in the CRF receptor binding sites in the frontal cortex, as well as a decrease in the mRNA expression of CRH1, pro-opiomelanocortin (POMC), and GR in the frontopolar cortex and anterior pituitary area, respectively.[71] The paradoxical findings of HPA axis dysfunction have been attributed to the groups studied, namely suicide attempters versus completed suicides.

While HPA dysregulation in suicide risk was invariably investigated in the context of mental disorders, other determinants of stress response have also been explored. Studies have examined the role of childhood trauma, abuse, and early life stress on suicide and SB. Early childhood trauma, stress, and adversity may negatively impact HPA axis activity and affect the development of brain structures via epigenetic alterations conferring a predisposition to SB.[65]

Polyamines

Polyamines are common aliphatic compounds with two or more amine (NH_2) groups. These include putrescine, spermidine, and spermine, which are endogenously generated in the brain, as well as agmatine, which can pass the blood–brain barrier. Endogenous polyamines interact with numerous transmembrane channels and influence neurotransmitter systems such as catecholamines, glutamate, GABA, and the nitric oxide system in the cell, while agmatine functions as a neurotransmitter. The spermidine/spermine N1-acetyltransferase 1 (SAT1) is a rate-limiting enzyme in the catabolism of polyamines and regulates intracellular concentration of polyamines. Polyamines, such as the HPA axis, are closely linked with stress response.[72]

Although studies are limited, they demonstrate decreased levels of putrescine, spermidine, and spermine in the hippocampal area, as well as decreased levels of putrescine in the nucleus accumbens of individuals who died by suicide. In addition, altered expression of spermine oxidase (SMOX) and spermine synthase (SMS), the enzymes responsible for the breakdown and synthesis of spermine, was also noted.[73]

Neuroinflammation Pathway

Microglia are brain-immune cells and identified to have important roles in moderating brain inflammation by releasing pro- and anti-inflammatory mediators such as cytokines and chemokines. Microglia by releasing a range of proinflammatory cytokines, such as interleukin (IL)-1, IL-6, tumor necrosis factor (TNF), and nitric oxide (NO), as well as anti-inflammatory cytokines, such as IL-10, insulin-like growth factor-1, transforming growth factor-β (TGF-β), and numerous neurotrophic factors, help with purging damaged or unnecessary neurons and synapses but also protect the CNS against stress-derived agents. However, chronic stress-induced activation of microglia has been linked to altered regulation of the tryptophan–kynurenine pathway, which results in altered production of neuroprotective and neurotoxic metabolites. The impaired release of inflammatory mediators causes the brain to maintain a chronic low-grade inflammatory state of neurotoxicity, excitotoxicity, and heightened glutamate release, which have been linked to psychiatric illnesses such as depression, schizophrenia, as well as suicide and SB.[74]

Elevated IL-6 levels have been consistently found in the CSF, blood, and postmortem brains of people with suicide and SB. However, findings pertaining to low plasma IL-2, IL-4, TNF, interferon-γ (IFN-γ), TGF-β, and soluble IL-2 receptors are mixed.[75] The studies have also demonstrated microglial activation in neuropathological studies of postmortem human brains of suicide victims. More than ten studies are published on KYN pathway metabolites in blood, but the results are mixed and inconclusive. Furthermore, only a few studies have corroborated the findings of greater levels of CSF quinolinic acid and lower levels of CSF kynurenic acid and picolinic acid in psychiatric patients with suicide attempts. While preliminary, this lends credibility to the potential involvement of the tryptophan–kynurenine pathway in suicide biology, possibly through stress-induced microglial activation in the brain.[76]

CELLULAR SIGNALING IN SUICIDE AND SB

Neurotrophic Factors in Suicide and SB

Neurotrophic factors, such as BDNF, nerve growth factor (NGF), neurotrophin (NT)-3, NT-4, play a prominent role in neurodevelopment and synaptic plasticity. The role of neurotrophic factors has been investigated extensively in psychiatric disorders and suicide. There is converging evidence that highlights the role played by them in suicide and SB. Consensus on the role of BDNF in suicide is unequivocal but remains to be understood more comprehensively.

A number of early studies found decreased expression of neurotrophic factors in hippocampus and PFC of patients who died

by suicide when compared to nonpsychiatric controls.[77,78] These findings were also replicated in a study from India which found lower mRNA and protein levels of BDNF, NGF, TrkA, and TrkB (tropomyosin receptor kinase activated by BDNF/NGF) in the hippocampus of patients who died by suicide.[79] Another study from India, which compared suicide attempters and age- and gender-matched healthy controls, also found lower levels of serum BDNF among suicide attempters.[80] Two recent meta-analyses compared peripheral BDNF levels in psychiatric patients with and without a history of a suicidal attempt and found that levels measured in plasma, but not serum or in pooled analysis, were significantly lower in patients with a history of suicidal attempt, indicating that BDNF levels could be a potential biomarker for SB.[81,82] The fact that known treatments for SB such as antidepressants and ketamine are known to increase levels of BDNF further reinforces its relevance in the pathophysiology of suicide.[83,84]

Signal Transduction Abnormalities in Suicide and SB

Signal transduction constitutes the series of steps by which extracellular signals are converted to intracellular signals, which ultimately trigger a cascade of events that alter cellular functions. The three well-established pathways for signal transduction are ligand-gated ion channels, G-protein-coupled receptors (GPCRs), and tyrosine kinase receptors. A majority of the neurotransmitters described in previous sections use these pathways to influence cellular functions.

Among them, GPCRs and associated downstream signaling have been studied the most in the context of suicide and SB. GPCRs activate two common second messenger pathways, namely the cyclic adenosine monophosphate (cAMP) pathway, which leads to increased activity of protein kinase A (PKA), and the phosphoinositide pathway which leads to increased activity of protein kinase C (PKC). These protein kinases in turn activate several transcription factors, including CREB (cAMP response element-binding protein) family and GSK-3β (glycogen synthase kinase-3β), which eventually lead to gene transcription and altered protein expression.

Studies have found decreased mRNA expression of different isoenzymes of PKC in the PFC and hippocampus of both depressed suicide and nonsuicide patients compared to controls in adolescents and adults.[36,85] cAMP binding, PKA activity, mRNA and protein expression of PKA subunits have also been found to be similarly decreased in PFC and hippocampus of patients with depression who died by suicide.[36]

NEUROIMAGING STUDIES IN SUICIDE AND SB

The identification of brain areas and networks that contribute to suicide and SB has been a major area of research.

Structural Magnetic Resonance Imaging Studies

Structural magnetic resonance imaging (MRI) studies typically employ T1- and T2-weighted scans to characterize brain morphological indices such as gray and white matter volumes and cortical thickness either in specific brain regions (region of interest/ROI-based analysis) or across the whole brain.

Early studies found evidence of gray and white matter hyperintensities in patients across the lifespan with depression and suicidal attempts compared to a matched group without a suicidal attempt.[86-89] In addition, lower gray matter volumes and cortical thickness in various brain regions such as prefrontal (including dorsolateral prefrontal, orbitofrontal) insular, cingulate, and temporal cortices[90-100] have also been identified. However, similar to findings from genetic studies, there has been a problem of replicability and inconsistent results, attributable to small sample sizes and phenotypic heterogeneity. This has been sought to be addressed through the formation of international neuroimaging consortia, which pool samples from different studies and conduct harmonized analyses.

An illustrative study from the ENIGMA-MDD working group pooled data from 18 international cohorts (N = 18,925) and identified 25 brain areas with statistically significant differences between groups.[101] Post hoc tests found bilateral thalamic and right pallidum reduced volume and a lower surface area of the left inferior parietal lobe. The pallidum is associated with reward responses and positive effect, while the thalamus, which has been traditionally viewed as a relay station, is a key component of cortico-striato-thalamo-cortical loops which play a crucial role in top-down regulation of impulses and urges.[101]

Diffusion Tensor Imaging Studies

Diffusion tensor imaging (DTI) studies use diffusion-weighted MRI scans to evaluate white matter tract integrity [using measures such as fractional anisotropy (FA) and mean diffusivity (MD)] within and between different brain areas.

Studies have consistently identified decreased frontal subcortical white matter connectivity in patients with MDD or BD with and without suicidality.[102-106] Impaired response inhibition mediated via the same might explain impulsivity noted in those with

SB, although findings have not been consistent across the literature.[107] In addition to the same, white matter abnormalities in the corpus callosum have also been implicated.[108,109]

These findings from cross-sectional studies were also replicated in a preliminary longitudinal evaluation where patients with MDD who attempted suicide during the 3 years follow-up period had decreased FA in the dorsomedial frontal, anterior limb of the internal capsule, and dorsal cingulate cortices at baseline and also had greater decreases over time in ventral and dorsal frontal FA indicating progressive deterioration in white matter integrity that contributes to impaired top-down modulation of responses to emotional stimuli.[110]

Conversely, findings seem to be distinct from patients with schizophrenia, where suicidal ideation has been associated with preserved integrity of white matter tracts as evidenced by higher FA and lower MD. This has been explained by the authors as being due to a possible association between white matter integrity, better cognitive function, and insight which may be responsible for greater depressive symptoms and suicidal ideation.[111]

Functional MRI Studies

Functional MRI (fMRI) uses the blood oxygen level-dependent (BOLD) signal, which is a ratio of oxygenated and deoxygenated hemoglobin, as a proxy measure for activation of brain structures and networks. This signal may be measured either during the performance of a task (task-based fMRI) or in the absence of any specific task (resting state fMRI). The analysis can focus either on specific brain areas or the whole brain.

A number of resting state fMRI studies have been conducted in recent years to identify neural signatures associated with suicide and SBs. These have implicated many brain areas and networks such as the orbitofrontal cortex (OFC),[112] anterior cingulate cortex (ACC),[113] insula,[114] amygdala and paracentral lobule/precuneus,[115,116] DMN,[117,118] and salience network (SN)[119] among others.

A large study investigated the neural correlates of transition from suicidal ideas to acts by comparing resting state activity and functional connectivity in patients with MDD with—a past suicidal attempt, suicidal ideas but no suicidal attempt, no suicidal ideas or attempts and healthy controls. It was seen that only those with a past attempt showed differences in functional connectivity in frontoparietal and subcortical networks.[120] These findings were also replicated in another study with a similar design,[121] suggesting that the subgroup of patients with MDD who attempt suicide have distinct neural signatures and that these may be used as a possible biological marker for vulnerability to suicide and SB.

Recent studies have also employed unsupervised machine learning (ML) algorithms on resting state fMRI parameters to classify risk of suicidal attempts in patients with depression[122] and schizophrenia,[123] with DMN and SN fluctuations being implicated. Reduced DMN functional connectivity is associated with difficulties with abstract thinking, planning, and social cognition, while reduced SN functional connectivity can be associated with impaired self-regulation, all of which may contribute to the etiology of suicide and SB. The ability to use ML-based methods in clinical settings is an intriguing prospect for suicide risk stratification in the future.

The findings from resting state fMRI studies have also been mirrored in task-based fMRI studies. A recent meta-analysis showed activation changes in the insula and fusiform gyrus in MDD patients with a history of suicide attempt. These changes were associated with the dysfunction of emotion regulation, processing negative information and self-awareness.[124]

In summary, imaging studies have identified both structural and functional abnormalities in areas of the brain such as PFC, insula, and amygdala, as well as networks such as the default mode, executive control, and SNs. These are associated with difficulties with executive control, including response inhibition, problem-solving, memory retrieval and decision-making, as well as emotional regulation contributing to an increased risk for suicide and SB.

IMPLICATIONS OF NEUROBIOLOGICAL CORRELATES OF SUICIDE IN THE PATIENT CARE AND MANAGEMENT

The identification and management of suicide and SB remain challenging. Existing findings allude to immunological, neurotransmitter, biochemical, brain region, neural network, cellular, molecular, epigenetic, as well as genetic biomarkers for suicide. Integrating these with clinical and behavioral findings may help in early identification of those vulnerable to suicide thereby permitting timely attenuation of risk. While currently, translational implications to management of suicide remain limited, the above-discussed preliminary findings hold great promise in offering opportunities to develop and deliver individually tailored interventions in the future.

CONCLUSION

Studies have identified neural substrates of suicide. These span from changes to brain architecture, aberrant neuronal networks, neuromodulator dysfunction, neurochemical dysregulation, imparied cellular and molecular signaling as well as alterations to gene expression and gene polymorphisms. However, exact mechanisms and the direction of these alterations are unclear. The findings from studies on stress, inflammation, neuroimmune system, neurotransmitters, neuroimaging, epigenetics and genetics confirm a distinct biological basis for SB, but remain to be understood comprehensively. Concerningly, despite the evident burden of suicide, there is an extreme paucity of neurobiological studies in the Indian setting. Using collaborative approaches could potentially overcome the same, thereby offering insights specific to the Indian context as well as furthering our understanding of the neurobiology of suicide.

Further unraveling the complexities of biological underpinnings warrants an integrated approach combining clinical, psychosocial, and biomarkers and exploring the same across the life span of individuals. This would be integral to developing accurate prediction models and formulating tailored treatment strategies, thereby effectively preventing suicide.

REFERENCES

1. deCatanzaro D. Human suicide: A biological perspective. Behav Brain Sci. 1980;3: 265-72.
2. Mann JJ, Arango V. Integration of neurobiology and psychopathology in a unified model of suicidal behavior. J Clin Psychopharmacol. 1992;12:2S-7S.
3. Vaquero-Lorenzo C, Vasquez MA. Suicide: Genetics and Heritability. Curr Top Behav Neurosci. 2020;46:63-78.
4. Brent DA, Melhem N. Familial transmission of suicidal behavior. Psychiatr Clin North Am. 2008;31:157-77.

5. O'Reilly LM, Kuja-Halkola R, Rickert ME, Class QA, Larsson H, Lichtenstein P, et al. The intergenerational transmission of suicidal behavior: An offspring of siblings study. Transl Psychiatry. 2020;10:1-11.

6. Kendler KS, Ohlsson H, Sundquist J, Sundquist K, Edwards AC. The sources of parent-child transmission of risk for suicide attempt and deaths by suicide in Swedish National samples. AJP. 2020;177:928-35.

7. Pedersen NL, Fiske A. Genetic influences on suicide and nonfatal suicidal behavior: Twin study findings. Eur Psychiatry. 2010;25:264-7.

8. Petersen L, Sørensen TIA, Kragh Andersen P, Mortensen PB, Hawton K. Genetic and familial environmental effects on suicide attempts: A study of Danish adoptees and their biological and adoptive siblings. J Affect Disord. 2014;155:273-7.

9. Petersen L, Sørensen TIA, Andersen PK, Mortensen PB, Hawton K. Genetic and familial environmental effects on suicide--an adoption study of siblings. PLoS One. 2013;8:e77973.

10. von Borczyskowski A, Lindblad F, Vinnerljung B, Reintjes R, Hjern A. Familial factors and suicide: An adoption study in a Swedish National Cohort. Psychol Med. 2011;41:749-58.

11. Kim CD, Seguin M, Therrien N, Riopel G, Chawky N, Lesage AD, et al. Familial aggregation of suicidal behavior: A family study of male suicide completers from the general population. Am J Psychiatry. 2005;162:1017-9.

12. McGirr A, Alda M, Séguin M, Cabot S, Lesage A, Turecki G. Familial aggregation of suicide explained by cluster B traits: A three-group family study of suicide controlling for major depressive disorder. Am J Psychiatry. 2009;166:1124-34.

13. Ballard ED, Cui L, Vandeleur C, Castelao E, Zarate CA Jr, Preisig M, et al. Familial aggregation and coaggregation of suicide attempts and comorbid mental disorders in adults. JAMA Psychiatry. 2019;76:826-33.

14. Mirkovic B, Laurent C, Podlipski MA, Frebourg T, Cohen D, Gerardin P. Genetic association studies of suicidal behavior: A review of the past 10 years, progress, limitations, and future directions. Front Psychiatry. 2016. 23;7:158.

15. Pasi S, Singh PK, Pandey RK, Kaur J. Evaluation of psychiatric and genetic risk factors among primary relatives of suicide completers in Delhi NCR region, India. Psychiatry Res. 2015;229:933-9.

16. Basu A, Chadda RK, Sood M, Kaur H, Kukreti R. A preliminary association study between serotonin transporter (5-HTTLPR), receptor polymorphisms (5-HTR1A, 5-HTR2A) and depression symptom-clusters in a north Indian population suffering from Major Depressive Disorder (MDD). Asian J Psychiatr. 2019;43:184-8.

17. Rawat S, Rajkumari S, Joshi PC, Kalasapati LK, Rao GLVC, Rao GP. Risk factors for suicide attempt: A population-based genetic study from Telangana, India. Curr Psychol. 2015;37(1):30-5.

18. Gupta G, Deval R, Mishra A, Shih MC. Re-testing reported significant SNPs related to suicide in a historical high-risk isolated population from north east India. Hereditas. 2020;157:31.

19. Strawbridge RJ, Ward J, Ferguson A, Graham N, Shaw RJ, Cullen B, et al. Identification of novel genome-wide associations for suicidality in UK Biobank, genetic correlation with psychiatric disorders and polygenic association with completed suicide. EBioMedicine. 2019;41:517-25.

20. Mullins N, Bigdeli TB, Børglum AD, Coleman JRI, Demontis D, Mehta D, et al. GWAS of suicide attempt in psychiatric disorders and association with major depression polygenic risk scores. Am J Psychiatry. 2019;176:651-60.

21. Docherty AR, Shabalin AA, DiBlasi E, Monson E, Mullins N, Adkins DE, et al. Genome-wide association study of suicide death and polygenic prediction of clinical antecedents. Am J Psychiatry. 2020;177:917-27.

22. Otsuka I, Akiyama M, Shirakawa O, Okazaki S, Momozawa Y, Kamatani Y, et al. Genome-wide association studies identify polygenic effects for completed suicide in the Japanese population. Neuropsychopharmacol. 2019;44:2119-24.

23. Monson ET, Pirooznia M, Parla J, Kramer M, Goes FS, Gaine ME, et al. Assessment of

whole-exome sequence data in attempted suicide within a bipolar disorder cohort. Mol Neuropsychiatry. 2017;3:1-11.

24. Tombácz D, Maróti Z, Kalmár T, Csabai Z, Balázs Z, Takahashi S, et al. High-coverage whole-exome sequencing identifies candidate genes for suicide in victims with major depressive disorder. Sci Rep. 2017;7:7106.

25. DiBlasi E, Shabalin AA, Monson ET, Keeshin BR, Bakian AV, Kirby AV, et al. Rare protein-coding variants implicate genes involved in risk of suicide death. Am J Med Genet B Neuropsychiatr Genet. 2021;186(8):508-20.

26. Moore LD, Le T, Fan G. DNA methylation and its basic function. Neuropsychopharmacol. 2013;38:23-38.

27. Cheung S, Woo J, Maes MS, Zai CC. Suicide epigenetics, a review of recent progress. J Affect Disord. 2020;265:423-38.

28. Guintivano J, Brown T, Newcomer A, Jones M, Cox O, Maher BS, et al. Identification and replication of a combined epigenetic and genetic biomarker predicting suicide and suicidal behaviors. AJP. 2014;171: 1287-96.

29. Rice L, Waters CE, Eccles J, Garside H, Sommer P, Kay P, et al. Identification and functional analysis of SKA2 interaction with the glucocorticoid receptor. J Endocrinol. 2008;198:499-509.

30. Haghighi F, Xin Y, Chanrion B, O'Donnell AH, Ge Y, Dwork AJ, et al. Increased DNA methylation in the suicide brain. Dialogues Clin Neurosci. 2014;16:430-8.

31. Schneider E, Hajj NE, Müller F, Navarro B. Epigenetic dysregulation in the prefrontal cortex of suicide completers. CGR. 2015;146:19-27.

32. Esteller M. Non-coding RNAs in human disease. Nat Rev Genet. 2011;12:861-74.

33. Pantazatos SP, Huang YY, Rosoklija GB, Dwork AJ, Arango V, Mann JJ. Whole-transcriptome brain expression and exon-usage profiling in major depression and suicide: Evidence for altered glial, endothelial and ATPase activity. Mol Psychiatry. 2017;22:760-73.

34. Lopez JP, Fiori LM, Gross JA, Labonte B, Yerko V, Mechawar N, et al. Regulatory role of miRNAs in polyamine gene expression in the prefrontal cortex of depressed suicide completers. Int J Neuropsychopharmacol. 2014;17:23-32.

35. Berger M, Gray JA, Roth BL. The expanded biology of serotonin. Annu Rev Med. 2009;60:355-66.

36. Pandey GN. Biological basis of suicide and suicidal behavior. Bipolar Disord. 2013;15:524-41.

37. Nordström P, Samuelsson M, Åsberg M, Träskman-Bendz L, Aberg-Wistedt A, Nordin C, et al. CSF 5-HIAA predicts suicide risk after attempted suicide. Suicide Life Threat Behav. 1994;24:1-9.

38. Palaniappan V, Ramachandran V, Somasundaram O. Suicidal ideation and biogenic amines in depression. Indian J Psychiatry. 1983;25:286-92.

39. Trivedi JK, Pandey S, Dalal PK, Dubey MP, Sinha PK. CSF 5—hiaa in violent and non-violent suicide attempters. Indian J Psychiatry. 1997;39:41-8.

40. Stanley M, Mann JJ. Increased serotonin-2 binding sites in frontal cortex of suicide victims. Lancet. 1983;1:214-6.

41. Pandey GN, Dwivedi Y, Rizavi HS, Ren X, Pandey SC, Pesold C, et al. Higher expression of serotonin 5-HT2A receptors in the postmortem brains of teenage suicide victims. AJP. 2002;159:419-29.

42. Stockmeier CA, Dilley GE, Shapiro LA, Overholser JC, Thompson PA, Meltzer HY. Serotonin receptors in suicide victims with major depression. Neuropsychopharmacology. 1997;16:162-73.

43. Gurevich I, Tamir H, Arango V, Dwork AJ, Mann JJ, Schmauss C, et al. Altered editing of serotonin 2C receptor pre-mRNA in the prefrontal cortex of depressed suicide victims. Neuron. 2002;34:349-56.

44. Molinoff PB, Axelrod J. Biochemistry of catecholamines. Annu Rev Biochem. 1971;40:465-500.

45. Roy A, Karoum F, Pollack S. Marked reduction in indexes of dopamine metabolism among patients with depression who attempt suicide. Arch Gen Psychiatry. 1992;49: 447-50.

46. Bowden C, Cheetham SC, Lowther S, Katona CL, Crompton MR, Horton RW, et al.

Reduced dopamine turnover in the basal ganglia of depressed suicides. Brain Res. 1997;769:135-40.

47. Ryding E, Lindström M, Träskman-Bendz L. The role of dopamine and serotonin in suicidal behaviour and aggression. Prog Brain Res. 2008;172:307-15.

48. Pitchot W, Hansenne M, Gonzalez Moreno A, Pinto E, Reggers J, Fuchs S, et al. Reduced dopamine function in depressed patients is related to suicidal behavior but not its lethality. Psychoneuroendocrinology. 2001;26:689-96.

49. Carballo JJ, Akamnonu CP, Oquendo MA. Neurobiology of suicidal behavior. An integration of biological and clinical findings. Arch Suicide Res. 2008;12:93-110.

50. Ernst C, Mechawar N, Turecki G. Suicide neurobiology. Prog Neurobiol. 2009;89:315-33.

51. Kopin IJ. Evolving views of the metabolic fate of norepinephrine. Endocrinol Exp. 1982;16:291-300.

52. Chandley MJ, Ordway GA. Noradrenergic dysfunction in depression and suicide. In: Dwivedi Y (Ed). The Neurobiological Basis of Suicide. Boca Raton (FL): CRC Press/Taylor & Francis; 2012.

53. Secunda SK, Cross CK, Koslow S, Katz MM, Kocsis J, Maas JW, et al. Biochemistry and suicidal behavior in depressed patients. Biol Psychiatry. 1986;21:756-67.

54. Arango V, Underwood MD, Mann JJ. Fewer pigmented locus coeruleus neurons in suicide victims: Preliminary results. Biol Psychiatry. 1996;39:112-20.

55. Biegon A, Fieldust S. Reduced tyrosine hydroxylase immunoreactivity in locus coeruleus of suicide victims. Synapse. 1992;10:79-82.

56. Nowak G, Ordway GA, Paul IA. Alterations in the N-methyl-D-aspartate (NMDA) receptor complex in the frontal cortex of suicide victims. Brain Res. 1995;675:157-64.

57. Furczyk K, Schutová B, Michel TM, Thome J, Büttner A. The neurobiology of suicide—a review of post-mortem studies. J Mol Psychiatry. 2013;1:2.

58. Anisman H, Merali Z, Poulter MO. Gamma-aminobutyric acid involvement in depressive illness interactions with corticotropin-releasing hormone and serotonin. In: Dwivedi Y (Ed). The Neurobiological Basis of Suicide. Boca Raton (FL): CRC Press/Taylor & Francis; 2012.

59. Korpi ER, Kleinman JE, Wyatt RJ. GABA concentrations in forebrain areas of suicide victims. Biol Psychiatry. 1988;23:109-14.

60. Gross-Isseroff R, Dillon KA, Israeli M, Biegon A. Regionally selective increases in μ opioid receptor density in the brains of suicide victims. Brain Res. 1990;530:312-6.

61. Gabilondo AM, Javier Meana J, García-Sevilla JA. Increased density of μ-opioid receptors in the postmortem brain of suicide victims. Brain Research. 1995;682:245-50.

62. Zalsman G, Molcho A, Huang Y, Dwork A, Li S, Mann JJ. Postmortem μ-opioid receptor binding in suicide victims and controls. J Neural Transm. 2005;112:949-54.

63. Stanley M. Cholinergic receptor binding in the frontal cortex of suicide victims. Am J Psychiatry. 1984;141:1432-6.

64. Hungund BL, Vinod KY, Kassir SA, Basavarajappa BS, Yalamanchili R, Cooper TB, et al. Upregulation of CB1 receptors and agonist-stimulated [35S]GTPgammaS binding in the prefrontal cortex of depressed suicide victims. Mol Psychiatry. 2004;9:184-90.

65. Berardelli I, Serafini G, Cortese N, Fiaschè F, O'Connor RC, Pompili M. The involvement of hypothalamus–pituitary–adrenal (HPA) axis in suicide risk. Brain Sci. 2020;10:653.

66. Alacreu-Crespo A, Olié E, Guillaume S, Girod C, Cazals A, Chaudieu I, et al. Dexamethasone suppression test may predict more severe/violent suicidal behavior. Front Psychiatry. 2020;11:97.

67. Mann JJ, Currier D. A review of prospective studies of biologic predictors of suicidal behavior in mood disorders. Arch Suicide Res. 2007;11:3-16.

68. Melhem NM, Keilp JG, Porta G, Oquendo MA, Burke A, Stanley B, et al. Blunted HPA axis activity in suicide attempters compared to those at high risk for suicidal behavior. Neuropsychopharmacology. 2016;41:1447-56.

69. Arató M, Bánki CM, Bissette G, Nemeroff CB. Elevated CSF CRF in suicide victims. Biol Psychiatry. 1989;25:355-9.

70. Szigethy E, Conwell Y, Forbes NT, Cox C, Caine ED. Adrenal weight and morphology in victims of completed suicide. Biol Psychiatry. 1994;36:374-80.

71. Jokinen J, Boström AE, Dadfar A, Ciuculete DM, Chatzittofis A, Åsberg M, et al. Epigenetic changes in the CRH gene are related to severity of suicide attempt and a general psychiatric risk score in adolescents. EBioMedicine. 2018;27:123-33.

72. Turecki G. Polyamines and suicide risk. Mol Psychiatry. 2013;18:1242-3.

73. Gross JA, Turecki G. Suicide and the polyamine system. CNS Neurol Disord Drug Targets. 2013;12:980-8.

74. Suzuki H, Ohgidani M, Kuwano N, Chrétien F, de la Grandmaison GL, Onaya M, et al. Suicide and microglia: Recent findings and future perspectives based on human studies. Front Cell Neurosci. 2019;13:31.

75. Gananança L, Oquendo MA, Tyrka AR, Cisneros-Trujillo S, Mann JJ, Sublette ME. The role of cytokines in the pathophysiology of suicidal behavior. Psychoneuroendocrinology. 2016;63:296-310.

76. Baharikhoob P, Kolla NJ. Microglial dysregulation and suicidality: A stress-diathesis perspective. Front Psychiatry. 2020;11:781.

77. Dwivedi Y, Rizavi HS, Conley RR, Roberts RC, Tamminga CA, Pandey GN. Altered gene expression of brain-derived neurotrophic factor and receptor tyrosine kinase B in postmortem brain of suicide subjects. Arch Gen Psychiatry. 2003;60:804-15.

78. Dwivedi Y, Mondal AC, Rizavi HS, Conley RR. Suicide brain is associated with decreased expression of neurotrophins. Biol Psychiatry. 2005;58:315-24.

79. Banerjee R, Ghosh AK, Ghosh B, Bhattacharyya S, Mondal AC. Decreased mRNA and protein expression of BDNF, NGF, and their receptors in the hippocampus from suicide: An analysis in human postmortem brain. Clin Med Insights Pathol. 2013;6:1-11.

80. Priya PK, Rajappa M, Kattimani S, Mohanraj PS, Revathy G. Association of neurotrophins, inflammation and stress with suicide risk in young adults. Clinica Chimica Acta. 2016;457:41-5.

81. Fusar-Poli L, Aguglia A, Amerio A, Amerio A, Bruno E, Placenti V, et al. Peripheral BDNF levels in psychiatric patients with and without a history of suicide attempt: A systematic review and meta-analysis. Prog Neuropsychopharmacol Biol Psychiatry. 2021;111:110342.

82. Salas-Magaña M, Tovilla-Zárate CA, González-Castro TB, Juárez-Rojop IE, López-Narváez ML, Rodríguez-Pérez JM, et al. Decrease in brain-derived neurotrophic factor at plasma level but not in serum concentrations in suicide behavior: A systematic review and meta-analysis. Brain Behav. 2017;7:e00706.

83. Ai M, Wang J, Chen J, Wang W, Xu X, Gan Y, et al. Plasma brain-derived neurotrophic factor (BDNF) concentration and the BDNF Val66Met polymorphism in suicide: A prospective study in patients with depressive disorder. Pharmgenomics Pers Med. 2019;12:97-106.

84. Sattar Y, Wilson J, Khan AM, Adnan M, Azzopardi Larios D, Shrestha S, et al. A review of the mechanism of antagonism of N-methyl-D-aspartate receptor by ketamine in treatment-resistant depression. Cureus. 2018;10:e2652.

85. Pandey GN, Sharma A, Rizavi HS, Ren X. Dysregulation of protein kinase C in adult depression and suicide: Evidence from postmortem brain studies. Int J Neuropsychopharmacol. 2021;24:400-8.

86. Ahearn EP, Jamison KR, Steffens DC, Cassidy F, Provenzale JM, Lehman A, et al. MRI correlates of suicide attempt history in unipolar depression. Biol Psychiatry. 2001;50:266-70.

87. Ehrlich S, Breeze JL, Hesdorffer DC, Noam GG, Hong X, Alban RL, et al. White matter hyperintensities and their association with suicidality in depressed young adults. J Affect Disord. 2005;86:281-7.

88. Pompili M, Ehrlich S, De Pisa E, Mann JJ, Innamorati M, Cittadini A, et al. White matter hyperintensities and their associations with suicidality in patients with major affective disorders. Eur Arch Psychiatry Clin Neurosci. 2007;257:494-99.

89. Hwang J-P, Lee T-W, Tsai S-J, Chen TJ, Yang CH, Lirng JF, et al. Cortical and subcortical abnormalities in late-onset depression with history of suicide attempts investigated with MRI and voxel-based morphometry. J Geriatr Psychiatry Neurol. 2010;23:171-84.

90. Giakoumatos CI, Tandon N, Shah J, Mathew IT, Brady RO, Clementz BA, et al. Are structural brain abnormalities associated with suicidal behavior in patients with psychotic disorders? J Psychiatr Res. 2013;47:1389-95.

91. Peng H, Wu K, Li J, Qi H, Guo S, Chi M, et al. Increased suicide attempts in young depressed patients with abnormal temporal-parietal-limbic gray matter volume. J Affect Disord. 2014;165:69-3.

92. Taylor WD, Boyd B, McQuoid DR, Kudra K, Saleh A, MacFall JR. Widespread white matter but focal gray matter alterations in depressed individuals with thoughts of death. Prog Neuropsychopharmacol Biol Psychiatry. 2015;62:22-8.

93. Colle R, Chupin M, Cury C, Vandendrie C, Gressier F, Hardy P, et al. Depressed suicide attempters have smaller hippocampus than depressed patients without suicide attempts. J Psychiatr Res. 2015;61:13-8.

94. van Heeringen K, Bijttebier S, Desmyter S, Vervaet M, Baeken C. Is there a neuroanatomical basis of the vulnerability to suicidal behavior? A coordinate-based meta-analysis of structural and functional MRI studies. Front Hum Neurosci. 2014;8:824.

95. Gosnell SN, Velasquez KM, Molfese DL, Molfese PJ, Madan A, Fowler JC, et al. Prefrontal cortex, temporal cortex, and hippocampus volume are affected in suicidal psychiatric patients. Psychiatry Res Neuroimaging. 2016;256:50-6.

96. Rizk MM, Rubin-Falcone H, Lin X, Keilp JG, Miller JM, Milak MS, et al. Gray matter volumetric study of major depression and suicidal behavior. Psychiatry Res Neuroimaging. 2019;283:16-23.

97. Wang P, Zhang R, Jiang X, Wei S, Wang F, Tang Y. Gray matter volume alterations associated with suicidal ideation and suicide attempts in patients with mood disorders. Ann Gen Psychiatry. 2020;19:69.

98. Wang L, Zhao Y, Edmiston EK, Womer FY, Zhang R, Zhao P, et al. Structural and functional abnormalities of amygdala and prefrontal cortex in major depressive disorder with suicide attempts. Front Psychiatry. 2019;10:923.

99. Besteher B, Wagner G, Koch K, Schachtzabel C, Reichenbach JR, Schlösser R, et al. Pronounced prefronto-temporal cortical thinning in schizophrenia: Neuroanatomical correlate of suicidal behavior? Schizophr Res. 2016;176:151-7.

100. Johnston JAY, Wang F, Liu J, Blond BN, Wallace A, Liu J, et al. Multimodal neuroimaging of frontolimbic structure and function associated with suicide attempts in adolescents and young adults with bipolar disorder. Am J Psychiatry. 2017;174:667-75.

101. Campos AI, Thompson PM, Veltman DJ, Pozzijr E, van Veltzenjr LS, Jahanshad N, et al. Brain correlates of suicide attempt in 18,925 participants across 18 international Cohorts. Biol Psychiatry. 2021;90:243-52.

102. Mahon K, Burdick KE, Wu J, Ardekani BA, Szeszko PR. Relationship between suicidality and impulsivity in bipolar I disorder: A diffusion tensor imaging study. Bipolar Disord. 2012;14:80-9.

103. Jia Z, Wang Y, Huang X, Kuang W, Wu Q, Lui S, et al. Impaired frontothalamic circuitry in suicidal patients with depression revealed by diffusion tensor imaging at 3.0 T. J Psychiatry Neurosci. 2014;39:170-7.

104. Olvet DM, Peruzzo D, Thapa-Chhetry B, Sublette ME, Sullivan GM, Oquendo MA, et al. A diffusion tensor imaging study of suicide attempters. J Psychiatr Res. 2014;51:60-7.

105. Myung W, Han CE, Fava M, Mischoulon D, Papakostas GI, Heo JY, et al. Reduced frontal-subcortical white matter connectivity in association with suicidal ideation in major depressive disorder. Transl Psychiatry. 2016;6:e835.

106. Fan S, Lippard ETC, Sankar A, Wallace A, Johnston JAY, Wang F, et al. Gray and white matter differences in adolescents and young adults with prior suicide attempts across bipolar and major depressive disorders. J Affect Disord. 2019;245:1089-97.

107. Reich R, Gilbert A, Clari R, Burdick KE, Szeszko PR. A preliminary investigation of impulsivity, aggression and white matter in patients with bipolar disorder and a suicide attempt history. J Affect Disord. 2019;247:88-96.

108. Zhang R, Jiang X, Chang M, Wei S, Tang Y, Wang F. White matter abnormalities of corpus callosum in patients with bipolar disorder and suicidal ideation. Ann Gen Psychiatry. 2019;18:20.

109. Wei S, Womer FY, Edmiston EK, Zhang R, Jiang X, Wu F, et al. Structural alterations associated with suicide attempts in major depressive disorder and bipolar disorder: A diffusion tensor imaging study. Prog Neuropsychopharmacol Biol Psychiatry. 2020;98:109827.

110. Lippard ETC, Johnston JAY, Spencer L, Quatrano S, Fan S, Sankar A, et al. Preliminary examination of gray and white matter structure and longitudinal structural changes in frontal systems associated with future suicide attempts in adolescents and young adults with mood disorders. J Affect Disord. 2019;245:1139-48.

111. Long Y, Ouyang X, Liu Z, Chen X, Hu X, Lee E, et al. Associations among suicidal ideation, white matter integrity and cognitive deficit in first-episode schizophrenia. Front Psychiatry. 2018;9:391.

112. Chen Z, Xia M, Zhao Y, Kuang W, Jia Z, Gong Q. Characteristics of intrinsic brain functional connectivity alterations in major depressive disorder patients with suicide behavior. J Magn Reson Imaging. 2021;54:1867-75.

113. Tian S, Zhu R, Chattun MR, Wang H, Chen Z, Zhang S, et al. Temporal dynamics alterations of spontaneous neuronal activity in anterior cingulate cortex predict suicidal risk in bipolar II patients. Brain Imaging Behav. 2021;15:2481-91.

114. Hu L, Xiao M, Cao J, Tan Z, Wang M, Kuang L. The association between insular subdivisions functional connectivity and suicide attempt in adolescents and young adults with major depressive disorder. Brain Topogr. 2021;34:297-305.

115. Stumps A, Jagger-Rickels A, Rothlein D, Amick M, Park H, Evans T. Connectome-based functional connectivity markers of suicide attempt. J Affect Disord. 2021;283:430-40.

116. Zhang R, Zhang L, Wei S, Wang P, Jiang X, Tang Y, et al. Increased amygdala-paracentral lobule/precuneus functional connectivity associated with patients with mood disorder and suicidal behavior. Front Hum Neurosci. 2020;14:585664.

117. Chase HW, Segreti AM, Keller TA, Cherkassky VL, Just MA, Pan LA, et al. Alterations of functional connectivity and intrinsic activity within the cingulate cortex of suicidal ideators. J Affect Disord. 2017;212:78-85.

118. Malhi GS, Das P, Outhred T, Bryant RA, Calhoun V, Mann JJ. Default mode dysfunction underpins suicidal activity in mood disorders. Psychol Med. 2020;50:1214-23.

119. Sobczak AM, Bohaterewicz B, Marek T, Fafrowicz M, Dudek D, Siwek M, et al. Altered functional connectivity differences in salience network as a neuromarker of suicide risk in euthymic bipolar disorder patients. Front Hum Neurosci. 2020;14:585766.

120. Wagner G, Li M, Sacchet MD, Richard-Devantoy S, Turecki G, Bär KJ, et al. Functional network alterations differently associated with suicidal ideas and acts in depressed patients: an indirect support to the transition model. Transl Psychiatry. 2021;11:100.

121. Stange JP, Jenkins LM, Pocius S, Kreutzer K, Bessette KL, DelDonno SR, et al. Using resting-state intrinsic network connectivity to identify suicide risk in mood disorders. Psychol Med. 2020;50:2324-34.

122. Dai Z, Shen X, Tian S, Yan R, Wang H, Wang X, et al. Gradually evaluating of suicidal risk in depression by semi-supervised cluster analysis on resting-state fMRI. Brain Imaging Behav. 2021;15:2149-58.

123. Bohaterewicz B, Sobczak AM, Podolak I, Wójcik B, Mętel D, Chrobak AA, et al. Machine learning-based identification of suicidal risk in patients with schizophrenia using multi-level resting-state fMRI features. Front Neurosci. 2020;14:605697.

124. Li H, Chen Z, Gong Q, Jia Z. Voxel-wise meta-analysis of task-related brain activation abnormalities in major depressive disorder with suicide behavior. Brain Imaging Behav. 2020;14:1298-308.

Epidemiology of Suicide in India: Gaps in Data

Varun S Mehta, Surendra Paliwal, Roshan V Khanande

ABSTRACT

India data in India is mostly derived from the figures released by the National Crime Records Bureau (NCRB) every year. The current chapter discusses latest NCRB data vis a vis figures reported by Million Death Study and Global Burden of Disease study. The gaps in data have been discussed and suggestions for improvement put forward.

Keywords: Suicide epidemiology; Suicide statistics.

■ BACKGROUND

Suicide has always been considered a serious global public health issue. Decreasing the suicide death rate (SDR) by one-third from 2015 to 2030 is one of the UN's sustainable development goals (SDG). India accounts for 18% of the world's population and has 42% of the population aged 15–39 years, so addressing suicides is imperative to make a global difference. In order to plan a successful suicide prevention policy, it is imperative to understand the demographic characteristics of individuals who completed suicide. We have relied upon four sources of data; one is a global initiative (1998–2016),[1] data released by WHO (2019),[2] and Million Death Study (MDS) data (1998–2014) from India,[3] along with reports released by the National Crime Records Bureau (NCRB)[4,5] in this chapter.

■ SUICIDE WORLDWIDE

Across the world, nearly 800,000 people die by suicide every year, more than the population of Bhutan or Maldives.[2] Nearly 80% of suicides occur in low- and middle-income countries. The WHO's Global Health Estimates (GHE) found that >1 in every 100 deaths (1.3%) in 2019 resulted from suicide. The global age-standardized SDR was 9.0 per 100,000 population for 2019. There were regional differences with suicide rates in the African (11.2 per 100,000), European (10.5 per 100,000), and South-East Asia (10.2 per 100,000) regions higher than the global average (9.0 per 100,000). Suicide is the second most common cause of death among young people aged 15–29 years of both sexes globally.[6] However, WHO's GHE relegates it to be the fourth leading cause of death after road injury, tuberculosis, and interpersonal violence. For females and males, suicide was the third and fourth leading cause of death in this age group.

Regarding gender, more males die than females by suicide globally, with the age-standardized SDR being 2.3 times higher in males than in females.[7] Males in high-income countries have the highest rate (16.5 per 100,000) compared to males in other income level groupings. However, females in lower-middle-income countries have the highest SDR (7.1 per 100,000) compared to females in other income level groupings.[2]

■ THE INDIAN DATA

Suicide rates are one of the highest globally and account for 26.6% of global suicide deaths. Using the Global Burden of Disease (GBD) study data, Dandona and colleagues estimated the national age-standardized SDR for 2016 was 17·9 per 100,000 population (2.35% for all deaths), with suicide being the ninth leading cause of death. The accidental deaths and suicides in India (ADSI) 2020 released by the NCRB in 2021 placed the national SDR at 11.3%, accounting for 153,052 deaths across the country, roughly six times the estimated maternal mortality (23,800) for the year 2020.[8] The national SDR for the previous year was 10.4% higher than the global SDR of 9% in 2019. This meant that the country witnessed 25.5% higher suicide rates in 2020 and 15.5% higher suicide rates during 2019 vis-à-vis global SDR 2019. Dwelling more profound into the NCRB report, the SDR for the last 3 years has steadily increased from 10.2% in 2018 to 11.3% in 2020, a 1.1% percentage points increase. The MDS appraises that 1 out of 77 Indians above the age of 15 years is at risk of suicide by the age of 80 years, the risk being high in men (1 in 59) and significantly higher in South India.

Demographic Correlates

Age

Suicide is the foremost cause of death in the age groups of 15–29 years and 15–39 years in the country compared with its second and third rank globally in these age groups, respectively.[1] The GBD study data also found a bimodal pattern with the young age and those 70 years above as the most susceptible unlike most other developed nations. Further, the peak in the younger ages was much more distinct in women than in men. The GHE by the WHO, 2019 also found suicide as the fourth most common cause of death in 15–29 years and 15–19 years. Besides, suicide was the third most common cause of death in girls aged 15–19 years. The ADSI 2020 report informs suicides among children under 18 years rose from 9,613 in 2019 to 11,396 in 2020, an 18.5% increase, the highest spike in the last 5 years. The report also mentions that persons aged 18 years to below 30 years are most vulnerable to suicide and account for 34.4% of total suicide, followed by the 30-below to 45 years age group, that account for 31.4% of total suicide. The rates in the age group 18–30 years also witnessed an 8% increase from the last year, the largest in the past 5 years. The MDS data also reveals that about 40% of male suicides and 56% of female suicides occur at ages 15–29 years.

Gender

The GBD study reveals that age-adjusted SDR was 14·7 and 21.2 for women and men in 2016, 2.1 times and 1.4 times higher than the global average in 2016. The states of Tamil Nadu, Karnataka, West Bengal, Tripura, Andhra Pradesh, and Telangana contributed to these disturbing numbers, along with Kerala and Chhattisgarh for males. Only three countries in the world had higher SDRs than these six states in 2016.[1] Disturbingly, the men-to-women SDR ratio was lower than the global ratio in 2016, which meant that the gap in the suicide rates between men and women in India is smaller than in the rest of the world. The same time, the age-adjusted SDR was 14.7% for men and 11.1% for women of all ages in 2019, according to WHO's GHE. According to the NCRB data, the male:female ratio of suicide victims for 2020, 2019, and 2018 were 70.9:29.1, 70.2:29.8, and 68.5:31.5, respectively. Thus, for every five men who die by suicide, two women die by suicide. However, this might not hold for ages below 18 years with females having a higher suicide rate over the past 6 years. The exact arguments for gender differences are challenging to put in place. However, some of the crucial reasons could be gender role differentiation and discrimination among the younger females and the methods of dealing with stress and conflict, help-seeking behaviors, domestic violence, early marriage, and lack of autonomy among married females. The excess male suicide rates are valid for every country, including China.

Marital Status

The ADSI 2020 reported that marriage related issues accounted for 5% of total suicide, including causes such as troubled marriages, divorce, dowry, and extramarital affairs. Throughout the NCRB data over the past 10 years (2011–2020), >65% of suicide victims were married. Married women account for the highest proportion of suicide deaths among women in the country.[9] In their analysis of gender differentials from the NCRB data over 10 years from 2001, Dandona and her colleagues identified "marriage related reasons" accounted for 8% of women's suicides and only 0.8% of men's suicide. Thus, marriage can no longer be considered a vital protective factor against suicide for women. The circumstances of arranged and early marriage, young motherhood, low social status, domestic violence, and economic dependence are the likely contributory factors.

Occupation

States with lower rates of male unemployment had a lower risk of suicide. The MDS data confirm these observations. These findings are consistent with the rest of the world, where increasing modernization is associated with higher suicide rates. Homemakers (housewives) accounted for approximately 15% of total suicide victims in 2020 and 2019. Students and unemployed accounted for 8.2% and 10.2% of suicides in 2020, higher than in 2019.

Literacy

States with the lowest literacy levels were associated with a lower risk of suicide in both genders.[9] ADSI 2020 revealed that 23.4% of suicide victims had educational qualifications up to matriculation, and 12.6% were illiterates, mainly similar to the reports for the previous 2 years. Although a high prevalence of suicide in a person with qualifications up to matriculation can be multi-factorial, it has been established that poor education qualification exposes an individual to a multitude of socio-economic adversity, which might increase the risk of attempting suicide.

Geographical Location

Like the global scenario, more economically developed states had almost four times higher age-standardized suicide rates for males and almost three times higher suicide rates for females than less economically developed states.[9] Females had higher agricultural employment levels for the states with high-suicide rates. Among Indian states, Maharashtra accounted for maximum suicide (>13% or more of total suicide) consecutively for the last 4 years (2017–2020).[5] Tamil Nadu, West Bengal, Madhya Pradesh, and Karnataka accounted for 50.1% of total suicide in 2020 and 49.5% of the total suicide in 2019. Despite being the most populous state, Uttar Pradesh reported 3.1% of the total suicides in 2020. In contrast, Delhi, the most populous Union Territory (UT), reported maximum suicide among all UTs in 2020. The levels of urbanization, literacy rate, and difference in literacy attainment between both genders could account for the regional variations.

Caste and Religion

States with lower proportions of the population with Hindu religion were associated with a lower risk of suicide.[9] However, analyzing the data obtained from the NCRB for the years 2014–2015, the highest suicide rates were observed among Christians (17.6 per 100,000), and the lowest rates were observed among Sikhs and Muslims, but the pattern was not uniform throughout the states. Similarly, suicide rates were lower among SC, ST, and OBC populations compared to the general population, not following a specific pattern across the states.[10] Given that elevated suicide rates have been documented among minority/underprivileged populations in other countries, these findings are surprising. However, there might not be much scientific evidence to highlight their issues; ample first-person accounts suggest the presence of societal discrimination and oppression based on caste triggering suicides.

Socioeconomic Correlates

The ADSI 2020 revealed that 63.3% of suicide victims had an annual income of <1 lakh, while 32.2% of suicide victims had an income of 1 lakh to <5 lakh. Likewise, in 2019 and 2018, 66.2% of suicide victims had an income of <1 lakh. Further, bankruptcy and indebtedness accounted for 3.4% of the total suicides. Unemployment and poverty resulted in 2.3% and 1.2% of the total suicides. Social, interpersonal, and cultural conflicts, substance abuse, lack of employment, economic adversity, and poor health have always been the fundamental reasons for suicide in India, irrespective of gender.[11]

Sociocultural Correlates

Prevailing stigma and cultural sanctions concerning suicide moderate the risk of suicide. From the ancient time of "sati tradition" in which widowed women had to end their life on the same pyre as their husbands to the still prevalent "santhara" (a practice of voluntarily starving to death in the Jain religion), there has been some implicit social acceptance for suicide in Indian culture. Nevertheless, there is a stigma attached to suicide in India. Culture might influence modes and means of suicide, which explains hanging in males and self-immolation in females as a common method of suicide in India. Stark regional variation in suicide rates across the country might also reflect the impact of culture in the community. Likewise, culture has also been implicated in mass and cluster suicide.

Beyond the economic and cultural correlates, family and interpersonal problems are among the leading causes of suicide in India. ADSI 2020 revealed that family problems accounted for 33.6% of total suicides, and love affairs contributed to 4.4% of suicides.

Suicide and Psychiatric Illness

There were 13,796 suicides due to mental illness in the ADSI 2020, increasing over 4 years. 7.5–9% of the suicide deaths are attributed to mental illness, and 5–6% of suicides are attributed to "alcohol addiction and drug abuse." This observation warrants attention as the contribution of mental illness to suicide is vastly low compared to the literature from western countries. Vijayakumar and Rajkumar (1999) reported that mood disorders accounted for nearly 25% of suicide deaths; the majority of the individuals attempted suicide in their first episode of depression. Among them, 60% of the suicides during an episode of depression had only reported mild to moderate symptoms. Moreover, only 10% of the suicides due to mental illness had sought medical consultation.[12] Alcohol dependence and abuse were reported for nearly 35% of the suicides. Thus, heavy alcohol use contributes to suicide, second to depression. It is also an essential factor in adolescent suicides, as the likelihood of considering suicide increases by two times under the effect of alcohol.[13] Among the suicide attempters admitted to the hospital, one in eight attempts was found to be under the influence of alcohol.[14] Schizophrenia accounts for 8% of the suicide in mental illness.[15]

Suicide and Physical Illness

The ADSI 2020 report mentions that 13,827 individuals died by suicide because of illnesses similar to the previous 3 years. The causes include AIDS/STD, cancer, paralysis, and other prolonged illnesses. The "other prolonged illness" category has the highest percentage of suicides. However, mental illness as a cause of death in the physically ill cannot be inferred from the available information. Srivastava et al. (2004)[16] cite chronic pain in the pelvic and abdominal region as one of the most familiar reasons for suicidal attempts in the physically ill. About one-fifth of suicide attempters had a physical illness. The other reasons were dysmenorrhoea, peptic ulcer disease, hypertension, bronchial asthma, and arthritis.

Methods of Suicide in India

There is a distinct difference in the modes opted for suicide in India than in the western world—especially in the US. The easy availability of firearms makes gunshot suicide (nearly 50%) the most commonly opted mode for suicide in the US, whereas hanging and self-poisoning predominate India's picture. The ADSI 2020 puts 57.8% of suicides by hanging, 25% by consuming poison (often ingestion of organophosphate pesticides), 5.2% by drowning, and 3% by self-immolation. These trends have been the same over the past decade. Thus, hanging and poisoning together account for 75% of deaths by suicide. In addition, there are gender-based differences, with self-immolation predominating among females, which is consistent with sex differences reported internationally. The likely reasons are the easy availability and accessibility of kerosene at home and the cultural sanction of fire as a purifier. Whereas in developed countries, women overdose with over-the-counter medications with low lethality; women in India who overdose with pesticides often die due to high lethality even if the intent is low.

■ SPECIAL POPULATION

Farmer Suicide

Agrarian suicide is preferred over farmer suicide as the former represents farmers and agricultural laborers. However, 83% of suicides occur in only 8 out of 17 states which produce >98% of domestic agricultural products in India, which are the central states (Gujarat, Maharashtra, Rajasthan, Madhya Pradesh, and Chhattisgarh) and southern states (Andhra Pradesh, Karnataka, Kerala, and Tamil Nadu).[17] The ADSI 2020 reports 10,677 suicides in the agriculture sector, accounting for 7% of the total suicides. Even though the percentage share has remained just over 7% in the past 3 years, an educated guess could mean that the numbers exceed three to four times the available data. The reasons for agrarian suicides are multifactorial. Slow output growth and low demand, noninstitutional credit sources, addiction, and relationship issues are some of the critical reasons.[18]

Armed Forces

The Central Armed Police Forces (CAPFs) has 9 lakh employees. 2019 witnessed 36 deaths due to suicide, higher than the previous year. For both the years, >35% of the suicides had "lingering family problems," and only a small number of victims reported "service-related problems." The ADSI 2020 report does not mention the armed forces.

In the defense forces, the number of suicide is more than CAPFs. 95 personnel died by suicide in 2019, with similar statistics over the past 3 years. The most common method was using a service firearm. The army accounts for most suicide deaths every year. Substance abuse, mental illness, and family problems are reasons behind suicides, contrary to the popular opinion that the stress and strain of serving at the frontier lead to suicide.[19]

Family Suicide

Taking note of the increasing number of family suicides, the Government of India started collecting related data since 2009. As a result, the ADSI 2020 mentions 272 such incidents, the maximum over the past 3 years. For most of the years, Andhra Pradesh and Tamil Nadu have reported the most family/mass suicides. Although reasons might be innumerable for such suicides, extreme poverty and debts, intractable ailments of family members, and superstitious beliefs are commonly reported.[20]

Suicides in the Medical Profession

Doctors have an 80% lower risk of suicide than other occupations, such as farmers but a higher risk than teachers. Nevertheless, suicide among physicians, trainee doctors, and residents has increased. Chahal et al. (2021)[21] reported that between 2010 and 2019, 358 suicides took place among physicians (128), medical students (125), and residents (105) by collating the information from published news and the online media articles. Further, 7 out of 10 died by suicide before 30, females being much younger than males. Among specialities, anesthesiology (22.4%) reported the highest rate of suicide after obstetrics-gynecology (16.0%). Hanging was the most preferred method. Academic stress and marital discord, followed by mental illness, were common reasons.

QUALITY OF DATA AND THE GAPS

Comparing both the datasets, the estimated number of suicide deaths reported by the NCRB was 37% lower per year than the rates reported by the GBD Study from 2005 to 2015, more so among the oldest and youngest age groups.[22] The difference results from underreporting female suicides among both age groups, amounting to 50% per year. Similarly, the numbers related to suicides from the MDS conducted from 1998 to 2014 also reveal that the NCRB numbers underestimated suicides among men by 25% and by 36% among women.[23]

The underreporting of suicides in the NCRB is well documented. The primary source of surveillance for suicides in India is the NCRB which remains the most comprehensive longitudinal source of suicides available at the state level. However, it is a passive surveillance system as the onus is on the reporting from the community, which can be unreliable. The police merely put together the first information reports (FIRs) provided to the NCRB. Thereby, the police do not have the primary responsibility to generate the data. The prevailing social stigma (consequences such as difficulty in getting married, ostracization of the family) attached to suicidal deaths and the criminalization of attempted suicide until recently are the likely reasons for the nonreporting of suicides. Misclassification of suicide as homicide and miscoding of information are other vital faultlines. For example, it is easy to misclassify suicide by pesticide poisoning as accidental death, just like drowning. However, it might be difficult to label hanging as accidental, due to which it might appear to be the most preferred method of suicide. Similarly, a farmer who suicides a day after beating his wife brutally in an intoxicated state is considered suicide due to a "marital dispute."

In addition, the division of categories for some of the demographic correlates is equally worrisome. For example, the "self-employed category" forms the largest collective group, including professionals, businesses, farms/agriculture, etc., making the singular analysis by occupation problematic. A very significant limitation is attributing a single cause to every suicide. For example, the ADSI 2020 mentions family problems as the most significant contributor (35%) of suicides under 18. Further, "marriage-related problems" and "love affairs" are separate categories. The reasoning behind the allocation of each category is fuzzy, and so are the definitions to represent these categories.

Furthermore, mentioning unknown/other reasons as the primary cause of suicide hides any reasonable understanding of the situation. Finally, an overdose of alcohol as a means of suicide does not seem plausible, further highlighting the need to improve data quality. Finally, we need to understand that suicides are multifactorial. Thus, for a young individual who faces family problems and subsequently dies by suicide after an examination failure, the decision to allot him the "right cause" is still unsettled.

The NCRB data representation might also selectively blind us to some disturbing events leading to suicide. For example, women exposed to violence in India are three to seven times more likely to attempt suicide. Similarly, WHO estimates that 64% of Indian women experience physical violence experience suicidal ideation. However, the ADSI reports fail to reflect any of these figures as "physical abuse" is included in a broad category of "personal/social" reasons for suicide.[24] Furthermore, the "Principal Offense Rule" could hide many domestic violence cases as each criminal incident is recorded as one crime. Thus, an incident involving dowry death and cruelty will be reported only as dowry death as it warrants the maximum punishment, thereby underreporting the number of cruelty cases by husbands or relatives.

There might also be some merit to doubt "hanging" as the most preferred method of suicide. However, the lack of representation of the vulnerable and marginalized population within the NCRB statistics is equally disturbing. For example, the NCRB started recording information on caste and religion of suicides for the first time in 2014 and 2015 but has not released the data in any of its reports to date.

The state-level data represented under the NCRB is very heterogenous and presented in tabulated formats making any meaningful interpretations difficult. For example, the NCRB does not report if suicides were in rural or urban areas, only in which state they occurred. It is amply clear that the NCRB does not do a detailed analysis of the data.

The GBD estimates, too, are not without their limitations. There is a possibility that specific causes of death might have been overestimated due to the reassignment of partially specified causes of death to specific causes of death.[25] Further, the lower SDRs in some states (e.g., Sikkim, Union Territories including Delhi) in the GBD estimates compared with the NCRB data also highlights possible underreporting. The data collection method is the significant difference between the GBD Study and the NCRB reports. The GBD Study primarily uses the Sample Registration System (SRS) data based on verbal autopsies and community surveillance programs. We also need to be acutely aware that the country suffers from poor death registration coverage and inadequate medical certification of the cause of death.[26]

ADDRESSING THE GAPS IN THE DATA

Though the reliability of suicide death statistics has been questioned in lower and higher-income countries, we need to focus on improving the quality of routinely collected and publicly available data. Efforts can be made to standardize data collection forms, clear guidelines to capture a specific type of data (e.g., reasons for suicide) to ensure comparability over time and area, and increased budgetary allocation and training of relevant staff. In addition, it would have been prudent for NCRB to release the anonymized individual data just like the Registrar General of India releases the raw census data. Overall, the quality and coverage of the death registration and assignment

systems must improve to have accurate mortality estimates. Finally, there is an urgent need to make the data available in a timely and periodic manner for the public good.

The vulnerable population deserve special attention. India is home to some of the highest female SDRs globally. The National Programs for elderly and adolescent health need to actively monitor the mental health issues and the reasons behind suicide. Similarly, the implementation of the Protection of Women from Domestic Violence Act can be tapped into the look into its effects on suicide prevention among young married women. Similarly, the decriminalization of suicide and adherence to media reporting guidelines could reduce the stigma and underreporting of suicides.

■ CONCLUSION

If we need to know that any suicide prevention program works, we need to have reliable data but evaluating the reliability of suicide statistics is an arduous task. The reviewed studies in this chapter differ in the data collection methods and administrative processes involved and the primary source of data gathering (e.g., verbal autopsies vs. registry records). Strengthening the quality of vital registration systems and mortality statistics is urgently needed. If the sample registration systems in India and China are considered sufficiently representative to provide information on their whole populations, then information on mortality is available for around 72% of the world's population.[27]

Despite the underreporting and the limitations of the available studies, the available information offers several insights into the nature and magnitude of the problem in India. Suicide disproportionately affects young women and is the leading cause of death. However, we do not know the many right reasons, so we urgently need to invest in a new credible and robust data monitoring system. Furthermore, the system should be clubbed with the registration system for accidents as there is a very high possibility that attempted suicides are misclassified as accidents. Also, the cause of death should not be determined by a police constable but by a psychological autopsy report. Meanwhile, we also need to work with the NCRB to improve its quality of data gathering, data representation, and data dissemination.

It is a well-established fact that a previous suicide attempt is the best predictor of future suicide. Nevertheless, we do not have any agency that collects data on suicide attempts. Therefore, the best guestimate would be 4–20 times the number of reported suicides. Going by the ADSI 2020, it would translate from 612,208 to 30,061,040 (roughly 30 million) attempted suicides. Despite these disturbing numbers, India is yet to develop a systematic response to suicide, and a comprehensive national suicide prevention strategy is urgently needed. The states of Kerala and Gujarat have a suicide prevention policy, and Chhattisgarh is the only state with a suicide prevention strategy but the ground level implementation has not been translated from paper.

It is a myth that suicide in India is purely due to mental health problems. Suicide is a multifactorial multidimensional phenomenon with complex interactions across the globe. An attempt to understand the interaction of sociodemographic and sociocultural determinants that drive suicide is equally paramount to gaining a holistic understanding, and so is getting the commitment of various stakeholders to address these drivers, more so in India.

Suicide is a public health crisis and should be considered a top health priority to save the females and the young generation from dying. The National Mental Health Policy (NMHP), 2014 mentions suicide prevention as one of the critical areas of action and rightly so for so many reasons.

■ REFERENCES

1. Dandona R, Kumar GA, Dhaliwal RS, Naghavi M, Vos T, Shukla DK, et al. Gender differentials and state variations in suicide deaths in India: the Global Burden of Disease Study 1990–2016. The Lancet Public Health. 2018;3(10):e478-89.
2. WHO. (2020). Global Health Estimates 2019: deaths by cause, age, sex, by country and by region, 2000–2019. [online] Available from: https://www.who.int/data/global-health-estimates [Last accessed October, 2022]
3. Patel V, Ramasundarahettige C, Vijayakumar L, Thakur JS, Gajalakshmi V, Gururaj G, et al. Suicide mortality in India: a nationally representative survey. The Lancet. 2012;23; 379(9834):2343-51.
4. National Crime Record Bureau. Accidental deaths and suicide in India. New Delhi: Government of India; 2019.
5. National Crime Record Bureau. Accidental deaths and suicide in India. New Delhi: Government of India; 2020.
6. World Health Organization. (2018b). Suicide data. [online] Available from: https://www. who.int/mental_health/prevention/suicide/ suicideprevent/en/ [Last accessed October, 2022].
7. Naghavi M. Global, regional, and national burden of suicide mortality 1990 to 2016: systematic analysis for the Global Burden of Disease Study 2016. BMJ. 2019;364:l94.
8. Meh C, Sharma A, Ram U, Fadel S, Correa N, Snelgrove JW, et al. Trends in maternal mortality in India over two decades in nationally representative surveys. BJOG: Int J Obstet Gynaecol. 2022;129(4):550-61.
9. Arya V, Page A, River J, Armstrong G, Mayer P. Trends and socio-economic determinants

of suicide in India: 2001–2013. Soc Psychiatry Psychiatr Epidemiol. 2018;53:269-8.

10. Arya V, Page A, Dandona R, Vijayakumar L, Mayer P, Armstrong G. The Geographic Heterogeneity of Suicide Rates in India by Religion, Caste, Tribe, and Other Backward Classes. Crisis: J Crisis Intervent Suicide Prevent. 2019;40:370-4.

11. Dandona R, Bertozzi-Villa A, Kumar GA, Dandona L. Lessons from a decade of suicide surveillance in India: who, why and how? Int J Epidemiol. 2017;46:983-93.

12. Vijayakumar L, Rajkumar S. Are risk factors for suicide universal? A case-control study in India. Acta Psychiatr Scand. 1999;99:407-11.

13. Jaisoorya TS, Beena KV, Beena M, Ellangovan K, Jose DC, Thennarasu K, et al. Prevalence and correlates of alcohol use among adolescents attending school in Kerala, India. Drug alcohol rev. 2016;35:523-9.

14. Ebenezer JA, Joge V. Suicide in Rural Central India: Profile of Attempters of Deliberate Self-harm Presenting to Padhar Hospital in Madhya Pradesh. Indian J Psychol Med. 2016;38:567-70.

15. Srinivasan TN, Thara R. Schizophrenia patients who kill themselves. In: Vijayakumar L (Ed). Suicide prevention. Hyderabad, India: Orient Longman; 2003. pp. 163-8.

16. Srivastava MK, Sahoo RN, Ghotekar LH, Dutta S, Danabalan M, Dutta TK, et al. Risk Factors Associated with Attempted Suicide: A Case Control Study. Indian J Psychiatry. 2004;46:33-8.

17. Nair SR. Agrarian suicides in India: Myth and Reality. Dev Policy Rev. 2021;39:3-21.

18. Das A. Farmers' suicide and agrarian crisis: Social policy and public mental health. Indian J Psychiatry. 2017;59:398-9.

19. Sinha A, Gupta S, Ray M, Kumar S, Gupta AK. Lessons learned from psychological autopsies in armed forces. Indian J Psychol Med. 2021;43:150-3.

20. Ponnudurai R. Suicide in India—changing trends and challenges ahead. Indian J Psychiatry. 2015;57:348-54.

21. Chahal S, Nadda A, Govil N, Gupta N, Nadda D, Goel K, et al. Suicide deaths among medical students, residents and physicians in India spanning a decade (2010–2019): an exploratory study using on line news portals and Google database. Int J Soc Psychiatry. 2021;1-11.

22. Arya V, Page A, Armstrong G, Kumar GA, Dandona R. Estimating patterns in the under-reporting of suicide deaths in India: comparison of administrative data and Global Burden of Disease Study estimates, 2005–2015. J Epidemiol Community Health. 2020:jech-2020-215260.

23. Tripathi A, Nadkarni A, Pathare S. Understanding Suicide. Who is dying of suicide (and Why)? In: Tripathi A, Nadkarni A, Pathare S (Eds). Life interrupted: Understanding India's Suicide Crisis,1st edition. India: Simon and Schuster; 2022. pp. 5-23.

24. Pathare S. Women and Suicide. In: Tripathi A, Nadkarni A, Pathare S (Eds). Life interrupted: Understanding India's Suicide Crisis, 1st edition. India: Simon and Schuster; 2022. pp. 52-62.

25. Bhalla K, Harrison JE. GBD-2010 overestimates deaths from road injuries in OECD countries: new methods perform poorly. Int J Epidemiol. 2015;44:1648-56.

26. Mikkelsen L, Phillips DE, Abou Zahr C, Setel PW, De Savigny D, Lozano R, et al. A global assessment of civil registration and vital statistics systems: monitoring data quality and progress. The Lancet. 2015;386(10001):1395-406.

27. Tøllefsen IM, Hem E, Øivind E. The reliability of suicide statistics: a systematic review. BMC Psychiatry. 2012;12:9.

Nonsuicidal Self-injury: Indian Perspective

Naresh Nebhinani, Swati Choudhary, Tanu Gupta

ABSTRACT

Nonsuicidal self-injury (NSSI) refers to the multitude of behaviors involving self-inflicted destruction of body tissues without suicidal intent. The research data suggests that a significant number of adolescents are either engaging or likely to engage in these behaviors, and this has been labeled as a "hidden pandemic" by a few of the researchers. There is growing evidence to suggest the increased risk of suicidal attempts in this population. The usual age of onset is early adolescence, and cutting is one of the most common NSSI behavior. Associated psychiatric disorders may be present, most commonly borderline personality disorders, depression, and anxiety disorders. Assessment requires a good therapeutic relationship and empathetic listening. Assessment scales can be used to determine the details regarding methods, frequency, and functions of NSSI; however, imminent risk of another NSSI or suicidal attempt must be evaluated first to ensure the safety of the individual. Considering the onset in adolescence, screening in schools and colleges might help in early intervention and identifying the individuals without any other apparent dysfunction. The first line of management includes psychological interventions such as cognitive behavioral therapy and dialectical behavior therapy. Brief motivational interviewing (MI) can help in the engagement with treatment and willingness to change. No conclusive evidence is available regarding pharmacological agents, except for individuals with comorbid psychiatric disorders.

Keywords: India; NSSI; Self-injury; Self-harm; Suicide.

■ INTRODUCTION

Nonsuicidal self-injury (NSSI) is an inexplicable and challenging to treat phenomenon that has increased evidently in the last few years. The underlying issues related to understanding the motivation and differentiating it from the suicide attempt pose greater challenges to the treating psychiatrists. NSSI works as a risk factor for suicide attempts later in life, and hence, it becomes pertinent to intervene for preventing the progression toward suicidal ideation or attempts. It also worsens the quality of life,

and many cases never even seek professional help.[1] Association of other mental disorders with NSSI is commonly seen, which further worsens the outcome. With limited mental health resources in our country, chances of such cases getting overlooked or inadequately treated are quite high. As per World Health Organization (WHO), 77% of the world suicides occur in middle- or low-income countries, which warrant the attention toward any self-injurious behavior.[2]

Nonsuicidal self-injury is defined as intentional destruction of one's body tissue without suicidal intent.[3] So far, it is not a diagnostic category in nosological system; however, it is included in Diagnostic and Statistical Manual of Mental Disorders, Fifth Edition (DSM-5) under the section of "Conditions for Further Study", which identifies NSSI as: *"intentional self-inflicted damage to the surface of his/her body, with the expectation that the injury will lead to only minor/moderate harm and there is no suicidal intent, on 5 or more days in past 1 year."*[4] Various terms have been used to describe and define self-injury in the available literature. Terms such as *deliberate self-harm* (DSH) and *parasuicide* have been used synonymously for both self-injury and NSSI. In available Indian literature, the term DSH has been used to describe two kinds of behavior, i.e., nonfatal suicidal behavior or suicide attempts[5,6] and NSSI-like behavior.[7]

The term, parasuicide, also has been used to describe two forms of behaviors: nonfatal, self-inflicted direct injury or self-poisoning.[8] However, WHO uses two terms to describe the nonsuicidal behaviors, i.e., NSSI and self-mutilation, which encompass all the behaviors which can be considered under NSSI.[9]

There has been an ever-ending debate over the concept of intent, whether it can be assessed reliably in individuals presenting with self-injurious behavior. The argument put forward regarding intent is that it is a dynamic construct, and most adolescents and young adults have an ambivalent suicidal intent. It is practically difficult to predict the change over intent from nonsuicidal to suicidal. The fact that most of the completed suicides were not receiving any mental healthcare highlights this fact further. So, it is suggested to evaluate any self-injurious behavior with the utmost care, irrespective of the intent. Because of the variable definition usage and difficulty in assessing various constructs of NSSI, the research in this area has got affected hugely.

■ EPIDEMIOLOGY

Due to different definitions, methodological issues, and heterogeneous study samples, variable prevalence rates are reported for NSSI as most of cross-sectional studies are conducted in college students, youth, or young adults.

On comparing profile of Indian young adults with Belgium data, it was found that age of onset of NSSI was higher in Indian sample. Self-bruising was more common in Indian sample, while cutting and scratching were more common in Belgian sample. Additionally, intrapersonal factors and identity confusion were more common in Belgian sample.[10]

A cross-sectional community survey conducted in India among 470 students from eight different colleges showed NSSI prevalence of 31% in the past year. Among these, 19.8% reported moderate/severe forms of NSSI.[11] In another cross-sectional survey, done among students, the rate of NSSI is reported to be 33.8%, with minor self-injury in 19.4% and moderate/severe forms in 14.6%.[12] The main method of self-harm was cutting in youth, which is similar to the findings from earlier research.[13]

Nevertheless, the authors found suicidal intent in 6.8% of these participants, which excludes the diagnosis of NSSI. Due to the methodological issues, overlapping terminologies and difficulties in interpreting intent, it has been challenging to report a reliable prevalence rate. In a review consisting of 38 Indian studies, only one study was stringently following the globally accepted definition for NSSI, where the lifetime prevalence is reported to be 31%.[14] These rates are higher than the global NSSI prevalence of 17.2% among adolescents, 13.4% among young adults, and 5.5% among adults, but the systematic review and meta-analysis found significant heterogeneity in prevalence estimates due to methodological factors.[15]

The average age of onset of NSSI is usually 15.9 years, which is in concurrence with the studies from other parts of the world.[16] For engaging in self-injury, the common reasons were reported as for feeling relaxed, controlling the situation, for stopping the bad feelings, and for punishing the self. Most individuals indulging in NSSI endorsed multiple methods; under the mild category, self-hitting was common, while under the moderate/severe category, majority cutting behaviors were seen. There were no significant gender differences in NSSI rates, whereas studies from the past have reported a higher prevalence in females. However, in current times, gender differences from major studies on NSSI are inconclusive.[11,15]

ETIOLOGICAL MODELS

Various factors, including social, psychological, and biological factors, play an imperative role in initiating and maintaining NSSI behaviors.

Biological Factors

Nonsuicidal self-injury patients report difficulties in the stress and emotion processing system, and emotional dysregulation has been considered a chief clinical feature in these patients.[17] Various biological explanations have been put forward to explain NSSI behaviors, such as general hyperactivity in amygdala, anterior cingulate cortex (ACC) and hippocampus regions of the brain,[18] reduction in volume in the ACC, dorsolateral prefrontal cortex (DLPFC), orbitofrontal cortex (OFC) and insula,[19-21] reduced control of prefrontal

areas over the limbic system, also known as the "frontolimbic disconnectivity model", was postulated as a possible underlying cause for NSSI.[22,23] Disturbance in emotional processing can be explained by limbic hyperreactivity and diminished recruitment of frontal brain regions.

Another theory that has been studied is that of "altered pain sensitivity", and it has been found that these individuals might benefit from the pain.[24,25] One of the key findings from studies was low physiological arousal before the painful stimuli and an increased one after the painful stimuli. It has also been argued that the simultaneous autonomic arousal and increase in cortisol levels may help in reducing negative affect and in counteracting the dissociative states, which support the postulated antisuicide function of NSSI by providing an outlet for difficult emotions.[24] There is an alteration in the stress response system in the individuals with NSSI, which reveals a higher cortisol awakening response in them when compared with healthy individuals and a reduced cortisol response with an in-vitro stressor.[26,27]

Psychological Factors

Psychological models are mainly discussed using the four functions of NSSI behavior via intrapersonal or interpersonal reinforcement.[28] It includes automatic positive and negative reinforcement where an individual indulging in NSSI gets helped in counteracting the dissociative state or occurrence of increased desired thoughts or feelings (intrapersonal positive reinforcement) and use self-injury as an escape from the negative affect such as anxiety, anger etc. (intrapersonal negative reinforcement). Similar reinforcements occur in social situations too, such as to gain attention as a tool for seeking help (social or interpersonal positive reinforcement) and avoid any kind of punishment (social or interpersonal negative reinforcement). Most agreed-upon functions of NSSI are to regulate the negative effect by avoiding it or by expressing the psychological distress.[29,30] **Flowchart 1** explains the self-injurious behavior using the experiential avoidance model.[29]

Social Factors

A wide range of adverse events and experiences such as physical and sexual abuse, family victimization and violence, emotional neglect, and bullying have been seen to be associated with NSSI. One of the strongest risk factors for the transition of suicidal ideation to attempt is experiencing/ witnessing self-harm by the near and dear ones; hence, this factor might also play a role in the manifestation of NSSI.[31]

As per one of the theoretical models (as shown in **Flowchart 2**), repetitive self-injury serves the function of regulating one's emotional experiences as well as social environment. Several intra- and interpersonal factors increase the risk of self-injury. Then, there are some factors specific to the risk of self-injury, which leads to engaging in such behaviors.[32]

LINK BETWEEN NSSI AND SUICIDAL BEHAVIOR

The NSSI is considered to be a gateway to suicide by many theorists. Compared to

Flowchart 1: Experiential avoidance model explaining the self-injurious behavior.

(NSSI: nonsuicidal self-injury)

Flowchart 2: Integrated model of the development and maintenance of self injury.[32]

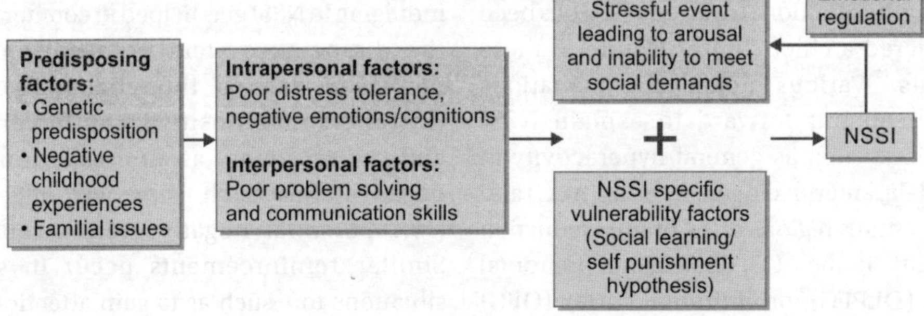

(NSSI: nonsuicidal self-injury)

subjects without history of NSSI, the subjects with history of NSSI are reported to have six times greater risk for suicidal plan, seven times greater risk for suicidal gestures, and nine times greater risk for suicidal attempts.[33] In other study after controlling for the presence of mental disorders, NSSI was associated with 2.8 times more risk of suicidal ideations, 3 times more risk of suicidal plan, and 5.5 times higher risk of a suicide attempt. Also, NSSI was associated with 1.7–2.1 times increased risk of transitioning from suicidal ideations to a plan and from plan to an attempt.[34]

The NSSI and suicidal behaviors lie on a continuum of self-harm behaviors, however, differ from each other in few aspects. In clinical practice, NSSI is seen more commonly, and it becomes pertinent to intervene so that to avoid the progression of this behavior towards lethal suicide attempts. As per the concept of NSSI, the individual does not intend to kill himself/herself and usually engages in behaviors such as cutting, burning which does not require medical attention on every occasion, but in due course, might enable an individual to attempt lethal methods. This continuum can be understood by Joiner's theory of suicide, where one of the factors leading to lethal attempts is the capability for suicide.[35] In general, humans fear from pain and suffering and try to avoid it as much as possible. But with repetitive self-injurious behaviors, even the non-significant ones, there is a possibility of acquiring the ability to overcome this fear, making them prone to try lethal methods, as depicted in **Figure 1**. NSSI behaviors are usually associated with some kind of personal or interpersonal distress, which also increases the risk of having suicidal ideations. Therefore, the individuals with NSSI are at greater risk for having suicidal ideations and acting on them with the acquired capability to indulge in painful and lethal methods. This makes the evaluation and intervention in such cases crucial.

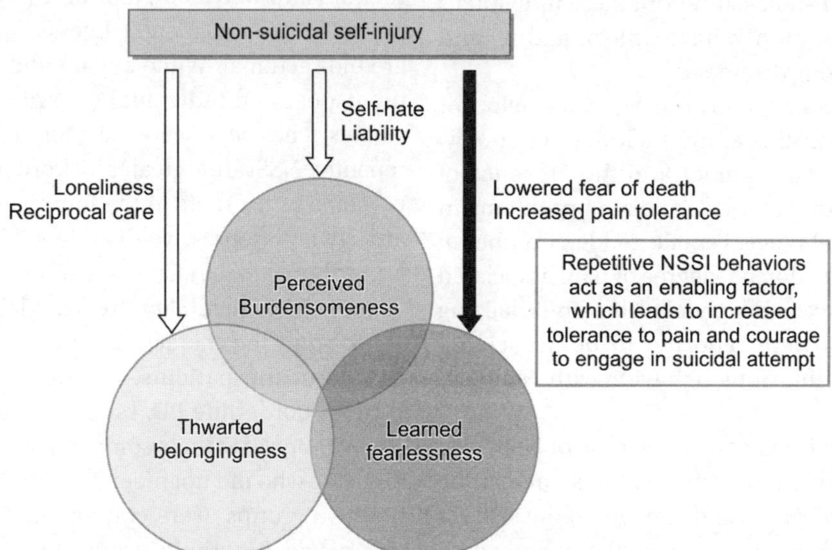

Fig. 1: Link between NSSI and suicide attempt, based on the interpersonal theory of suicidal behavior.[14,36]
(NSSI: nonsuicidal self-injury)

RISK FACTORS AND PREDICTORS OF NSSI

The complex interplay between the NSSI behaviors and suicide attempts has been studied in few studies for India. As per available western data, predictors of suicide attempt include severe forms of self-injury,[16,37-39] different way of self-injury,[40] and depressed individuals.[41] A longitudinal study was done among Chinese adolescents,[42] in which authors found an association between the presence of depressive symptoms and the occurrence of self-injurious behaviors in a 2-year follow-up study. Other risk factors, which make an individual vulnerable to suicidal behaviors, are self-injury performed when alone drug use, duration of NSSI, multiple methods of self-injury, and absence of injury-related physical pain.[15,43]

In Indian studies,[12] higher suicidal intent was associated with a higher number of self-injury methods and the use of moderate-to-severe methods, such as cutting/carving skin, self-tattooing, and scraping skin. As per youth and adult self-report, these individuals more commonly have internalizing and externalizing disorders.

Predictors for any self-injurious behavior reported in this study included age below 18 years, male gender and the presence of internalizing and externalizing problems in the clinical range. Female gender, number of methods endorsed, degree of pain associated with the act, and higher levels of internalizing problems were reported to be associated with self-injurious behavior with "suicidal intent."[12]

Protective factors in the case of NSSI also hold prime importance as the same can be used to safeguard and strengthen the skills of these individuals. It is seen that people with high self-esteem are less likely to indulge in NSSI behaviors, and similarly targeted interventions to enhance self-esteem can be used.[44] In a study done on college students, factors related to life satisfaction and its meaning and spirituality/religiosity, such as support, hope, and direction in life, were acting as a protective factor from self-injuring.[45] NSSI behaviors are seen less in individuals who experience lesser negative emotions and often know how to handle these emotions.[46] Family and social supports also have been studied in relation to suicidal behavior; however, the data regarding NSSI remains inconclusive. Studies from India have not focused on the protective factors against NSSI and hence, these remain an area for future research.

COMORBIDITY WITH OTHER DISORDERS

In clinical practice, NSSI may often serve as a proxy marker of underlying mental health disorders; therefore, identifying these cases might hasten the treatment process. However, there is a dearth of research about the relationship between NSSI and psychiatric patients. NSSI and mental illness associations are bidirectional. While any mental disorder predisposes an individual towards NSSI, in studies, it has been seen that adolescents with repetitive NSSI are at greatest risk of developing psychiatric disorders in the future, especially anxiety and depressive disorders.[47] This can be attributed to the shared environmental risk factors and vulnerability stress model.

To study the characteristics of NSSI, three groups of the patients, classified as NSSI without borderline PD, borderline PD (with and without NSSI), or a comparison condition for those who did not meet the criteria for the first two groups, were compared. The NSSI group had functional impairment similar to that of the BPD group, but most of the patients from the NSSI group did not exhibit subthreshold BPD or not otherwise specified personality disorder symptoms. This study concluded that the NSSI disorder group has high depressive symptoms, anxiety, suicidality, and had lower functionality when compared to individuals with mood/anxiety disorders. This finding also supports the need for a separate diagnostic entity for NSSI.[48]

Mood disorders, especially a recurrent major depressive disorder, and personality disorders, particularly the borderline syndrome, are closely reported with NSSI. Self-injury is also frequently seen in anxiety and substance use disorders. Externalizing disorders in the adolescent age group are also reported with NSSI.[49]

About half of the patients presenting with self-harm behavior at emergency department of tertiary care centers are found to have psychiatric disorders, more commonly depression and substance use disorders.[50,51]

■ ASSESSMENT

Identifying and assessing the patients indulging in NSSI are of primary importance. A respectful curiosity along with a nonjudgmental and empathetic stance is required on behalf of the treating physician. It can be done verbally or with a written form completed by the patient or healthcare professional. Age-appropriate questioning must be done like direct approach can be used with young adults while indirect questioning is preferred in younger age groups. For example, rather than asking a direct question such as "Do you intentionally hurt yourself?", questions such as "I've had some knowledge that some people hurt themselves by biting or cutting whenever they feel stressed. Has this ever happened to someone you know or may be to you?" can be asked to the younger individuals. The crucial thing is respect and sensitivity **(Box 1)**.

> **BOX 1:** Assessment of nonsuicidal self-injurious (NSSI) behaviors.
>
> *Basic assessment of NSSI should include:*
> - General physical examination should be done and immediate medical/surgical (dressing, suturing, etc.) treatment should be given
> - Immediate risk of self-harm should be assessed, and supervision should be ensured
> - Complete mental health assessment with an emphasis on suicidal intent/planning
> - Methods and frequency should be assessed
> - Factors likely to be associated with NSSI, such as home environment, peer relationship, should be evaluated
> - Specific assessment scales for NSSI and possible comorbid psychiatric disorders can be used

Few mnemonic devices have been suggested for the primary care physicians to facilitate the crucial assessment required at this first level of contact, e.g., "STOPS FIRE" (*S*uicidal ideation, *T*ypes, *O*nset, *P*lace/location, *S*everity of damage, *F*unctions self-injury serves for patient, *I*ntensity of self-injury urges, *R*epetition, *E*pisodic frequency)[52] and "SOARS" (*S*uicidal ideation, *O*nset, frequency, and methods, *A*ftercare, *R*easons, *S*tage of change).[53] Both of which evaluate the degree of suicidality, duration, type of self-injury, motivations, and readiness for change.

Formal screening assessment tools are also available, but none has been validated for the Indian population. The most commonly used scales are depicted in **Table 1**.

Other assessment tools include—the Brief Non-Suicidal Self-Injury Assessment Tool (BNSSI-AT), Deliberate Self-Harm Inventory, Ottawa Self-Injury Inventory, the Risk-Taking and Self-Harm Inventory for Adolescents (RTSHIA), Self-Harm Inventory, Skin, Links, Injury, Culture, Environment (SLICE), Self-Injury Questionnaire (SIQ), Self-Mutilative

TABLE 1: Assessment scales for nonsuicidal self-injurious (NSSI) behaviors.

Scale	Authors	Assessment areas
Inventory of statements about self-injury (ISAS)[54]	Klonsky ED, Glenn CR	Thirteen items assessing functions of NSSI behaviors; 12 methods and their frequency
Nonsuicidal self-injury assessment tool (NSSI-AT)[55]	Whitlock J, Exner-Cortens D, Purington A	Primary and secondary NSSI characteristics, functions, recency and frequency, age of onset and cessation, wound locations, initial motivations, severity, practice patterns, habituation and perceived life interference, NSSI disclosures, NSSI treatment experiences, personal reflection, and advice
Functional assessment of self-mutilation (FASM)[38]	Lloyd-Richardson EE, Perrine N, Dierker L, Kelley ML	• Eleven methods, classifying them as "moderate/severe" and "minor" and possible reasons for these behaviors • Twenty-two statements for assessing the functions as per the four function model of NSSI[27] • Nature of behaviors—suicidal or nonsuicidal; the concurrent use of substance; the degree of impulsivity and pain experienced and the age of onset of NSSI

Behaviors Interview, and Youth Risk Behavior Surveillance Survey (YRBSS).[52] NSSI is a risk factor for suicide, so the assessment of any suicidal thoughts or past suicide attempts is essential.

PREVENTION

A number of school-based prevention programs for NSSI have been implemented, which did not show any change in the help-seeking behavior of the study population.[56] In the large European Saving and Empowering Young Lives in Europe (SEYLE) program, significant effect was found on preventing suicidal ideations and suicidal attempts, but not on preventing NSSI.[57] Similarly, other trials replicated the same findings.[58]

Sign of self-injury (SOSI) is another school-based prevention program that utilizes ACT model (acknowledge the signs, cares for the person, and tell the trustworthy adult) to train school staff and students to help the peers presenting with NSSI. Preliminary result of the pilot study found to increase awareness and competence to deal with NSSI; however, the study did not comment upon the help-seeking behavior of students engaging in NSSI.[56]

"Happyles" is another school-based prevention program that utilizes principles of positive psychology, cognitive behavior therapy, and problem-solving to enhance general well-being and social connectedness. The program has shown to reduce the high-risk group's internalizing problems; however, effectiveness for reducing the NSSI has not been established.[59] Another study extended the current "Happyles" program to "Happylesplus" by adding the component of NSSI as the target of intervention and found the program effective for increasing the help-seeking behavior of school students who are indulging in NSSI.[60]

Indian literature is scarce on the prevention of NSSI; however, lessons can be taken from the global evidence available that suggests implementing universal preventive interventions to enhance the awareness about the available sources of help along with NSSI and a positive attitude toward help seeking. Peers and families can be trained for identifying and providing the initial support for individuals with NSSI. General life skills to enhance resilience and thriving can be incorporated at various curriculum levels in school to prevent the occurrence of NSSI as coping. Children and youth are encouraged to think about different coping alternatives available for a given problem situation.[61] There should be more emphasis on parent family connectedness, positive school climate and peer relations, and emotional regulation, with building psychological flexibility, self-esteem, positive personality traits, virtues, and character strengths.[62]

■ TREATMENT

Treatment of NSSI includes a multimodal approach where nonpharmacological/psychological management takes precedence over pharmacological management.

Psychological Management of NSSI

Psychological interventions are the mainstream treatment for NSSI in all age groups. Though Indian data is scarce about the management of NSSI, however, the clinician mostly utilizes general strategies no harm contract, high-risk management, safety plan, relaxation techniques etc. along with specific techniques of cognitive behavioral therapy and dialectical behavior therapy. Depending upon the case presentation, psychologists assess various developmental, familial, and interpersonal factors contributing to NSSI to draw upon a comprehensive case formulation. If trauma, abuse, and neglect are the major contributors

then components of trauma-focused interventions are also incorporated to address the underlying phenomenon.

Intervention usually starts with psycho-education about NSSI and discussion of case formulation with the patient. NSSI is a complex phenomenon; patients present with feelings of ambivalence about their recovery from NSSI as they have been using it as a coping strategy to deal with overwhelming emotions. Therefore, motivational interviewing (MI) techniques are used to assess the stage of change as per the transtheoretical model of change (precontemplation, contemplation, preparation, action, and maintenance). Empathy, reflective listening, validation of emotions, encouragement, enhancing self-efficacy, and therapeutic alliance are the commonly used techniques of MI interventions.[63]

The treatment plan is individualized as per the need of the targeted patient; however, various components of DBT such as mindfulness, emotional regulation, distress tolerance, and interpersonal skills have shown promising outcomes for patients with NSSI. At the core, patients with NSSI struggle with managing their emotions and indulge in experiential avoidance. Therefore, emotional regulation skills that incorporate identification of emotions, acknowledgement of associated distress, and different handling emotions are pertinent to learning for patients with NSSI. Mindfulness encourages acceptance of emotions and experiences without judgment, which further pave the way for compassion for self and others. Distress tolerance skills incorporate distraction, radical acceptance, and self-soothing skills to overcome the emotionally overwhelming situation. In addition, various behavioral skills such as removing access to means, learning to deal with environmental triggers, and positive feedback for one's efforts can be utilized as crucial factors toward behavioral change. Furthermore, adaptive coping skills are encouraged in place of maladaptive coping.[64]

Pharmacological Treatment

Pharmacological treatment of NSSI is used as an adjunct to the psychological approach. Studies are lacking on the pharmacological treatment for NSSI. Pharmacological agents can be used in cases where comorbid psychiatric disorders are diagnosed, as per the indication. In the available Cochrane review for borderline personality disorder, pharmacological treatments are not effective on self-injury.[65] Few studies have demonstrated the benefits of atypical antipsychotics, selective serotonin reuptake inhibitors (SSRIs), serotonin–noradrenaline reuptake inhibitors (SNRIs), and naltrexone in reducing NSSI, which can be explained with the implicated neurobiology of disrupted serotonergic, dopaminergic, and opioid systems.[66] In the Cochrane review for pharmacological interventions for self-harm in adults, no significant treatment effect on repetition of NSSI was found for antidepressants [e.g., tricyclic antidepressants (TCAs), SSRIs], low-dose fluphenazine, mood stabilizers, or natural products (omega-3 essential fatty acids).[67] A significant reduction in NSSI repetition was found in a single trial of the antipsychotic flupenthixol, but the quality of evidence was very low. However, the sample size of these studies was not sufficiently large to make any recommendation. There is also a general lack of research for clinical decision-making, which poses difficulty in choosing a medication.

Nevertheless, in the cases of severe restlessness and urge to self-harm, sedatives can be used after other strategies have already been tried. Benzodiazepines can be used under supervision by family or hospital staff after weighing the risk–benefit ratio. Therefore, the use of pharmacological agents is based on the individual's characteristics, preference, treatment setting, comorbid physical and psychiatric disorders.[68] Treatment algorithm for subjects presenting with NSSI is depicted in **Flowchart 3**.

RISK OF NSSI AND MITIGATION STRATEGIES IN COVID PANDEMIC

The worldwide situation of the coronavirus disease 2019 (COVID-19) pandemic and associated lockdown has led to a change in daily routine and social engagements. The adolescents, who are at the highest risk of NSSI, cannot attend schools/colleges, and the social interaction is limited to social media. Also, the lockdown has led to increase in the conflict situation among families. So clearly, this situation has led to an increased demand for emotional regulation in the absence of protective factors such as social support. Also, there has been limited access to professional help.[69] In this scenario, psychiatrists shall continue regular and emergency treatment as much as feasible to tackle the negative consequences of the prevailing situation. Innovative approaches through telepsychiatry can also be used for delivering mental health services.[70]

ETHICAL AND LOGISTIC ISSUES IN NSSI-RELATED RESEARCH

One major challenge in this field is the overlap between the various terminologies given for these behaviors and different concepts used in various researches. The majority of the studies have been conducted in adolescent and young adult age groups where similar

Flowchart 3: Treatment algorithm for individuals presenting with NSSI.[68]

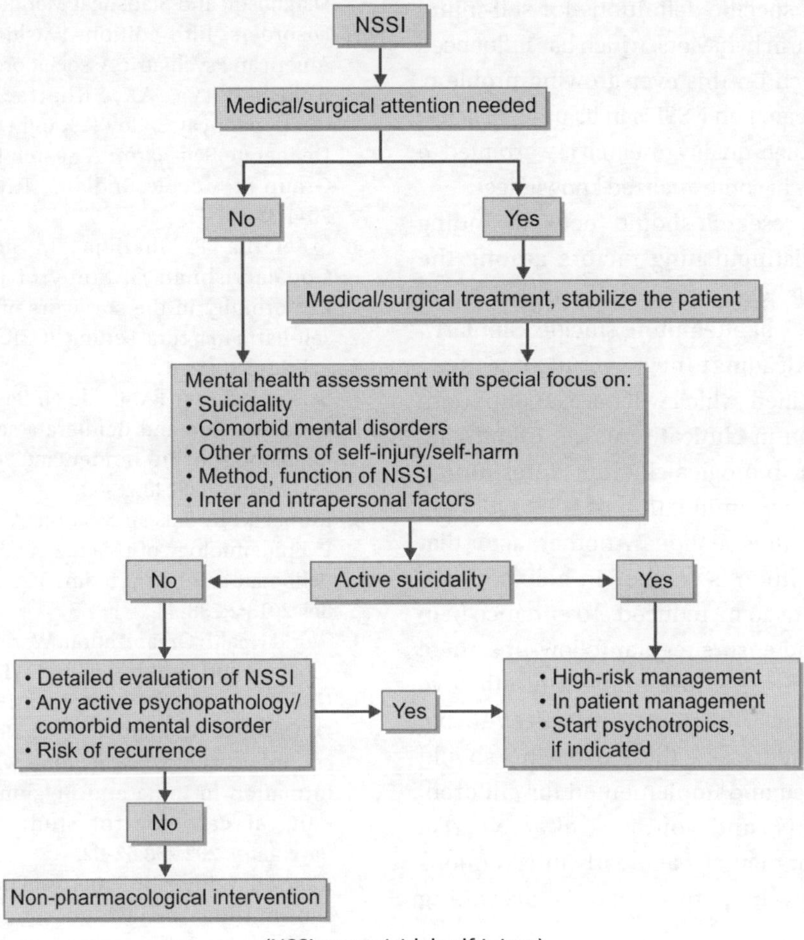

(NSSI: nonsuicidal self-injury)

criteria regarding consent have been used without taking assent from younger kids and consent from their parents. Relevant rules and regulations should be considered while designing any study. Similarly, it becomes relevant to specify the process of assessing and managing the imminent risk of suicide for ethical purposes. In current times, a good amount of research is being done through online platforms, but the researchers are not trained about the ethics in internet-based research. With the possible risk of suicide in individuals with NSSI, the assessment regarding suicidal ideation, depression levels, and frequency, form, and timing of NSSI behavior must be done along with appropriate management.[71]

General practitioners (GPs) are generally the first point of contact for patients presenting with self-harm. Their positive attitude, with comprehensive risk assessments, and collaborative individualized care are vital for the holistic approach.[72]

To conclude, NSSI has increased significantly in the clinical as well as community population, mostly among adolescents and young adults. There is a lack of consensus for the use of specific definitions for self-injury and self-harm behaviors, which has influenced the research on this ever-growing problem. Indian research on NSSI is in its nascent stage; therefore, high-quality research is warranted to fill the gaps in contextualized knowledge.

Future research should focus on finding out the distinguishing factors among the individuals who only indulge in NSSI and those at risk of attempting suicide. Similarly, risk factors leading to negative outcomes need to be identified, which will have an important implication in clinical practice. Identifying social and biological factors determining remission or continuation of NSSI will help to plan the interventions. Another factor that needs attention is barriers in help seeking, which needs to be reduced. To enhance help seeking and ensure regular follow-ups, there is a need for the development of effective therapeutic interventions. Preventive strategies addressing these behaviors should be designed and implemented for children, adolescents, and youth as effective risk assessment methods and early interventions might only help to curb this prevailing situation.

■ REFERENCES

1. Ougrin D, Tranah T, Leigh E, Taylor L, Asarnow JR. Practitioner review: Self-harm in adolescents. J Child Psychol Psychiatry. 2012;53:337-50.
2. World Health Organization. Preventing Suicide: A Global Imperative. Geneva: WHO; 2014a.
3. Nock MK, Favazza AR. Nonsuicidal self-injury: Definition and classification. Understanding nonsuicidal self-injury: Origins, assessment, and treatment. Washington, DC, US: American Psychological Association; 2009. pp. 9-18.
4. American Psychiatric Association (APA). Diagnostic and Statistical Manual of Mental Disorders, fifth edition. Washington, DC: American Psychiatric Association; 2013.
5. Bhattacharya AK, Bhattacharjee S, Chattopadhyay S, Roy P, Kanji D, Singh OP. Deliberate Self-harm: A Search for Distinct Group of Suicide. Indian J Psychol Med. 2011;33:182-7.
6. Sreelatha P, Shailaja B, Sushma VI, Gopalakrishnan G. Study of psychiatric comorbidity in the survivors of deliberate self-harm in a rural setting. IOSR J Dent Med Sci. 2014;13:53-6.
7. Sarkar P, Sattar FA, Gode N, Basannar DR. Failed suicide and deliberate self-harm: A need for specific nomenclature. Indian J Psychiatry. 2006;48:78-83.
8. Kumar KPK, Sukesh Kakunje A, Bhagavath P. Epidemiology of psychiatric disorders in deliberate self-harm victims. J Evol Med Dent Sci. 2013;2:738-44.
9. World Health Organization. World Report on Violence and Health. Geneva: WHO; 2002.
10. Gandhi A, Luyckx K, Adhikari A, Parmar D, Desousa A, Shah N, et al. Non-suicidal self-injury and its association with identity formation in India and Belgium: A cross-cultural case-control study. Transcult Psychiatry. 2021;58:52-62.
11. Kharsati N, Bhola P. Patterns of non-suicidal self-injurious behaviours among college students in India. Int J Soc Psychiatry. 2015;61:39-49.
12. Bhola P, Manjula M, Rajappa V, Phillip M. Predictors of non-suicidal and suicidal self-injurious behaviours, among adolescents and young adults in urban India. Asian J Psychiatry. 2017;29:123-8.
13. Klonsky ED, Muehlenkamp JJ. Self-injury: A research review for the practitioner. J Clin Psychol. 2007;63:1045-56.
14. Gandhi A, Luyckx K, Maitra S, Claes L. Non-suicidal self-injury and other self-directed violent behaviors in India: A review of definitions and research. Asian J Psychiatry. 2016;22:196-201.
15. Swannell SV, Martin GE, Page A, Hasking P, John NJS. Prevalence of nonsuicidal

self-injury in nonclinical samples: Systematic review, meta-analysis and meta-regression. Suicide Life Threat Behav. 2014;44:273-303.

16. Whitlock J, Muehlenkamp J, Eckenrode J. Variation in nonsuicidal self-injury: Identification and features of latent classes in a college population of emerging adults. J Clin Child Adolesc Psychol. 2008;37:725-35.

17. Linehan MM. Dialectical behavior therapy for treatment of borderline personality disorder: Implications for the treatment of substance abuse. NIDA Res Monograph. 1993;137:201.

18. Plener PL, Bubalo N, Fladung AK, Ludolph AG, Lulé D. Prone to excitement: Adolescent females with non-suicidal self-injury (NSSI) show altered cortical pattern to emotional and NSS-related material. Psychiatry Res Neuroimaging. 2012;203:146-52.

19. Whittle S, Chanen AM, Fornito A, McGorry PD, Pantelis C, Yücel M. Anterior cingulate volume in adolescents with first-presentation borderline personality disorder. Psychiatry Res Neuroimaging. 2009;172:155-60.

20. Brunner R, Henze R, Parzer P, Kramer J, Feigl N, Lutz K, et al. Reduced prefrontal and orbitofrontal gray matter in female adolescents with borderline personality disorder: Is it disorder specific? Neuroimage. 2010;49:114-20.

21. Goodman M, Hazlett EA, Avedon JB, Siever DR, Chu KW, New AS. Anterior cingulate volume reduction in adolescents with borderline personality disorder and co-morbid major depression. J Psychiatr Res. 2011;45:803-7.

22. Westlund Schreiner M, Klimes-Dougan B, Begnel ED, Cullen KR. Conceptualizing the neurobiology of non-suicidal self-injury from the perspective of the Research Domain Criteria Project. Neurosci Biobehav Rev. 2015;57:381-91.

23. Westlund Schreiner M, Klimes-Dougan B, Mueller BA, Eberly LE, Reigstad KM, Carstedt PA, et al. Multi-modal neuroimaging of adolescents with non-suicidal self-injury: Amygdala functional connectivity. J Affect Disord. 2017;221:47-55.

24. Koenig J, Brunner R, Fischer-Waldschmidt G, Parzer P, Plener PL, Park J, et al. Prospective risk for suicidal thoughts and behaviour in adolescents with onset, maintenance or cessation of direct self-injurious behaviour. Eur Child Adolesc Psychiatry. 2017;26:345-54.

25. Rinnewitz L, Koenig J, Parzer P, Brunner R, Resch F, Kaess M. Childhood adversity and psychophysiological reactivity to pain in adolescent nonsuicidal self-injury. Psychopathology. 2018;51:346-52.

26. Reichl C, Heyer A, Brunner R, Parzer P, Völker JM, Resch F, et al. Hypothalamic-pituitary-adrenal axis, childhood adversity and adolescent nonsuicidal self-injury. Psychoneuroendocrinology. 2016;74: 203-11.

27. Kaess M, Hille M, Parzer P, Maser-Gluth C, Resch F, Brunner R. Alterations in the neuroendocrinological stress response to acute psychosocial stress in adolescents engaging in nonsuicidal self-injury. Psychoneuroendocrinology. 2012;37:157-61.

28. Nock MK, Prinstein MJ. A functional approach to the assessment of self-mutilative behavior. J Consult Clin Psychol. 2004;72:885-90.

29. Chapman AL, Gratz KL, Brown MZ. Solving the puzzle of deliberate self-harm: The experiential avoidance model. Behav Res Ther. 2006;44:371-94.

30. Walsh B. Clinical assessment of self-injury: A practical guide. J Clin Psychol. 2007;63:1057-68.

31. Mars B, Heron J, Klonsky ED, Moran P, O'Connor RC, Tilling K, et al. What distinguishes adolescents with suicidal thoughts from those who have attempted suicide? A population-based birth cohort study. J Clin Child Adolesc Psychol. 2019;60:91-9.

32. Nock MK. Self-injury. Annu Rev Clin Psychol. 2010;6:339-63.

33. Whitlock J, Knox KL. The relationship between self-injurious behavior and suicide in a young adult population. Arch Pediatr Adolesc Med. 2007;161:634-40.

34. Kiekens G, Hasking P, Boyes M, Claes L, Mortier P, Auerbach RP, et al. The associations between non-suicidal self-injury and first onset suicidal thoughts and behaviors. J Affect Disord. 2018;239:171-9.

35. Joiner T. Why People Die By Suicide. Cambridge, US: Harvard University Press; 2007.

36. Joiner TE, Ribeiro JD, Silva C. Nonsuicidal self-injury, suicidal behavior, and their co-occurrence as viewed through the lens of the interpersonal theory of suicide. Curr Dir Psychol Sci. 2012;21:342-7.

37. Favaro A, Ferrara S, Santonastaso P. Self-injurious behavior in a community sample of young women: Relationship with childhood abuse and other types of self-damaging behaviors. J Clin Psychiatry. 2007;68: 122-31.

38. Lloyd-Richardson EE, Perrine N, Dierker L, Kelley ML. Characteristics and functions of non-suicidal self-injury in a community sample of adolescents. Psychol Med. 2007;37:1183-92.

39. Tang J, Yu Y, Wu Y, Du Y, Ma Y, Zhu H, et al. Association between non-suicidal self-injuries and suicide attempts in Chinese adolescents and college students: A cross-section study. PloS One. 2011;6:e17977.

40. Turner BJ, Layden BK, Butler SM, Chapman AL. How often, or how many ways: Clarifying the relationship between non-suicidal self-injury and suicidality. Arch Suicide Res. 2013;17:397-415.

41. Anestis MD, Anestis JC. Suicide rates and state laws regulating access and exposure to handguns. Am J Public Health. 2015;105: 2049-58.

42. You J, Leung F. The role of depressive symptoms, family invalidation and behavioral impulsivity in the occurrence and repetition of non-suicidal self-injury in Chinese adolescents: A 2-year follow-up study. J Adolesc. 2012;35:389-95.

43. Nock MK, Joiner TE Jr, Gordon KH, Lloyd-Richardson E, Prinstein MJ. Non-suicidal self-injury among adolescents: Diagnostic correlates and relation to suicide attempts. Psychiatry Res. 2006;144:65-72.

44. Lin MP, You J, Ren Y, Wu JY, Hu WH, Yen CF, et al. Prevalence of nonsuicidal self-injury and its risk and protective factors among adolescents in Taiwan. Psychiatry Res. 2017;255:119-27.

45. Kress VE, Newgent RA, WhitlockJ, Mease L. Spirituality/religiosity, life satisfaction, and life meaning as protective factors for nonsuicidal self-injury in college students. J Coll Couns. 2015;18:160-74.

46. Klonsky ED, Victor SE, Saffer BY. Nonsuicidal self-injury: What we know, and what we need to know. Can J Psychiatry. 2014;59:565-8.

47. Wilkinson PO, Qiu T, Neufeld S, Jones PB, Goodyer IM. Sporadic and recurrent non-suicidal self-injury before age 14 and incident onset of psychiatric disorders by 17 years: Prospective cohort study. Br J Psychiatry. 2018;212:222-6.

48. Selby EA, Bender TW, Gordon KH, Nock MK, Joiner TE Jr. Non-suicidal self-injury (NSSI) disorder: A preliminary study. Personal Disord. 2012;3:167-75.

49. Nitkowski D, Petermann F. Non-suicidal self-injury and comorbid mental disorders: A review. Fortschr Neurol Psychiatr. 2011; 79:9-20.

50. Grover S, Sarkar S, Bhalla A, Chakrabarti S, Avasthi A. Demographic, clinical and psychological characteristics of patients with self-harm behaviours attending an emergency department of a tertiary care hospital. Asian J Psychiatr. 2016;20:3-10.

51. Singh S, Kumar S, Deep R. Patients with deliberate self-harm attended in emergency setting at a tertiary care hospital: A 13-month analysis of clinical-psychiatric profile. Int J Psychiatry Med. 2019;54:363-76.

52. Kerr PL, Muehlenkamp JJ, Turner JM. Nonsuicidal self-injury: A review of current research for family medicine and primary care physicians. J Am Board Fam Med. 2010;23:240-59.

53. Westers N, Muehlenkamp J, Lau M. SOARS model: Risk assessment of nonsuicidal self-injury. Contemp Pediatr. 2016;33:25-31.

54. Klonsky ED, Glenn CR. Assessing the functions of non-suicidal self-injury: Psychometric properties of the Inventory of Statements About Self-injury (ISAS). J Psychopathol Behav Assess. 2009;31: 215-9.

55. Whitlock J, Exner-Cortens D, Purington A. Assessment of nonsuicidal self-injury:

Development and initial validation of the non-suicidal self-injury-assessment tool (NSSI-AT). Psychol Assess. 2014;26: 935-46.

56. Muehlenkamp JJ, Walsh BW, McDade M. Preventing non-suicidal self-injury in adolescents: The signs of self-injury program. J Youth Adolescence. 2010;39:306-14.

57. Wasserman D, Carli V, Wasserman C, Apter A, Balazs J, Bobes J, et al. Saving and Empowering Young Lives in Europe (SEYLE): A randomized controlled trial. BMC Public Health. 2010;10:192.

58. Calear AL, Christensen H, Freeman A, Fenton K, Busby Grant J, van Spijker B, et al. A systematic review of psychosocial suicide prevention interventions for youth. Eur Child Adolesc Psychiatry. 2016;25:467-82.

59. van der Zanden R, Kramer J, Gerrits R, Cuijpers P. Effectiveness of an online group course for depression in adolescents and young adults: A randomized trial. J Med Internet Res. 2012;14:e86.

60. Baetens I, Decruy C, Vatandoost S, Vanderhaegen B, Kiekens G. School-based prevention targeting non-suicidal self-injury: A pilot study. Front Psychiatry. 2020; 11:437.

61. Whitlock J, Rodham K. Understanding nonsuicidal self-injury in youth. School Psychology Forum. 2013;7:93-110.

62. Nebhinani N, Singhai K. Protective factors against suicidality in childhood and adolescence. J Indian Assoc Child Adolesc Ment Health. 2021;17:1-11.

63. Meheli S, Bhola P, Murugappan NP. From self-injury to recovery: A qualitative exploration with self-injuring youth in India. J Psychosoc Rehabil Ment Health. 2021;8:147-58.

64. Kruzan KP, Whitlock J. Processes of change and nonsuicidal self-injury: A qualitative interview study with individuals at various stages of change. Glob Qual Nurs Res. 2019;6:2333393619852935.

65. Stoffers JM, Völlm BA, Rücker G, Timmer A, Huband N, Lieb K. Psychological therapies for people with borderline personality disorder. Cochrane Database Syst Rev. 2012;2012:CD005652.

66. Plener PL, Libal G, Nixon MK. Use of medication in the treatment of nonsuicidal self-injury in youth. In: Nixon MK, Heath NL (Eds). Self-injury in youth: The essential guide to assessment and intervention. New York (NY): Routledge/Taylor & Francis Group; 2009. pp. 275-308.

67. Hawton K, Witt KG, Taylor Salisbury TL, Arensman E, Gunnell D, Hazell P, et al. Pharmacological interventions for self-harm in adults. Cochrane Database Syst Rev. 2015;(7):CD011777.

68. Plener PL, Brunner R, Fegert JM, Groschwitz RC, In-Albon T, Kaess M, et al. Treating nonsuicidal self-injury (NSSI) in adolescents: Consensus-based German guidelines. Child Adolesc Psychiatry Ment Health. 2016;10:46.

69. Plener PL. COVID-19 and nonsuicidal self-injury: The pandemic's influence on an adolescent epidemic. Am J Public Health. 2021;111:195-6.

70. Fegert JM, Vitiello B, Plener PL, Clemens V. Challenges and burden of the Coronavirus 2019 (COVID-19) pandemic for child and adolescent mental health: A narrative review to highlight clinical and research needs in the acute phase and the long return to normality. Child Adolesc Psychiatry Ment Health. 2020;14:20.

71. Singhal N, Bhola P. Ethical practices in community-based research in non-suicidal self-injury: A systematic review. Asian J Psychiatr. 2017;30:127-34.

72. Bellairs-Walsh I, Perry Y, Krysinska K, Byrne SJ, Boland A, Michail A, et al. Best practice when working with suicidal behaviour and self-harm In primary care: A qualitative exploration of young people's perspectives. BMJ Open. 2020;10:e038855.

8

Psychiatric Disorders and Suicide in India

Om Prakash Singh, Seshadri Sekhar Chatterjee

ABSTRACT

The current chapter deals with suicide in relation to various psychiatric disorders globally with special emphasis on the Indian context. The chapter highlights how the psychiatric disorders as a cause of suicide shows lower figures in India compared to the West. A brief update on Indian research is provided at the end.

Keywords: Psychiatric disorder; Suicide; Bipolar disorder; Depression.

"If you cry because the sun has gone out of your life, your tears will prevent you from seeing the stars"

—**Rabindranath Tagore**

◼ INTRODUCTION

There are about 800,000 suicides every year, with more than three quarters happening in low- and middle-income countries (LMICs). Suicide rates have increased alarmingly consistently since the last decade, with isolated dips in the middle. Blame it on cultural factors, globalization, open economy, economic disparity, and what not, India reported a suicide rate of 12 (per lakh population) in 2021, an increase of 6.2% from 2020, which is alarming.[1]

In India, like many other LMIC countries, suicide research is hindered by many factors such as underreporting, social taboos, a lack of a centralized list, and a lack of cross-departmental collaboration. The Mental Healthcare Act (MHCA) 2017 has ushered in several progressive steps, but the challenges are also increasing exponentially.[2] Nevertheless, many recent studies have focused on these topics. And when we dig deeper in these studies, some unique differences are evident.

▌ EVALUATION OF CONCEPT AND NOSOLOGY

The World Health Organization (WHO) defines *suicide* as a deliberate act of killing oneself. *Suicide attempt* is defined as any nonfatal suicidal behavior, such as intentional self-inflicted poisoning, injury, or self-harm, which may or may not have a fatal intent or outcome. The term "suicidal behavior" has been used in the WHO Suicide Report to refer to the entire spectrum of suicidal phenomena; "suicidal behavior refers to a range of behaviors that include thinking about suicide (or ideation), planning for suicide, attempting suicide, and suicide itself".[3] This definition implies that nonfatal self-harm without suicidal intent is included under this term, which is problematic due to the possible variations in related interventions (WHO, 2014). *Suicide behavior disorder* (SBD) was introduced in DSM-5 (Diagnostic and Statistical Manual of Mental Disorders, Fifth Edition) as a disorder for further consideration and potential acceptance into the diagnostic criteria list in future.[4]

PSYCHIATRIC DISORDERS AND SUICIDE—CONTEXT SETTINGS

Mental disorders are the strongest individual risk factors of SB. In fact, the increased suicide risk is one of the main reasons why people with mental disorders live 15–20 years less than the average person. Around 90% of suicide attempters have a comorbid psychiatric diagnosis, if not more, and it increases further when subsyndromic and milder versions are added. Most inpatient suicides take place within the first week of admission.[5]

A suicidal high-risk period ensues in the first days and months following discharge, especially in the first week, when the risk is up to 102-fold (for men) and 246-fold (for women), when compared to a background population without previous admissions.[6] The following clinical factors have been associated with an increased risk: history of suicide attempt, depressed mood, feelings of hopelessness or worthlessness, suicidal ideations expressed at admission, family history of suicide, diagnosis of schizophrenia, and having been prescribed antidepressant medication.[7]

HOW INDIAN DATA IS DIFFERENT

Psychiatric disorders may play a less prominent role in suicidal behavior in India when compared to global data. From Freud's "cry for help" hypothesis to Durham's Social Theory, these explanations are too simplistic for a heterogeneous, diverse population such as India. In fact, there are arguments that basic behaviors of suicidal act itself are different in India.[8] In high-income countries (HICs), 80–90% of suicides and 92% of suicide attempts have a background psychiatric disorder.[9] According to studies from LMIC, psychiatric morbidity in suicidal behavior ranges from 10 to 88%.[10] As compared to Western countries, Indian studies indicate that there are fewer diagnosable psychiatric disorders and a greater number of psychosocial problems.[11] This observation may be contested but warrants clarification. Impulsiveness, to mention again, has a significant role in suicide in the Indian context. This is more evident when it is superimposed on other mental disorders. Additionally, it explains the unique correlation between pesticides and suicide rates in rural areas. This is a great example of how trend analysis backed by robust clinical data and resultant policy changes can have enormous positive social impact.[12]

According to a study done in Chennai, although 25% of individuals were diagnosed with depression, 60% only suffered from mild-to-moderate depression. The majority attempted suicide during their first episode.[13] The prevalence of alcohol-use disorders and impulsive personality traits in Asia is higher than in the West. In HIC, mental disorders (especially depression and alcohol-use disorders) play a major role in suicide. However, impulsivity plays a crucial role in India.[8]

Understanding the relationship between psychiatric disorders and suicidal behavior is essential to ensuring that the limited resources in India are used appropriately.

MOOD DISORDERS

Undeniably, mood disorders are the leading cause of suicide worldwide, and India is not an exception. The majority of patients with mood disorders in psychiatric settings have attempted suicide or have significant suicidal ideation.[14] Patients with bipolar disorder (BD) types I and II are more likely to attempt suicide than those with major depressive disorder (MDD). Associated comorbidities and alcohol dependence increase the risk further.

In contrast to the general population, patients with BD have a much lower ratio of suicide attempts to suicide deaths (i.e., the lethality index).[15] This ratio has been reported in one study to be 35:1 for the general population and 3:1 for BD patients. The incidence of suicidal attempt among patients with major depression that had suicidal ideation was 16.6%.[16] Suicidal attempt also correlated positively with depression severity. There is a greater incidence of dysthymia in India than in the West.[17] In their seminal review, Knipe et al. found that mood disorders constituted the most prevalent diagnoses for both fatal and nonfatal suicidal behavior (25% and 21%, respectively) in LMIC countries. This is much lower than previous estimates of suicide and nonfatal suicidal behavior (43–59%).[10]

A synthesis of the evidence suggests that psychiatric disorders may be less common among suicidal individuals in India.[18] Because of the wide range of estimates and the high degree of heterogeneity between study estimates, this result needs to be interpreted cautiously. Disempowered members of the community (e.g., women and young people) may use suicidal behavior as a form of communication in India.[19,20] In light of this explanation, it may again be less likely to be associated with psychiatric morbidity. A culturally specific expression of psychiatric symptoms may be missed by diagnostic criteria such as the ICD and DSM.[21,22]

Suicidal acts are conceptualized in the paradigmatic stress-disease model as the outcome of a balance between trait- and state-related predisposing and protective factors. Time-varying risk factors should be explicitly considered in this context, including not only symptoms' presence and severity, but also the duration of the high-risk states. In general, and for depression-related suicidal behavior in particular, traits of impulsiveness and aggression play a major role. Despite the fact that suicidal acts among patients with mood disorders almost always occur in the presence of a major mood episode and are preceded by suicidal ideation, these traits likely play a major role in determining which patients will act on their urges.

▌ SCHIZOPHRENIA AND RELATED DISORDER

Schizophrenia patients often die much earlier than expected. Suicide and unnatural deaths account for up to 40% of this excess premature mortality.[23]

Sixty-percent of people with schizophrenia who commit suicide do so within the first 4–10 years after being diagnosed. First psychotic episodes are associated with a significantly increased risk of suicide. Comorbid depression and a history of suicidal behavior are substantial contributors to suicide risk in patients with schizophrenia. A 12-fold increase in all-cause death and a 37-fold increase in suicide rates are observed after discharge from the hospital after the first episode of schizophrenia without antipsychotics. Researchers have linked insight and stigma to this increase in suicide mortality.[24]

The duration of untreated psychosis (DUP), multiple hospitalizations, immediate postdischarge period, a family history of schizophrenia and suicide, a previous suicide attempt, presence of positive symptoms, and depressive symptoms all contribute to suicidal behavior.[25]

There is well-established evidence that clozapine has antisuicidal properties. Schizophrenia-specific suicide risk factors include recurrent relapses, significant severity of the disorder, a decline in social and occupational functioning, and a true and realistic understanding of the disease's impact. Patients with the paranoid subtype of schizophrenia are eight times more likely to die by suicide in comparison with patients with the deficit subtype of schizophrenia. A research report indicates that suicidal behavior in schizophrenia is associated with delusions. Hostility at hospital admission is also associated with long-term suicidal behaviors. Antipsychotic medications have yielded inconclusive results. According to some evidence, poor adherents are at increased risk while some studies have found a significant connection between akathisia and suicidality in first-episode psychosis and also in the long term.

Indian studies in this area are scarce. Recently in a cross-sectional study on 140 sample size, it has been reported that about 25% have past history of suicidal attempt and 30% have ongoing suicidal ideation. Suicide attempts in the past, family history of mental illness, and the history of suicide and substance abuse all significantly predicted the current suicidal ideation. A significant correlation has also been found between ideation and comorbid depression and the positive, negative, emotional, and excitement domains of schizophrenia.[26]

■ ANXIETY DISORDER

Evidence of anxiety disorder in suicide and SI is emerging, despite it being under-researched. In particular, social anxiety disorder has been linked to an increase in SI in adolescence emerging in adulthood and older adults as well.[27] Indeed, it can be explained in light of the interpersonal theory of suicide. Here to mention, the symptoms of SAD are often accompanied by alcohol-abuse disorders or have subsequent associations with them.[28]

In a study conducted on 545 patients with obsessive compulsive disorder (OCD), Viswanath et al. report that OCD when comorbid with MDD is associated with higher suicidal risk.[29]

■ FURTHER INDIAN STUDIES

On searching in PubMed with the MeSH (medical subject heading) terms such as "psychiatric disorder" or "psychiatric morbidity" and "suicide" and "India" and other related words, 146 results came, most of which are reviews. The Indian Journal of Psychiatry's (IJP) first publication on suicide was in 1967. Till now, there are 572 results. In Indian Journal of Psychological Medicine, the number of articles with the search word "suicide" is 503.

Bagadia et al.[30] conducted a study on 521 patients admitted for suicidal behavior and found that depression (39.73%), schizophrenia (24.4%), and hysteria (14%) were the most common psychiatric diagnoses made.

Gupta and Singh[31] reported psychiatric disorders in 62% with 58% having abnormal personalities. Mahla et al.[32] investigated attempted cases of self-immolation and reported that the behavior was associated with the presence of psychiatric and personality disorders. Another study also found that 37.5% of the suicide attempters had a diagnosis of depression.[33] Khan et al. identified the presence of psychiatric illness and stressful life events as the two most important reasons for completing suicide.[34]

In the 1980s, a study found a positive and significant correlation between depressive illness, suicidal ideation with early parental deprivation, recent bereavement, and positive family history of suicide.[35] Recent studies and systematic reviews back these evidences further.[36,37]

Even before that, in the 1970s, investigation on attempted suicides in psychiatric inpatients reported that during a 1-year period, out of 1,881 admissions 126 had made suicidal attempts. Patients with schizophrenia accounted for 64% of the attempted suicides.[38] Another 2-year follow-up study of patients who had attempted suicide with schizophrenia and depression reported that 51.8% of the suicide attempters had a personality disorder, 42% had neurotic symptoms during childhood, and 23.5% had a history of drug dependence. During the follow-up period 17.1% of the schizophrenia patients had attempted suicide again with one completing suicide, compared to 19% of the depressed patients.[39]

In a study of attempted suicide, 11.6% had a psychiatric diagnosis with alcohol dependence followed by depression being the most common diagnoses; schizophrenia, conduct disorder, and personality disorder comprised the rest.[16] In their study on patients with MDD, they reported that 17% of patients with suicidal ideation attempted suicide. The risk factors identified were being below 30 years of age, having higher education, and being a single male or a married woman or a student. Suicide attempters also had more suicidal ideation, agitation, and paranoid symptoms.

Rates of psychiatric diagnosis as high as 46.7%,[40] 59.7%,[41] 57%,[33] and even 93%[42] have been described among suicide attempters.

Mood disorders, particularly depressive disorders, were the most common diagnosis followed by alcohol abuse. Neurotic, stress-related, and somatoform disorders were diagnosed in 14.5%.[33]

In a study of patients with major depressive disorder with suicidal ideation, the incidence of suicidal attempt was 16.6%; all attempters were <30 years old. Suicidal attempts have also been found to be positively correlated with the severity of depression.[43]

In a study of 1,560 patients with schizophrenia, the rate of attempted suicide was 4.7%. These patients did not differ in illness duration from patients with depression who had attempted suicide.[39] In an interesting study, researchers found a diagnosis of schizoaffective disorder and history of depression to be significantly associated with suicide attempts in the US sample but not in the Indian sample.[44]

■ LAST 10 YEARS' UPDATE

In a study conducted on 827 patients attending primary care OPD, it was found that the prevalence of current depression was 81% (severe depression, 61%) in patients reporting past suicide attempts.[45] A verbal autopsy study on 100 suicidal deaths from rural India found A DSM-III—revised (R) diagnosis was associated with 37 of the suicide deaths. The most common categories were alcohol dependence (16%) and adjustment disorders (15%). Schizophrenia, mania, and dysthymia all had prevalence rates of 2%.[46]

There are other studies from Kashmir[47] that explore the association of suicide with depression, among BD type 1[48] in schizophrenia patients[49] and among injectable drug abusers.[50]

One study from Delhi among schizophrenia patients revealed that one-fourth of schizophrenia patients reported self-harm including suicide attempt with a prevalence of suicide attempts of 10%.[51] Further exploration revealed significant association with lipid profile and impulsivity affecting suicidality among schizophrenia patients.[52] In an international collaboration study, carried out on a total 3,711 OCD patients among which 802 were from India, suicidal ideation was noted as 6.4% in the last month and 9% in lifetime.[53]

■ CONCLUSION

An unsurmountable personal tragedy and a perpetually confusing psychosocial dilemma, suicide is and will always be the last thing a doctor and a victim's family will ever expect. In the last 2 decades, India has produced a multitude of studies. However multicenter, planned, analytical, level-1 studies are still lacking. Demographics, risk factors, disease characteristics, management priorities, policy-making, and media role[54]—the total discourse behind suicide is very different in India from Western countries. Hence, it poses unique challenges.[55] It is therefore essential to conduct more comprehensive research and more robust data in order to move toward a "zero suicide policy".[56]

■ REFERENCES

1. Singh OP. Startling suicide statistics in India: Time for urgent action. Indian J Psychiatry. 2022;64(5):431-2.
2. Sarkhel S. Mental health insurance and attempted suicide: Need for a reappraisal. Indian J Psychiatry. 2021;63(6):624-5.
3. World Health Organization. Preventing Suicide: A Global Imperative. Geneva: WHO; 2014.
4. Fehling KB, Selby EA. Suicide in DSM-5: current evidence for the proposed suicide behavior disorder and other possible improvements. Front Psychiatry. 2021;11:499980.
5. Madsen T, Agerbo E, Mortensen PB, Nordentoft M. Predictors of psychiatric inpatient suicide: a national prospective register-based study. J Clin Psychiatry. 2012;73:144-51.
6. Madsen T, Egilsdottir E, Damgaard C, Erlangsen A, Nordentoft M. Assessment of Suicide Risks During the First Week Immediately after Discharge From Psychiatric Inpatient Facility. Front Psychiatry. 2021;12:643303.
7. Large M, Smith G, Sharma S, Nielssen O, Singh SP. Systematic review and meta-analysis of the clinical factors associated with the suicide of psychiatric in-patients. Acta Psychiatr Scand. 2011;124:18-29.
8. Radhakrishnan R, Andrade C. Suicide: An Indian perspective. Indian J Psychiatry. 2012;54(4):304-19.
9. Hawton K, Saunders K, Topiwala A, Haw C. Psychiatric disorders in patients presenting to hospital following self-harm: a systematic review. J Affect Disord. 2013;151(3):821-30.
10. Knipe D, Williams AJ, Hannam-Swain S, Upton S, Brown K, Bandara P, et al. Psychiatric morbidity and suicidal behaviour in low- and middle-income countries: A systematic review and meta-analysis. PLoS Med. 2019;9;16(10):e1002905.
11. Bhatia MS, Aggarwal NK, Aggarwal BB. Psychosocial profile of suicide ideators, attempters and completers in India. Int J Soc Psychiatry. 2000;46(3):155-63.
12. Bonvoisin T, Utyasheva L, Knipe D, Gunnell D, Eddleston M. Suicide by pesticide poisoning in India: a review of pesticide regulations and their impact on suicide trends. BMC Public Health. 2020;20(1):251.
13. Vijayakumar L, Rajkumar S. Are risk factors for suicide universal? A case-control study in India. Acta Psychiatr Scand. 1999;99(6):407-11.
14. Isometsä E. Suicidal behaviour in mood disorders—who, when, and why? Can J Psychiatry. 2014;59(3):120-30.
15. Dome P, Rihmer Z, Gonda X. Suicide Risk in Bipolar Disorder: A Brief Review. Medicina (Kaunas). 2019;55(8):403.
16. Srivastava AS, Kumar R. Suicidal ideation and attempts in patients with major depression: Socio demographic and clinical variables. Indian J Psychiatry. 2005;47:225-8.

17. Chandrasekaran R, Gnanaseelan J, Sahai A, Swaminathan RP, Perme B. Psychiatric and personality disorders in survivors following their first suicide attempt. Indian J Psychiatry. 2003;45(2):45-8.
18. Bansal P, Gupta A, Kumar R. The Psychopathology and the Sociodemographic Determinants of Attempted Suicide Patients. J Clin Diagn Res. 2011;5(5):917-20.
19. Kumar CTS, Mohan R, Ranjith G, Chandrasekaran R. Gender differences in medically serious suicide attempts: a study from south India. Psychiatry Res. 2006;144(1):79-86.
20. Vishnuvardhan G, Saddichha S. Psychiatric comorbidity and gender differences among suicide attempters in Bangalore, India. Gen Hosp Psychiatry. 2012;34(4):410-4.
21. Chatterjee S, Kadam M. Study of psychiatric comorbidity and psychosocial stress factors in patients attempting suicide. Indian J Psychiatry. 2015;1:S78.
22. Kulkarni RR, Nagaraja Rao K, Begum S. Clinical profile of first suicide attempters in a general hospital. Indian J Psychiatry. 2013;55:S56.
23. Sher L, Kahn RS. Suicide in Schizophrenia: An Educational Overview. Medicina (Kaunas). 2019;55(7):361.
24. Pompili M, Amador XF, Girardi P, Harkavy-Friedman J, Harrow M, Kaplan K, et al. Suicide risk in schizophrenia: learning from the past to change the future. Ann Gen Psychiatry. 2007;6:10.
25. Barrett EA, Sundet K, Faerden A, Nesvåg R, Agartz I, Fosse R, et al. Suicidality before and in the early phases of first episode psychosis. Schizophr Res. 2010;119(1-3):11-7.
26. Nath S, Kalita KN, Baruah A, Saraf AS, Mukherjee D, Singh PK. Suicidal ideation in schizophrenia: A cross-sectional study in a tertiary mental hospital in North-East India. Indian J Psychiatry. 2021;63(2):179-83.
27. Herres J, Shearer A, Kodish T, Kim B, Wang SB, Diamond GS. Differences in Suicide Risk Severity Among Suicidal Youth With Anxiety Disorders. Crisis. 2019;40(5):333-9.
28. Buckner JD, Lemke AW, Jeffries ER, Shah SM. Social anxiety and suicidal ideation: Test of the utility of the interpersonal-psychological theory of suicide. J Anxiety Disord. 2017;45:60-3.
29. Viswanath B, Narayanaswamy JC, Rajkumar RP, Cherian AV, Kandavel T, Math SB, et al. Impact of depressive and anxiety disorder comorbidity on the clinical expression of obsessive-compulsive disorder. Compr Psychiatry. 2012;53(6):775-82.
30. Bagadia VN, Abhyankar RR, Shroff P, Mehta P, Doshi J, Chawla P. Suicidal behavior: A clinical study. Indian J Psychiatry. 1979;21:370-5.
31. Gupta SC, Singh H. Psychiatric illness in suicide attempters. Indian J Psychiatry. 1981;23:69-74.
32. Mahla VP, Bhargava SC, Dogra R, Shome S. The psychology of self-immolation in India. Indian J Psychiatry. 1992;34:108-13.
33. Jain V, Singh H, Gupta SC, Kumar S. A study of hopelessness, suicidal intent and depression in cases of attempted suicide. Indian J Psychiatry. 1999;41(2):122-30.
34. Khan FA, Anand B, Devi MG, Murthy KK. Psychological autopsy of suicide-a cross-sectional study. Indian J Psychiatry. 2005;47(2):73-8.
35. Badrinarayana A. Study of suicidal risk factors in depressive illness. Indian J Psychiatry. 1980;22:81-3.
36. Ahmed HU, Hossain MD, Aftab A, Soron TR, Alam MT, Chowdhury MWA, et al. Suicide and depression in the World Health Organization South-East Asia Region: A systematic review. WHO South East Asia J Public Health. 2017;2017;6(1):60-6.
37. Rane A, Nadkarni A. Suicide in India: a systematic review. Shanghai Arch Psychiatry. 2014;26(2):69-80.
38. Satyavati K. Attempted suicide in psychiatric patients. Indian J Psychiatry. 1971;13:37-48.
39. Gupta SC, Singh H, Trivedi JK. Evaluation of suicidal risk in depressives and schizophrenics: A 2-year follow-up study. Indian J Psychiatry. 1992;34:298-310.
40. Sharma RC. Attempted suicide in Himachal Pradesh. Indian J Psychiatry 1998;1998;40(1):50-4.

41. Unni SK, Mani AJ. Suicidal ideators in the psychiatric facility of a general hospital—a psychodemographic profile. Indian J Psychiatry. 1996;38:79-85.
42. Latha KS, Bhat SM, D'Souza P. Suicide attempters in a general hospital unit in India: their socio-demographic and clinical profile—emphasis on cross-cultural aspects. Acta Psychiatr Scand. 1996;1996;94(1):26-30.
43. Srivastava S, Kulsreshtha N. Expression of suicidal intent in depressives. Indian J Psychiatry. 2000;42:184-7.
44. Bhatia T, Thomas P, Semwal P, Thelma BK, Nimgaonkar VL, Deshpande SN. Differing correlates for suicide attempts among patients with schizophrenia or schizoaffective disorder in India and USA. Schizophr Res. 2006;1;86(1-3):208-14.
45. Indu PS, Anilkumar TV, Pisharody R, Russell PS, Raju D, Sarma PS, et al. Prevalence of depression and past suicide attempt in primary care. Asian J Psychiatr. 2017;27:48-52.
46. Manoranjitham S, Rajkumar A, Thangadurai P, Prasad J, Jayakaran R, Jacob K. Risk factors for suicide in rural South India. Br J Psychiatry. 2010;196(1):26-30.
47. Shoib S, Islam SM, Arafat SY, Hakak SA. Depression and suicidal ideation among the geriatric population of Kashmir, India. Int J Soc Psychiatry. 2021;67(6):651-5.
48. Kattimani S, Subramanian K, Sarkar S, Rajkumar RP, Balasubramanian S. History of lifetime suicide attempt in bipolar I disorder: its correlates and effect on illness course. Int J Psychiatry Clin Pract. 2017;21(2):118-24.
49. Verma D, Srivastava MK, Singh SK, Bhatia T, Deshpande SN. Lifetime suicide intent, executive function and insight in schizophrenia and schizoaffective disorders. Schizophr Res. 2016;178(1-3):12-6.
50. Armstrong G, Jorm AF, Samson L, Joubert L, Singh S, Kermode M. Suicidal ideation and attempts among men who inject drugs in Delhi, India: psychological and social risk factors. Soc Psychiatry Psychiatr Epidemiol. 2014;49(9):1367-77.
51. Jakhar K, Beniwal RP, Bhatia T, Deshpande SN. Self-harm and suicide attempts in Schizophrenia. Asian J Psychiatry. 2017;30:102-6.
52. Kavoor AR, Mitra S, Kumar S, Sisodia AK, Jain R. Lipids, aggression, suicidality and impulsivity in drug-naïve/drug-free patients of schizophrenia. Asian J Psychiatr. 2017;27:129-36.
53. Brakoulias V, Starcevic V, Belloch A, Brown C, Ferrao YA, Fontenelle LF, et al. Comorbidity, age of onset and suicidality in obsessive-compulsive disorder (OCD): an international collaboration. Compr Psychiatry. 2017;76:79-86.
54. Chatterjee SS, D'cruz M. Imitative Suicide, Mental Health, and Related Sobriquets. Indian J Psychol Med. 2020;42(6):560-5.
55. Vijayakumar L. Challenges and opportunities in suicide prevention in South-East Asia. WHO South East Asia J Public Health. 2017;6(1):30-3.
56. Pisani AR, Murrie DC, Silverman MM. Reformulating Suicide Risk Formulation: From Prediction to Prevention. Acad Psychiatry. 2016;40(4):623-9.

Substance Abuse and Suicide in India

Nidhi Sharma, Vikas Sharma, Debasish Basu

ABSTRACT

Suicidal behaviors are associated with significant morbidity and mortality in both short and long term and hence pose a major global challenge. It is 10th leading cause of mortality across the globe. In India, >1.5 lakh persons lost their lives due to suicides in 2020 and country has witnessed a rise of about 15% in number of deaths due to suicides as compared to previous decade. Substance use disorders (SUDs) have been regarded as important risk factors for both attempted and completed suicides. Persons with SUDs including alcohol have 10–14 times greater risk of dying by suicide than general population. In India, SUDs are third leading cause of suicides. Impact of SUDs on suicidality has been substantiated by various cohort and psychological autopsy studies as well as by meta-analysis. It is estimated that only one out of twenty suicidal attempts turn out to be completed suicides, thus suicidality significantly contributes to morbidity as well. In addition to SUDs, few psychotropic agents and alcohol may be randomly consumed to facilitate suicides. Prevention of suicide is one of the most challenging tasks of healthcare system worldwide. Identifying at-risk population and evaluating risk of suicidality using validated tools while avoiding stigmatization play a key role. Careful identification and redressal of risk factors including SUDs may be effective in preventing both attempted and completed suicides. Integrated treatment of suicidality and SUDs may prove beneficial in reducing the underdiagnosis and improving treatment outcome.

Keywords: Suicide; Substance use disorders; Substance abuse; India; Alcohol; Opioids; Management.

■ INTRODUCTION

Suicidal behaviors pose a major global challenge as they are associated with significant morbidity and mortality in both short and long term. It is 10th leading cause of mortality across the globe. As per National Crime and Research Bureau (NCRB) data, every year, more than 1.3 lakh lives are lost due to suicides in our country. In 2020, 1.53 lakh suicides were reported in India, which were 10% more as compared to the previous year. Among these, nearly two-thirds were of economically productive age group (18–45 years).[1] Worldwide, suicides are second leading cause of mortality among adolescents (15–29 years).[2] Even in our country, deaths due to suicides are rising by nearly 15% as compared to previous decade, and, hence, there is an urgent need for efficient suicidal prevention plan.[3]

Risk factors associated with suicidality are too complex and interwoven. They influence each other in nonadditive and unpredictable manner. Substance use disorders (SUDs) have been regarded as important risk factors for both attempted and completed suicides. Persons with

SUDs including alcohol have 10–14 times greater risk of dying by suicide than general population.[4] Impact of SUDs on suicidality has been substantiated by various cohort and psychological autopsy studies as well as by meta-analysis.[4,5] In NCRB report 2020, SUDs were third leading cause of suicides in India after family problems and illnesses and directly contributed to 6% suicides. Alcohol and drugs contributed to at least one suicide every hour in India. As compared to 2019, there was a sharp rise of 16.65% in suicides due to alcohol and drug addiction in 2020 in India.[1] Influence of psychiatric comorbidities, age and gender differences, and highly vulnerable subpopulations such as sexual minorities on suicide and SUDs needs a special mention. Coronavirus disease 2019 (COVID-19) pandemic has further complicated the situation as lockdowns and hampered services in the hospitals compromised both availability of psychotropic substances and access to psychiatry and deaddiction services.

It is estimated that only one out of twenty suicide attempts turns out to be completed suicides, thus, suicidality significantly contributes to morbidity as well. Prevention of suicide is one of the most challenging tasks of healthcare system worldwide. Identifying at-risk population and evaluating risk of suicidality using validated tools while avoiding stigmatization play a key role. Careful identification and redressal of risk factors including SUDs may be effective in preventing both attempted and completed suicides. Integrated treatment of suicidality and SUDs may be a breakthrough.

SUBSTANCE ABUSE AND SUICIDE

Alcohol and other substance use increases the suicidal behavior by impairing judgment and increasing impulsivity. Lately, physiological and psychological stresses also contribute to this phenomenon. SUDs also cause unemployment and social stigma that may indirectly lead to suicides. Association of suicidality and SUDs has been substantiated by various cohort and psychological autopsy studies. In a meta-analysis, Wilcox et al. estimated the risk of suicide by calculating standardized mortality ratios (SMRs). SMR was highest for mixed drug use (1685) followed by intravenous (IV) drugs (1,373), opioids (1,351), and alcohol (979). Opioid and IV drug users thus have more risk of dying from suicide than those using alcohol. Lifestyle of patients with SUDs and neuropharmacological effects of these agents may contribute to this increased phenomenon.[4]

In India, nearly 5.6% suicides are directly attributed to alcohol and other SUDs.[1] However, this may be an underestimate as NCRB data relies on self-reporting and hospital data. In a hospital study in North India ($N = 300$), patients who had SUDs as per Diagnostic and Statistical Manual of Mental Disorders, Fifth Edition (DSM-5) criteria were assessed using deliberate self-harm inventory. About 32.7% of the participants reported self-harm at least once in their lifetime. Being single, unemployed, use of injectable drugs and high-risk sexual behaviors were the factors associated with SUD and self-harm.[6] Cannabis dependence, severity of SUD, and being caught for unlawful activities were also found to influence deliberate self-harm in this hospital-based Indian study.[6]

Alcohol

It is widely known that alcohol use leads to increased suicidality. Alcohol is said to contribute to every fifth suicide directly or indirectly.[7] Lifetime risk of mortality due to suicide in persons with alcohol dependence is 8%.[5] Younger age of onset of alcohol use disorder (AUD), binge drinking, and severe AUD have strong association with suicidal behaviors. Risk of dying from suicide is five times more in heavy drinkers than those who consume alcohol intermittently.[8] Since elderly people often consume alcohol to alleviate pain and mood symptoms, AUD is one of the most common factors associated with elderly suicide.[9]

Besides disinhibition and impulsive behavior associated with alcohol, there are other factors that may be associated with alcohol-related suicidality. Alcohol consumption may be used as means to increase courage to act upon one's suicidal thoughts or may be used as method of committing suicide itself.[10]

Both alcohol intoxication and AUD have been linked with suicidality. Breet et al. did a systematic review to explore association of SUD and suicidality in low- and middle-income countries. Out of ten studies investigating association of suicidality with alcohol intake, six showed a positive association. Majority of these studies were done on adolescent population. Similarly, there was a positive association of suicidality and AUD as well.[11] Due to methodological limitations, most of alcohol-related suicidality studies focus on suicidal intent or attempts and not on completed suicides. Sreelatha et al. ($N = 175$) studied the relationship between alcohol and suicidality in South India. 38.3% subjects among suicide attempters had AUD, whereas 18.3% consumed alcohol prior to suicidal act in order to facilitate the same. Further, the number of lethal attempts was higher in those who consumed alcohol in order to facilitate suicide. Most of these facilitators were males, who were married and belonged to rural and low socioeconomic background.[12] In another Indian study, Bhattacharjee et al. ($N = 200$) subdivided study population who

consumed alcohol into three categories (some alcohol consumption; enough alcohol consumption—enough to impair judgment; and intentional alcohol intake—in order to facilitate suicide). Most of the enough alcohol consumption groups comprised of illiterate and unskilled workers; whereas, those who consumed alcohol to facilitate suicide were either students or educated at least up to high school. Enough alcohol intake also increased lethality of suicidal attempts.[13] Hence, socioeconomic and family-related factors play a significant role in alcohol-related suicidality in countries such as India.

In a systematic review, Rane et al. have shown that AUD is one of the most important risk factors for suicides in India and this is in contrast to developed and high-income countries where affective disorders such as depression, mania, and substance abuse comprise major mental disorders associated with suicides. Alcohol consumption [odds ratio (OR) = 4.5], chronic alcohol abuse in self (OR = 23.4), chronic alcohol abuse in spouse (OR = 6.1), and alcohol dependence (OR = 2.8) have been found to be strongly associated with suicides in India.[14]

Opioids

Increased suicide rates among persons with opioid dependence are well known. Proportion of deaths due to suicide among these ranges from 3 to 35% in various studies. In a meta-analysis, death rate due to suicide was 14 times more in heroin users as compared to normal population.[15] In a community study on people who inject drugs (PWID) ($N = 420$), which was conducted in Delhi, more than half of participants reported suicidal ideation and a substantial proportion among these (65%) had attempted to kill themselves at least once.[16] In contrast to western data, social factors such as being single, poor family relationships, homeless, beaten up by someone, or forced into sex are important factors influencing suicidality among patients having opioid dependence in India.[16] In addition, comorbid alcohol was significantly associated with suicidal attempts in PWID in India.[16] Suicidality is also influenced by duration of IV drug use and is three times more common in persons injecting drugs for more than 21 years than those injecting for less than 10 years.[16]

In a study from North India that was done in context of human right abuses among PWID, the prevalence of suicidal ideation was nearly 50%. Further, there was a positive correlation between human rights violation and suicidal thoughts among PWID.[17]

People who inject drugs with suicidal thoughts are more likely to have high-risk sexual behaviors such as multiple sexual partners and unprotected sexual intercourse with paid partners.[18] Comorbid poor mental health, physical and sexual abuse, lack of homes, lower education status, SUD in parents, and social isolation are important factors contributing to suicidality in patients of opioid dependence.[18] Family disruption is a known phenomenon among patients having opioid dependence and has been described in Indian setting too.[19] As family system is core of Indian social structure, strained family relationships due to social stigma and shame associated with substances of abuse further contribute to poor mental health. This, in turn, is responsible for poor family relationships, marital conflicts, poor adherence to treatment protocols, and suicidality.

Cannabinoids

Most commonly used illicit substance worldwide is cannabis. It is widely believed that cannabis use increases risk of both attempted and completed suicides. This fact has been substantiated by various studies in past. In a prospective cohort study, more than 2,000 adolescents were followed for a period of 13 years. Although, in early adolescence, no association was found between cannabis use and suicidality, a significant association was seen when same cohort entered in their twenties (OR = 2.9). Significantly, cannabis use was by itself did not lead to depression.[20] In another twin study, suicidal attempts were 2.9 times more common in cannabis users than nonusers.[21] Although cannabis use is thought to increase the suicidal behavior through depressive symptoms, some case reports have suggested that occasional cannabis use may also induce suicidal ideas through paranoid thoughts and panic symptoms.[22] Naji et al. reported that although there was no gender difference with respect to suicidality in cannabis use disorder, heaviness of cannabis use did influence suicidality in men.[23]

However, in a large longitudinal study of more than 50,000 males, association of cannabis use with suicidality was eliminated after confounding factors were taken into consideration.[24] Even in a systematic review, this association could not be established.[25] There is no Indian data that specifically addresses this issue.

Other Substances of Abuse

Lifetime cocaine use has been associated with suicidality and posttraumatic stress disorder (PTSD).[26] A large number of individuals having cocaine dependence, currently abstinent, were interviewed for suicidality in past. About 43.5% of them attempted suicide at least once. Factors such as childhood abuse and neglect, concurrent alcohol dependence, and comorbid depression were strongly associated with cocaine-related suicidality.[27] In a multisite longitudinal study, cocaine as substance of abuse has been regarded as important predictor of future suicidal attempts even after abstinence.[28]

In US National Epidemiologic Survey on Alcohol and Related Conditions (NESARC), suicidal ideations were present in more than two-thirds of inhalant users and nearly 20% attempted suicide at least once in their lifetime. Risk of suicidality was highest among inhalant users who were either having dependence or were women.[29] Similarly, in a Brazilian study, there was a significant association of suicidality with both inhalants and cocaine use.[30]

There is a need of further studies to substantiate these results in different parts of world including India.

■ COMORBID MENTAL DISORDERS

Nearly 100% individuals who attempted suicides have some mental disorder. OR for suicide is highest among patients with bipolar disorder (7.77). Since impulsivity is predominant symptom both in bipolar disorder and in SUD and also an important aspect of psychopathology associated with suicidality, comorbid bipolar disorder and SUD exhibit highest risk of suicide.[31] Other psychiatric disorders too increase risk of suicides and the presence of SUD further increases suicidality among them.

However, this enhanced effect on suicidality is less clear in people with comorbid PTSD. While a Turkish study did predict enhanced suicidality in patients with alcohol dependence as well as PTSD, same was not seen in a study done on US-war veterans.[31] An additive effect of comorbid SUD on suicide-related mortality among patients discharged with a diagnosis of mental disorders was demonstrated in a Danish study.[32]

In Indian literature, sociocultural and economic factors play a significant role in

suicidal ideation and suicidal attempts.[16] In a community study of PWID in North India, mental disorders such as depression and anxiety were significantly associated with suicidal ideation but not with suicidal attempts.[16] Similarly, in a nation-wide population survey in Australia, social factors such as unemployment and relationship difficulties were associated with suicide attempts.[33] However, in developed world, many studies have found an association between suicidal attempts and psychological distress such as anxiety and depressive symptoms.[34] As persons with SUD are at extreme social disadvantage, especially in developing nations such as India, social factors may influence suicidality to great extent. It can also be concluded that, whereas psychological distress influences suicidal thoughts, both suicidal attempts and completed suicides are determined by socioeconomic factors to a great extent.

In Indian study by Bhattacharjee et al., dysthymic disorder was present in 66.66% of those who consumed alcohol prior to suicide attempt either enough to impair judgment or to facilitate suicide. More than one-third of those who consumed alcohol to facilitate suicide had intermittent explosive disorder as well.[13]

Hence, it can be concluded that comorbid psychiatric disorders enhance SUD-related suicidality.

■ SPECIAL SUBGROUPS

Adolescents

Adolescent suicidal behaviors pose a significant challenge, as suicide is one of the leading causes of mortality among this population. In 2014, 54,100 adolescents (aged 15–29 years) lost their lives due to suicides in India. This amounts to an economic loss of 378.7 billion rupee, thus significantly affecting economy of our country.[2] SUDs are among major risk factors that contribute in adolescent suicidal behaviors. Early onset of alcohol and tobacco use, cannabis, and other substance use or dependence is best predictors of suicidality in younger population.[31] Though suicides do not constitute top five causes of mortality in early adolescents, there is steep rise of suicides in late adolescence (15–19 years age group) where it becomes second most common cause of mortality worldwide.[35]

Among adolescents, estimated lifetime suicidal attempts among males and females are 1.3–3.8% and 1.5–10.1%, respectively. This gender difference is most likely due to different psychiatric comorbidities that influence suicidality synergistically. Whereas adolescent females are more likely to have internal distress and depression, adolescent males more commonly exhibit violence and antisocial behavior. Further, adolescent females with substance abuse are more likely to engage in high-risk sexual activities than males. As a result, suicidal and self-harm events are more common in adolescent females, whereas males are more likely to indulge in violent and completed suicides.[31]

Women

There is dearth of knowledge about gender differences in this phenomenon. Lower suicide rates among women in developed countries and tendency to exclude women in earlier studies may have led to meager data on this issue. Suicides are often unreported, as it is often treated as illegal in most of countries. Suicides are more common among men, whereas nonfatal suicidal events are more prevalent among women. These are responsible for paucity of studies investigating suicidality and SUD in women.

In a review by Wilcox et al., they have demonstrated that SMR due to suicide by alcohol is significantly higher for women as compared to men (1690 vs. 483). Both reviews by Harris and Barraclough and Wilcox et al. have concluded that association between suicidality and AUD is stronger in women.[4] Naji et al. merged the data of two studies and studied gender differences in suicidal behaviors among cannabis use disorder patients. Unlike general population, no significant difference was seen in suicidal behavior among men and women who had cannabis use disorder.[23]

Sexual Minorities

Lesbian–gay–bisexual (LGB) and commercial sexual workers (CSW) are major subgroups among sexual minorities. They suffer from increased stress and social isolation. A large study comprising of >12,000 LGB youth reported that the lifetime risk of suicidal attempts in this subpopulation is 2.5 times higher than their heterosexual counterparts. Similarly, alcohol and other SUDs were 1.5 times higher in LGB subgroup.[36] Approaching this subgroup is very difficult. Most of them either do not disclose their sexual preferences or are not sure of their sexual preferences. So, healthcare providers must pay extra attention to their needs. Prospective studies to identify their needs and problems are need of hour. Among persons with SUD and PWID, forced sex and sexual abuse have been regarded as important contributors for both suicidality and suicidal attempts.[16,36]

COVID-19 AND SUD-RELATED SUICIDALITY

The COVID-19 pandemic is bound to cause negative impact on mental health through fear of uncertainty, social isolation, and economic losses. Earlier too, disasters have contributed to increased mood and anxiety disorders and suicidal behaviors. This is more pronounced among people with SUD.[37] Those with SUD may experience change in drug use pattern either as increased consumption as reactive behavior to negative impact of pandemic or shift to some other substance as a part nonavailability. They may also experience relapse in view of poor access to medical facility and may experience fatal overdoses as well. These factors are bound to increase stress and in-turn suicidality in people with SUD.[38] In India, increased suicides due to nonavailability of alcohol have been reported from several southern states during lockdown in March–May, 2020. More flexible take-home medication programs, increased access to telemedicine services, and behavioral therapies must be encouraged all over.

■ MANAGEMENT

In our country, mortality due to suicide is twice that of HIV/AIDS. However, it has got less public attention.[39] Suicides not only lead to loss of life but causes significant mental and emotional stress to family and close ones. As only one in twenty suicidal attempts results in completed suicide, need for effective suicidal prevention strategies cannot be undermined. Persons with SUDs are at greater risk of both attempted and completed suicides. Whereas depression and other psychiatric disorders are important contributors of suicide, socioeconomic factors such as homelessness, unemployment, exposure to violence, violation of human rights, sexual abuse, and poor family support have been identified as important factors associated with suicide among people who abuse drugs in India. Hence, in addition to strengthening mental health services, protection of basic human rights needs special attention.[16,17]

It is very important to design strategies that maximize the accurate assessment of high-risk individuals. Further reducing suicidal thoughts and attempts in these high-risk populations remain a challenge as exact efficacy of different interventions is not easy to predict and has not been studied across the globe. Since both suicidality and SUDs are most prevalent in adolescents and young adults, this subgroup should receive maximum focus. Patients with SUDs in general and high-risk subgroups such as adolescents, sexual minorities, and those with comorbid mental disorders must be assessed time-to-time by validated assessment scales while avoiding stigmatization. Since many of these patients are suffering from "dual diagnosis" (psychiatry illness comorbid with SUD), both mental health and deaddiction services must be integrated and all patients must be managed holistically.

Evidence regarding role of psychosocial interventions such as cognitive behavioral therapy (CBT) and dialectical behavior therapy (DBT)-based interventions in reducing future self-harm episodes is low-to-moderate quality only.[40] Cannabis youth treatment study was one of the largest trials that studied efficacy of psychosocial interventions in SUDs. Although five sessions of motivational enhancing therapy and CBT were found to be efficacious and cost-effective in treatment of SUDs, whether these would have any suicide-lowering effect too—is difficult to predict.[41]

Although many strategies are available for suicide prevention and treatment, it is seen throughout the world that most of those who complete suicide were not in contact with mental health services in recent past. Hence, awareness and exposure of youth through various media sources; screening programs at school, college, community levels in a nonjudgmental environment; motivating and encouraging for referral to primary care and also to mental health and deaddiction services; and retention in these services may carry a substantial impact in the strategies toward suicide prevention.

■ REFERENCES

1. National Crime and Research Bureau (NCRB), Govt. of India. Suicides in India in Accidental Deaths and Suicides in India. 2020;2:196-208.
2. Mathew A, Suja MK, Priya V. Critical overview of adolescent suicides in India; A public health concern. Medico Legal Update. 2020;20:1351-8.
3. Kamalja KK, Khangar NV. A statistical study of suicidal behaviour of Indians. Egyptian J Forensic Sci. 2017;7:12.
4. Wilcox HC, Conner KR, Caine ED. Association of alcohol and drug use disorders and completed suicide: An empirical review of cohort studies. Drug Alcohol Depend. 2004;76:S11-9.
5. Schneider B. Substance use disorders and risk for completed suicide. Arch Suicide Res. 2009;13:303-16.
6. Gupta R, Narnoli S, Das N, Sarkar S, Balhara YPS. Patterns and predictors of self-harm in patients with substance-use disorder. Indian J Psychiatry. 2019;61:431-8.
7. WHO. Global status report on alcohol and health 2014. Geneva: World Health Organization; 2014.
8. Esang M, Saeed A. A closer look at substance use and suicide. Am J Psychiatry Resid J. 2018;13:6-8.
9. Blow FC, Brockmann LM, Barry KL. Role of alcohol in late-life suicide. Alcohol Clin Exp Res. 2004;28:S48-56.
10. Pompili M, Serafini G, Innamorati M, Dominici G, Ferracuti S, Kotzalidis GD, et al. Suicidal behavior and alcohol abuse. Int J Environ Res Public Health. 2010;7: 1392-431.
11. Breet E, Goldstone D, Bantjes J. Substance use and suicidal ideation and behaviour in low- and middle-income countries: A systematic review. BMC Public Health. 2018;18:549.
12. Sreelatha P, Haritha G, Ryali VS, Janakiraman RP. Alcohol dependence syndrome in suicide attempters: A cross-sectional study in a rural tertiary hospital. Arch Med Health Sci. 2019;7:195-200.
13. Bhattacharjee S, Bhattacharjee A, Thakurta RG, Ray P, Singh OP. Putative effect of alcohol on suicide attempters: An evaluative study in a tertiary medical college. Ind J Psychol Med. 2012;34:371-5.
14. Rane A, Nadkarni A. Suicide in India: A systematic review. Shanghai Arch Psychiatry. 2014;26:69-79.
15. Harris EC, Barraclough B. Suicide as an outcome for mental disorders. A meta-analysis. Br J Psychiatry. 1997;170:205-28.
16. Armstrong G, Jorm AF, Samson L, Joubert L, Singh S, Kermode M. Suicidal ideation and attempts among men who inject drugs in Delhi, India: Psychological and social risk factors. Soc Psychiatry Psychiatr Epidemiol. 2014;49:1367-77.
17. Sarin E, Samson L, Sweat M, Beyrer C. Human rights abuses and suicidal ideation among male injecting drug users in Delhi, India. Int J Drug Policy. 2011;22:161-6.
18. Armstrong G, Jorm AF, Samson L, Joubert L, Nuken A, Singh S, et al. Association of depression, anxiety, and suicidal ideation with high-risk behaviors among men who inject drugs in Delhi, India. J Acquir Immune Defic Syndr. 2013;64:502-10.
19. Mattoo SK, Nebhinani N, Kumar BA, Basu D, Kulhara P. Family burden with substance dependence: A study from India. Indian J Med Res. 2013;137:704-11.
20. Pedersen W. Does cannabis use lead to depression and suicidal behaviours? A population-based longitudinal study. Acta Psychiatr Scand. 2008;118:395-403.
21. Lynskey MT, Glowinski AL, Todorov AA, Bucholz KK, Madden PA, Nelson EC, et al. Major depressive disorder, suicidal ideation, and suicide attempt in twins discordant

for cannabis dependence and early-onset cannabis use. Arch Gen Psychiatry. 2004;61:1026-32.

22. Raja M, Azzoni A. Suicidal ideation induced by episodic cannabis use. Case Rep Med. 2009;2009:321456

23. Naji L, Rosic T, Dennis B, Bhatt M, Sanger N, Hudson J, et al. The association between cannabis use and suicidal behavior in patients with psychiatric disorders: An analysis of sex differences. Biol Sex Differ. 2018;9:1-8.

24. Price C, Hemmingsson T, Lewis G, Zammit S, Allebeck P. Cannabis and suicide: Longitudinal study. Br J Psychiatry. 2009; 195:492-7.

25. Calabria B, Degenhardt L, Hall W, Lynskey M. Does cannabis use increase the risk of death? Systematic review of epidemiological evidence on adverse effects of cannabis use. Drug Alcohol Rev. 2010;29:318-30.

26. Roy A. Characteristics of cocaine dependent patients who attempt suicide. Arch Suicide Res. 2009;13:46-51.

27. Narvaez JC, Jansen K, Pinheiro RT, Kapczinski F, Silva RA, Pechansky F, et al. Psychiatric and substance-use comorbidities associated with lifetime crack cocaine use in young adults in the general population. Compre Psychiatry. 2014;55:1369-76.

28. Britton PC, Conner KR. Suicide attempts within 12 months of treatment for substance use disorders. Suicide Life Threat Behav. 2010;40:14-21.

29. Howard MO, Perron BE, Sacco P, Ilgen M, Vaughn MG, Garland E, et al. Suicide ideation and attempts among inhalant users: Results from the national epidemiologic survey on alcohol and related conditions. Suicide Life Threat Behav. 2010;40:276-86.

30. Zubaran C, Foresti K, Thorell MR, Franceschini P, Homero W. Depressive symptoms in crack and inhalant users in southern Brazil. J Ethn Subst Abuse. 2010;9:221-36.

31. Vijayakumara L, Kumarb MS, Vijayakumar V. Substance use and suicide. Curr Opin Psychiatry. 2011;24:197-202.

32. Christiansen E, Jensen BF. Suicide attempts after psychiatric care. Nord J Psychiatry. 2009; 63:132-9.

33. Fairweather AK, Anstey KJ, Rodgers B, Butterworth P. Factors distinguishing suicide attempters from suicide ideators in a community sample: Social issues and physical health problems. Psychol Med. 2006;36:1235-45.

34. Darke S, Ross J, Williamson A, Mills KL, Havard A, Teesson M. Patterns and correlates of attempted suicide by heroin users over a 3-year period: Findings from the Australian treatment outcome study. Drug Alcohol Depend. 2007;87:146-52.

35. Patton GC, Coffey C, Sawyer SM, Viner RM, Haller DM, Bose K, et al. Global parameters of mortality in young people: A systematic analysis of population health data. Lancet. 2009;374:881-92.

36. Havens JR, Strathdee SA, Fuller CM, Ikeda R, Friedman SR, Des Jarlais DC, et al. Correlates of attempted suicide among young injection drug users in a multi-site cohort. Drug Alcohol Depend. 2004;75:261-9.

37. Petterson S, Westfall J, Miller BF. Projected deaths of despair during the coronavirus recession. Well Being Trust. 2020;8:2020.

38. Chiappini S, Guirguis A, John A, Corkery JM, Schifano F. COVID-19: The hidden impact on mental health and drug addiction. Front Psychiatry. 2020;11:767.

39. Patel V, Ramasundarahettige C, Vijayakumar L, Thakur JS, Gajalakshmi V, Gururaj G. Suicide mortality in India: A nationally representative survey. Lancet. 2012;379:2343-51.

40. Padmanathana P, Hallb K, Morana P, Jonesa HE, Gunnella D, Carlislec V, et al. Prevention of suicide and reduction of self-harm among people with substance use disorder: A systematic review and meta-analysis of randomised controlled trials. Compr Psychiatry. 2020;96:152135.

41. Dennis M, Titus JC, Diamond G. The Cannabis youth treatment (CYT) experiment: Rationale, study design and analysis plan. Addiction. 2002;99(Suppl 1):16-34.

Personality Disorders and Suicide in India

Shubh Mohan Singh, Chandrima Naskar

ABSTRACT

Suicide is an act of deliberate self-murder. The epidemiology of suicide in India suggests that it is a public health crisis. However, good-quality data regarding the quantum and nature of in suicide is scarce. Existing epidemiological data suggests that suicide in India has some meaningful differences from that seen in the west. This is seen in the extent of suicide in youth and women, and in the role of stress in precipitating suicide. Personality factors and disorders may play an important role in explaining these differences. However, this line of inquiry is hampered by lack of epidemiological data regarding the prevalence of personality disorders and traits, and the emphasis on the study of severe mental illness in suicidology. The authors suggest possible mechanisms explaining this connection and how it may be influenced by social, cultural, and environmental factors. Considering the possibilities of suicide prevention based on modulation of personality factors, there is an urgent need to increase the evidence base in this area.

Keywords: Personality disorders; Suicide; Borderline.

■ INTRODUCTION

Suicide is an event with complex psychosocial and biological antecedents, which culminates in an act of deliberate self-murder. Suicide is often (though not invariably) preceded by suicidal behaviors. Suicidal behaviors can be understood as actions that have the potential to lead to the death of the perpetrator. These can vary in severity on continuums of intentionality and lethality.[1] Given the close correlations between the two, especially in a country such as India, we have expanded the scope of inquiry from suicide alone to suicide and suicidal behaviors for the purpose of this chapter.

It may be safe to say that suicidal behaviors are often meant to be symbolic of psychological distress and may act as a cry for help. Most suicidal behaviors do not culminate in completed suicide. However, as suicide ends in the death of an individual, unless previous psychiatric or medical records are available, it becomes difficult to conclude about pre-existing psychiatric morbidity with any certainty.

Popular and scientific literature emphasizes the role of severe mental illness (mostly depression and schizophrenia), substance abuse, and the role of stressors in the genesis of suicide.[2] However, another less apparent and less discussed factor that may underlie much of suicide and suicidal behaviors is that of personality factors and disorders of personality.[3,4]

Personality can be understood as individual, characteristic, and enduring patterns of behavior, thinking, and feeling. It is considered to be the product of experience and genetic predisposition and is taken to be crystallized by the beginning of adulthood. Characteristic traits of personality are often apparent even in childhood. Personality factors and traits may be understood as specific parts or patterns of personality which are well defined and measurable, are based on a specific theoretical construct (for example based on the 5-factor theory), and are consistent and stable.[5]

While there are various definitions and theories about personality, it is probably easier to define a personality disorder (PD). A PD can be understood as an enduring pattern of inner experience and behavior that deviates markedly from the expectations of the individual's culture, is pervasive and inflexible, has an onset in adolescence or early adulthood, is stable over time, and leads to distress or impairment.[6] International Classification of Diseases 10th Revision (ICD-10) describes PDs as conditions that comprise deeply ingrained and enduring behavior patterns that manifest themselves as inflexible responses to a broad range of personal and social situations.[7] The ICD-11 brings a paradigm shift in the classification and diagnosis of PDs; in that, it completely does away with subtyping unlike earlier.[8] As nosological systems are atheoretical, these do not follow the variables as defined in the theories such as the 5-factor theory but make do with clinical descriptions instead. These PDs can be further usefully grouped into Cluster A (odd and eccentric), Cluster B (dramatic, unpredictable, and emotionally unstable), and Cluster C (anxious, fearful, and avoidant).

The mandate of this chapter is to discuss the association between suicide and PDs in India. A narrative literature review and analysis of data in this area exploring different aspects of the association was carried out and is presented below. In this chapter, we would mostly discuss the relationship between various subtypes of PDs (as per ICD-10 and DSM-IV (Diagnostic and Statistical Manual of mental Disorders-IV); 8 and 10 subtypes, respectively), personality traits, and suicide and suicidal behavior.

■ LITERATURE REVIEW

Prevalence of Personality Disorders with an Emphasis on Indian Data

Good-quality epidemiological data regarding the prevalence of PDs in India is scarce. There are very few studies from India that have assessed the prevalence of PDs in either hospital or the general population. The available studies show a much lower weighted prevalence of 0.6% compared to the Western data.[9] The National Mental Health Survey done across India in 2015–2016 did not include any assessment for PDs.[10] Also, no recent study has tried to assess the prevalence of different PDs. The International Pilot Study of Personality Disorders (IPSPD) done in 1997 included a cohort of a clinical sample at Bangalore and found the prevalence to be schizotypal (19.1%) and borderline (14.7%) according to the DSM-III-R system; and emotionally unstable (8.6%) according to the ICD-I0 system.[11]

On the other hand, the most recent systematic review and meta-analysis completed in 2020 assessed 46 epidemiological studies across the six continents, reported a global pooled prevalence of 7.8% [95% confidence interval (CI) 6.1–9.5]. However, heterogeneity in results and study design acted as a significant confounding factor. Although studies from China (overall prevalence of PDs ~4%) and Bangladesh (overall prevalence of PDs ~0.5%) were included in this review, it is telling that no Indian studies were included. Also, this study noted that there was a large difference between the prevalence of PDs in Western and Asian countries.[12] Globally, the prevalence of cluster A, B, and C PDs was reported to be around 3.8% (95% CI: 3.2, 4.4%), 2.8% (1.6, 3.7%), and 5.0% (4.2, 5.9%), respectively.[12]

Thus, it is apparent that while PDs are relatively well researched and quantified in many other countries, there is very little good-quality data with regards to the prevalence of PDs in India. Whatever data exists suggests that there is a low prevalence of PDs in India and South Asia. This may be because of a genuinely low prevalence of PDs or an apparently low prevalence of PDs due to an overemphasis on severe mental illness and normalization of deviant behavior as result, or an underemphasis and undercounting of subsyndromal PDs.

We could not find any population-based surveys of personality traits in India as are available in some other parts and countries of the world. The most common model that is employed in population studies of personality traits and suicide research is the 5-factor model.[13,14] In addition, traits such as anger, hostility, and impulsivity have also been studied.[15,16]

However, as discussed below, there are indications and hints in Indian data about suicide that suggest a role of PDs and personality factors.

The Association of Suicide and Suicidal Behaviors and PDs

The usual methods for determining the prevalence of PDs and personality traits in suicide and suicidal behaviors are by determining the presence of these attributes in people who have exhibited suicidal behavior by diagnostic exercises in the latter or by psychological autopsy in those who have died by suicide.

Worldwide, a host of personality factors have been consistently identified to be associated with suicide and suicidal behaviors. These include factors such as high levels of neuroticism, low levels of extraversion, hostility, and social introversion, irritability, hostility, avoidant and obsessive–compulsive personality traits, impulsivity, self-criticism, among others.[16-18] However, these traits are difficult to compare as they are often products of different schools of theories of personality or classificatory systems.

Borderline PD and other cluster B PDs (antisocial, histrionic, and narcissistic) have been identified as consistent risk factors for suicide in various longitudinal studies done across the world.[19] In fact, suicidal behavior is a diagnostic criterion for borderline PD.

Psychological autopsies can provide valuable data. For instance, a meta-analysis of 27 psychological autopsy studies conducted worldwide showed that 87.3% of suicides had a psychiatric diagnosis, most commonly affective disorders.[20] PDs accounted for 16.2% of diagnoses, with the risk for PDs higher in male than female suicides, indicating the possibility of gender-specific clinical risk factors for suicide.[10,11] Thus, PDs and especially borderline PD confer an elevated risk for dying by suicide or suicidal behavior when compared to the normal population. However, it has been reported that the method of psychological autopsy, although quite effective in detecting axis I psychopathology, might not be sensitive enough to lead to a retrospective diagnosis of PDs, thus resulting in a possible underestimation of their role as a suicide risk factor.[21,22]

Tables 1 and 2 present the data with regards to these attributes in the Indian population. One needs to keep in mind, however, that data regarding the actual

TABLE 1: How suicide in India is different from the rest of the world.

Study	Population assessed	Completed suicide/suicide attempt/ideation	Findings	Conclusions	Finding relevant to personality disorders (PDs)
Rane and Nandkarni, 2014[23]	Systematic review (Indian population)	Completed	• 82–95 per 100,000 population • Highest in 20–29 years of age • Female > male in below 30 years of age; opposite in ≥30 years • Hanging and ingestion of op: most common methods • Among women, self-immolation is relatively common • Lower socio-economic status (LSES), mental illness (especially alcohol misuse), and interpersonal difficulties are the factors that are most closely associated with suicide	Compared to suicides in high-income countries, suicide in India is more prevalent in women (particularly young women), is much more likely to involve ingestion of pesticides is more closely associated with poverty and is less closely associated with mental illness	OR of PD and suicide (9.5, 95% CI = 2.3–84.1)[24]
Bernier et al., 2014[25]	Systematic review (Asian population)	Completed, attempt, and ideation	4 highest results from the 11 (52–87.1%) all came from suicidal cohorts, one was retrospective and examined cases of completed suicide	Highest rates of PD were found in suicidal cohorts within the various countries	

Contd…

Study	Population assessed	Completed suicide/suicide attempt/ ideation	Findings	Conclusions	Finding relevant to personality disorders (PDs)
Accidental deaths and suicides in India 2019, National Crime Records Bureau (NCRB)[26]	Data on suicides from police recorded suicide cases, Projected population from census	Completed	• Incidence: 10.4/lakh in 2019 • "family problems" (32.4) and "illness" (17.1) were the major causes • "Drug abuse/addiction" (5.6%), "marriage-related issues" (5.5%), "love affairs" (4.5%), "bankruptcy or indebtedness" (4.2%), "failure in examination" and "unemployment" (2.0% each), "professional/career problem" (1.2%) and "property dispute" (1.1%) • 30–45 years most vulnerable • Male:female ~2.5:1; in <18 years, f>m • Higher incidence among LSES, lesser education years • Cities > rural	—	No assessment of personality disorders associated with suicide
Radhakrishnan and Andrade, 2012[27]	Review of current literature; Only about 25% of deaths are registered And only about 10% are medically certified; thus NCRB has major under-reporting of suicide	Completed, attempt, ideation	Highest rate in 15–29 years age group (38 per 100,000 population) Among young people, suicidal behavior related to females, not attending school or college, lack of independent decision making, premarital sex, physical abuse at home, lifetime experience of sexual abuse, and probable common mental disorders	• Marital status is not necessarily protective • Female:male ratio in the rate of suicide is higher	• Multiple suicide attempts of low intentionality and lethality associated with maladaptive coping and impulsivity • Rate of PDs in attempted suicide in India ranges from 7 to 50% in various studies[28,15] • Most common diagnoses are schizoid, borderline, and antisocial personality disorders[29] • Among first attempters, the most common diagnoses: anankastic and histrionic personality disorder[15]

Contd…

Contd…

Study	Population assessed	Completed suicide/suicide attempt/ideation	Findings	Conclusions	Finding relevant to personality disorders (PDs)
Mythri and Ebnezar, 2016[30]	Systematic review	Completed	2 peaks in the age-specific suicide rates, one at 15–24 years and another around 65 years. F>M in younger age group	• Alcohol use disorders, financial problems, interpersonal problems, and academic or romantic failures form important issues causing psychological distress • Mental illness diagnosed in 3.8–25.4%: Much lesser than the global average	Impulsive personality trait reported as one of the major contributors to suicide in Indian studies; unlike the West, alcohol use disorders and impulsive personality traits are seen more often than specific psychiatric disorders such as depressive disorder
National Mental Health Survey, 2015–16[10]	Population survey (N = 34,748)	Suicidality	0.3% had at least one suicide attempt in the past month Prevalence of overall suicidality F>M; Highest in 40–49 years in females	LSES, depressive disorder, and alcohol use disorder had significant association with higher suicidality	No data on PD

Contd…

Contd…

Study	Population assessed	Completed suicide/suicide attempt/ideation	Findings	Conclusions	Finding relevant to personality disorders (PDs)
Kulkarni et al., 2013[31]	Case-control study between 100 first time suicide attempters and healthy controls	Suicide attempt	• 52% cases had PDs and 24% of controls had PD • Most common: Cluster-B (impulsive), then, cluster-A (schizoid) and cluster-C (anankastic) • In the attempter group, higher prevalence of multiple comorbid PDs, especially a combination of (dissocial and impulsive) and (paranoid, borderline, and anankastic)	Survivors of first suicide attempt are at 19 times increased odds of having psychiatric morbidity and/or comorbidity, especially with PD	Suicide attempters had significantly higher prevalence of PDs
Menon et al., 2015[32]	Chart review of 156 consecutive suicide attempters, Impact of gender on personality traits and suicide	Suicidality on Beck Suicide Intent Scale	Significant differences between men and women w.r.t. age ($p = 0.001$), formal employment ($p < 0.001$), the method of attempt ($p = 0.003$), and the attempt being under intoxication ($p < 0.001$)		Impulsivity did not differ significantly between men and women, but aggressiveness and past feelings and acts of violence were significantly higher in males

(CI: confidence interval)

TABLE 2: Insights obtained from psychological autopsies (PAs).

Study	Population assessed	Findings	Conclusions	Effect of personality disorders (PD) on suicide
Chavan et al., 2008[33]	101 suicides	59.4% between 20 and 29 years; 57.4% males; in 72.2% psychosocial stressors in 60.3% psychiatric illness in 33.6%	57.4% of the suicides were in migrants	No mention of PD or personality traits in the assessment
Milner et al., 2012[34]	Systematic review of PA studies from 2000 onwards, across China, Hong Kong, Taiwan, Bali, India, and Pakistan, Italy, Germany, Sweden, Hungary, UK, Canada, USA, Colombia	In non-Western countries, higher proportion of suicide is due to causes other than axis I or axis II disorder	In China and India, a higher proportion of suicides without a diagnosis than studies based in Europe, North America, or Canada	Only 1/3 of the studies assessed PDs in the PA.
Sinha et al., 2021[35]	16 PAs in suicide in individuals in armed forces	• 12 cases were having significant stressors and 10 cases had personal stressors • Failed love affair/conflict with a partner was the most common stressor (7 cases)	3 had a family history of mental illness, 3 had a known history of mental illness	None had diagnosed personality disorder; Premorbid personality was assessed, whether it had any effect on the suicide is not reported in the study
Menon et al., 2020[20]	Overview of all Indian studies on PAS till February 2020	Major risk factor for suicide in the Indian setting was stressful life events	This review suggests impulsivity/emotional instability/violence or aggression/resourcefulness/ tendency to conceal emotions/coping skills/ attitudes to suicide needs to be assessed as part of a PA	Only 2 studies: Gururaj et al., 2004 and Kulkarni et al., 2015 clearly state about assessing personality in PAs: Gururaj et al. found 20% prevalence of PD among 269 PAs that they did[36]

prevalence of suicide in India may be inaccurately reported due to low registration rates of death and misreporting of suicidal deaths as of accidental or natural causes. Thus, assessing the factors contributing to completed suicides is always a challenge.[27] As is obvious from the tables, a handful of studies from India have identified associations between suicide attempts and certain PDs or traits. PDs tend to be a risk factor for repetitive suicidal behaviors with low lethality and intent. Based on the different methodologies of assessment, different Indian studies report a range of 7–50% prevalence of PDs among those who exhibit suicidal behaviors. One study reported the most associated PDs with attempted suicide are schizoid, borderline, and antisocial disorders.[29] Another study assessed PDs among first-time suicide attempters and reported the most common diagnoses to be anankastic and histrionic disorders.[15] Indian and Asian studies have repeatedly reported a strong association of high impulsivity, low frustration tolerance, and psychosocial stressors with suicide attempts by self-immolation.[27]

Personality factors may be an important determinant of suicide and suicidal behavior.[16,37] The association of personality factors is inconsistent across studies. However, commonly implicated as per the five-factor theory are high levels of neuroticism and low levels of extraversion. In addition, there is a consistent association with aggression, hostility, and impulsivity.[37]

A recent systematic review to assess the epidemiological patterns of suicide in India concludes that unlike the Western data, where severe mental disorders are a major contributor to completed suicides, in India, impulsive personality traits and psychosocial stressors act as major contributors to completed suicides in India.[30] It is also evident from the handful of epidemiological studies on suicide that are available in India, higher prevalence of completed suicide in among younger population (15–24 years), higher prevalence among the females in the age group of 15–24 years (male > female in other age groups) as well as in those with alcohol use disorders, financial problems, interpersonal problems, and academic or romantic failures form important issues causing psychological distress and leading to a suicide attempt and completion.[30]

With regards to psychological autopsies in India, Menon et al. recently conducted a narrative review of 34 studies on psychological autopsies done in various kinds of suicidal death across India.[20] Only one case-control study looked into PDs as a contributing factor to the completed suicide and found out that 20% of individuals out of 269 had a history suggestive of PD at the time of their death by suicide.[36] The review found that the presence of mental illness, prior suicide attempts, interpersonal conflicts, substance use, financial loss, stressful life events, and solitary living arrangement were the seven most reported risk factors across the studies. The prevalence of mental illness among the deceased varied widely from 37 to 88% and was noted to be higher in the studies that employed a structured diagnostic instrument than those without. Overall, stressful life events were also a significant contributor to suicides in all these studies. Personality assessment was done in a handful of studies to conduct the psychological autopsy by using NEO-FFI (NEO Five-Factor Inventory) or Standardized Personality Assessment Scale, but they did not reflect as important contributor to the death as reported by the studies.[20] The occurrence of stressful life events immediately before the attempt came out to be a common factor among the majority of attempters.[20]

In addition, there are reports of copycat suicides, suicides in response to deaths, and suicides of prominent personalities such as film stars and political leaders, and methods of suicide that may be socially and culturally determined such as self-immolation or drowning which are not seen as often in other parts of the world.[38-41] Though older articles reiterate the cultural determinants playing an important role in suicide, we found that relatively lesser new articles have taken up this aspect.

■ DISCUSSION

It is well known that different regions differ at a population level about psychological characteristics. Thus, it is certainly feasible that this may be true for India and different regions in India. This is especially reflected in the differential epidemiology of suicide in India and in different regions in India. However, it is difficult to draw definitive conclusions about PDs and suicide, either individually or together in India based upon the quality and quantity of data available.

When we examine the reported low prevalence of PDs in India and Southeast Asia, we first need to examine why this is so. Is this a reflection of the real situation based on cultural explanations as speculated above or is there more to it? It is possible that PDs, by their very nature, attract less interest as compared to severe mental illness. Thus, the lack of research interest may itself be one of the reasons for the reported low prevalence due to lack of good-quality evidence. In addition, many disruptive and deviant behaviors may be culturally and socially determined and thus be different from that seen in the west and thus not be counted in standard checkbox methods of surveys. Finally, it is possible that rather than PDs, it is personality traits or subsyndromal PDs that

do not reach the threshold of "caseness" but are nevertheless important.

Personality is conceptualized as a product of nature (genes) and nurture (environment and culture) and determines how we respond to the world around us in the inner and outer space. Suicide is usually a deeply personal choice and act. There is evidence that suicide and suicidal behaviors are consistently associated with specific personality traits and disorders. So even though there is a dearth of evidence, we need to examine the issue of suicide and personality in the Indian context in some detail.

It is certain that the prevalence of suicide and suicidal behaviors in India is substantial and qualifies to be called a public health crisis. It is also clear that the epidemiological pattern of suicide in India is meaningfully different from that seen in the West. The nature of suicides in India suggests that a substantial quantum is brought about by stressful life events rather than severe mental illness. These stressful events are mostly encountered by and reacted to by young people and hence the preponderance of suicide in this age group. The methods employed for suicide and suicidal behaviors also exhibit peculiarities that are in all probability reflective of social and cultural influences rather than the accessibility of lethal means of self-harm. Further, the phenomenon of copycat suicides, suicides in temporal association with deaths of political leaders or movie stars, and suicide as a means of protest are also more common in the Indian context. How do we explain this difference? Various authors have pointed out the multiple etiologies of suicide and suicidal behaviors. The peculiarities of suicidal behavior in India suggest a role of culture and personality factors. While culture and environment provide a context in the sense of role models and legitimization of a certain course of action in response to a

Flowchart 1: Hypothesized model of how personality disorders/traits affect suicide and suicidal behavior.

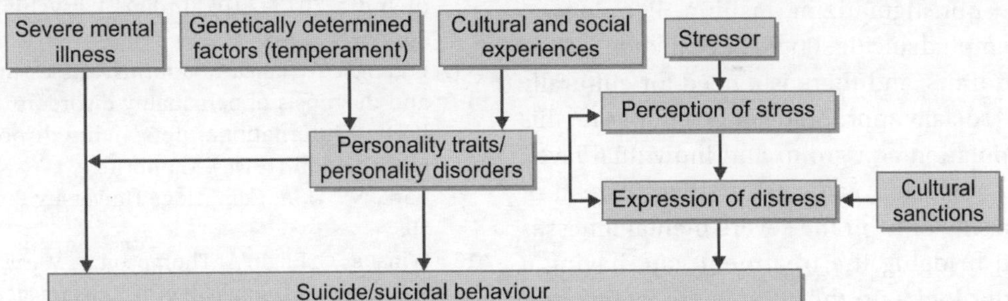

specific stressor, personality traits such as neuroticism and impulsivity can provide the necessary impetus to psychologically process the stressor into being responded to by self-harm and to create the motivation and indeed the recklessness and courage to take the step. Thus, it is possible that PDs and personality-related factors may play an important role in explaining this connection. This is illustrated in **Flowchart 1**.

As discussed above, personality factors determine the habitual and characteristic ways of responding to the demands of life in an individual. Whenever these characteristic ways are sufficiently deviant from whatever is considered normal for society, these qualify for being classified as PDs. PDs as well as certain personality traits have been regarded as risk factors for both suicidal behaviors and completed suicide. The degree of association and contribution is difficult to ascertain reliably and validly.[42] The contribution of PDs to suicide can follow multiple trajectories. These can include PDs acting as a risk factor for deliberate self-harm and completed suicide. This is exemplified by a host of data that suggest certain PDs such as borderline and antisocial are independently associated with suicide via personality traits such as identity disturbance, chronic feelings of emptiness, and frantic efforts to avoid abandonment.[19] PDs can also be comorbid with severe mental disorders,

affecting its course and treatment response, leading to suicide. This is especially so in mood disorders, eating disorders, substance abuse, and anxiety disorders. All of these are characterized by an elevated risk of suicide. PDs and traits can also make individuals more vulnerable to suicidal behavior and completed suicide. This is especially so in borderline PD and antisocial PD.[3]

The implications of the discussion above are potentially far-reaching. Firstly, recognition of personality factors in suicidal behavior and suicide are likely to be important from a preventive point of view. This can be at a universal, selective, and indicated level. Since each act of suicide is the result of an unique interaction of various sociodemographic, economic, cultural, and health-related factors in a larger ecological context, suicide prevention requires a clearer understanding of this interaction.[43] Universal methods of prevention can include media campaigns that seek to emphasize that suicide in India is associated with youth and stressful life situations and that young people often take recourse to self-harm. Also, media campaigns can focus on healthier ways of coping, seeking social support in addition to seeking help only for mental illnesses. Family members, teachers, and community can be made aware of traits impulsivity and neuroticism and can engage with people who have shown such traits in a nonjudgmental and nonstigmatizing fashion. People who attempted suicide should be evaluated for PDs and traits, and there is a need for culturally and socially appropriate interventions for this population at a group and individual level. In conclusion, we can say that, instead of focusing only on the severe mental illnesses and bridging the treatment gap, having a better look into the personality factors as a driving force of suicide seems essential.

■ REFERENCES

1. DeBastiani S, De Santis JP. Suicide lethality: A concept analysis. Issues Ment Health Nurs. 2018;39(2):117-25.
2. Brådvik L. Suicide risk and mental disorders. Int J Environ Res Public Health. 2018;15(9):2028.
3. Krysinska K, Heller TS, De Leo D. Suicide and deliberate self-harm in personality disorders. Curr Opin Psychiatry. 2006;19(1):95-101.
4. Bi B, Liu W, Zhou D, Fu X, Qin X, Wu J. Personality traits and suicide attempts with and without psychiatric disorders: Analysis of impulsivity and neuroticism. BMC Psychiatry. 2017;17(1):294.
5. Chmielewski MS, Morgan TA. Five-factor model of personality [Internet]. In: Gellman MD, Turner JR (Eds). Encyclopedia of Behavioral Medicine. New York, NY: Springer New York; 2013. pp. 803-4.
6. American Psychiatric Publishing. Diagnostic and statistical manual of mental disorders: DSM-5™, 5th edition. Arlington, VA, US: American Psychiatric Publishing, Inc.; 2013.
7. World Health Organization. (2004). ICD-10: International Statistical Classification of Diseases and related Health Problems: Tenth Revision. [online] Available from https://apps.who.int/iris/handle/10665/42980. [Last accessed July 2022].
8. Mulder RT. ICD-11 Personality Disorders: Utility and Implications of the New Model. Front Psychiatry. 2021;12:655548.
9. Sharan P. An overview of Indian research in personality disorders. Indian J Psychiatry. 2010;52(Suppl1):S250-4.
10. Murthy RS. National Mental Health Survey of India 2015–2016. Indian J Psychiatry. 2017;59(1):21-6.
11. Loranger AW, Janca A, Sartorius N. Assessment and diagnosis of personality disorders: the ICD-10 international personality disorder examination (IPDE). Cambridge, UK; New York, NY, USA: Cambridge University Press; 1997.
12. Winsper C, Bilgin A, Thompson A, Marwaha S, Chanen AM, Singh SP, et al. The prevalence of personality disorders in the community: A global systematic review and meta-analysis. Br J Psychiatry. 2020;216(2):69-78.
13. McCann SJH. Suicide, big five personality factors, and depression at the American state level. Arch Suicide Res. 2010;14(4):368-74.
14. Blüml V, Kapusta ND, Doering S, Brähler E, Wagner B, Kersting A. Personality factors and suicide risk in a representative sample of the German general population. PLOS One. 2013;8(10):e76646.
15. Chandrasekaran R, Gnanaseelan J, Sahai A, Swaminathan RP, Perme B. Psychiatric and personality disorders in survivors following their first suicide attempt. Indian J Psychiatry. 2003;45(2):45-8.
16. Kumar PNS, Rajmohan V, Sushil K. An exploratory analysis of personality factors contributed to suicide attempts. Indian J Psychol Med. 2013;35(4):378-84.
17. Schneider B, Schnabel A, Wetterling T, Bartusch B, Weber B, Georgi K. How do personality disorders modify suicide risk? J Pers Disord. 2008;22(3):233-45.
18. Yen S, Shea MT, Sanislow CA, Skodol AE, Grilo CM, Edelen MO, et al. Personality traits as prospective predictors of suicide attempts. Acta Psychiatr Scand. 2009;120(3):222-9.
19. Yen S, Peters JR, Nishar S, Grilo CM, Sanislow CA, Shea MT, et al. Association of borderline personality disorder criteria with suicide attempts: Findings from the collaborative longitudinal study of personality disorders over 10 years of follow-up. JAMA Psychiatry. 2021;78(2):187-94.
20. Menon V, Varadharajan N, Bascarane S, Subramanian K, Mukherjee MP, Kattimani S. Psychological autopsy: Overview of Indian

evidence, best practice elements, and a semi-structured interview guide. Indian J Psychiatry. 2020;62(6):631.

21. Arsenault-Lapierre G, Kim C, Turecki G. Psychiatric diagnoses in 3275 suicides: A meta-analysis. BMC Psychiatry. 2004;4:37.

22. Ernst C, Lalovic A, Lesage A, Seguin M, Tousignant M, Turecki G. Suicide and no axis I psychopathology. BMC Psychiatry. 2004;4(1):7.

23. Rane A, Nadkarni A. Suicide in India: A systematic review. Shanghai Arch Psychiatry. 2014;26(2):69-80.

24. Vijayakumar L, Rajkumar S. Are risk factors for suicide universal? A case-control study in India. Acta Psychiatrica Scandinavica. 1999;99(6):407-11.

25. Bernier G-L de, Kim Y-R, Sen P. A systematic review of the global prevalence of personality disorders in adult Asian populations. Personal Ment Health. 2014;8(4):264-75.

26. National Crime Records Bureau. (2019). Accidental Deaths & Suicides in India—2019. [online] Available from https://ncrb.gov.in/en/accidental-deaths-suicides-india-2019. [Last accessed July 2022].

27. Radhakrishnan R, Andrade C. Suicide: An Indian perspective. Indian J Psychiatry. 2012;54(4):304.

28. Latha KS, Bhat SM, D'Souza P. Suicide attempters in a general hospital unit in India: their socio-demographic and clinical profile-emphasis on cross-cultural aspects. Acta Psychiatr Scand. 1996;94(1):26-30.

29. Gupta SC, Singh H, Trivedi JK. Evaluation of suicidal risk in depressives and schizophrenics : A 2-year follow-up study. Indian J Psychiatry. 1992;34(4):298-310.

30. Mythri SV, Ebenezer JA. Suicide in India: Distinct epidemiological patterns and implications. Indian J Psychol Med. 2016;38(6):493-8.

31. Kulkarni RR, Rao KN, Begum S. Comorbidity of psychiatric and personality disorders in first suicide attempters: A case-control study. Asian J Psychiatr. 2013;6(5):410-6.

32. Menon V, Sarkar S, Kattimani S. Association between personality factors and suicide intent in attempted suicide: Gender as a possible mediator? Personal Ment Health. 2015;9(3):220-6.

33. Chavan BS, Singh GP, Kaur J, Kochar R. Psychological autopsy of 101 suicide cases from northwest region of India. Indian J Psychiatry. 2008;50(1):34.

34. Milner A, Sveticic J, De Leo D. Suicide in the absence of mental disorder? A review of psychological autopsy studies across countries. Int J Soc Psychiatry. 2013;59(6):545-54.

35. Sinha A, Gupta S, Ray M, Kumar S, Gupta AK. Lessons learned from psychological autopsies in armed forces. Indian J Psychol Med. 2021;43(2):150-3.

36. Gururaj G, Isaac MK, Subbakrishna DK, Ranjani R. Risk factors for completed suicides: A case-control study from Bangalore, India. Inj Control Saf Promot. 2004;11(3):183-91.

37. Singh PK, Rao VR. Explaining suicide attempt with personality traits of aggression and impulsivity in a high-risk tribal population of India. PLoS One. 2018;13(2):e0192969.

38. Vijayakumar L, John S. Is Hinduism ambivalent about suicide? Int J Soc Psychiatry. 2018;64(5):443-9.

39. Kannapiran T, Haroon AE, Vivekanandan S, Arunagiri S. Personality profiles of self-immolators. Indian J Psychiatry. 1997;39(1):37-40.

40. Maharajh HD, Abdool PS. Cultural aspects of suicide. Sci World J. 2005;5:736-46.

41. Menon V, Kar SK, Marthoenis M, Arafat SY, Sharma G, Kaliamoorthy C, et al. Is there any link between celebrity suicide and further suicidal behaviour in India? Int J Soc Psychiatry. 2021;67(5):453-60.

42. Duberstein PR, Conwell Y. Personality disorders and completed suicide: A methodological and conceptual review. Clin Psychol. 1997;4(4):359-76.

43. Patel V, Gonsalves PP. Suicide prevention: Putting the person at the center. PLoS Med. 2019;16(9):e1002938.

Medical Illness and Suicide in India

Pankaj Kumar, Rajeev Ranjan, Nidhi Varghese, Farheen Fatma

ABSTRACT

Medical illness is an important factor associated with suicide particularly among >50 years of age group. Suicide is significantly related to chronic, functionally disabling, life-threatening and terminal illness. The data regarding prevalence and risk factors are significantly lacking in Indian context. There is no policy, program, or identified suicide prevention strategies in medical illness in India. A large number of patients suffering from physical illness do commit suicide or exhibit suicide behaviors across life course of physical illness. However, they are not being identified, screened or managed at each level of healthcare system in our country. In this chapter, the prevalence and risk factors of suicide in physical illness will be described with focus on Indian scenario. The important physical illness and suicide patterns will also be described. The suicide risk assessment, management, and prevention strategies are proposed which will be suitable keeping in mind the Indian context. The suicide issue in terminally ill and palliative care setting is an important emerging area which requires attention so far as suicide behavior is increasing in such population. The gap in research in this area in Indian context is also being highlighted in this chapter. The prevention of suicide in physically ill population is an important area of public safety concern and this chapter is proposing a suicide prevention model to tackle this concern.

Keywords: Medical illness; Physical illness; Suicide.

■ INTRODUCTION

Suicide poses a significant health-risk worldwide. This risk is magnified in patients being treated for long-term physical illnesses. Medical illness is an important factor in 50 and 70% of suicidal behavior in age group of 50 years and 70 years, respectively.[11] According to NCRB (National Crime Records Bureau) in India, 21% of the 1.8 million suicides from 2001 to 2015 were because of their identified illnesses, of which 237,000 died by suicide because of chronic illnesses.[17]

Despite having clear evidence that suicide is linked to physical ailments especially chronic and functionally disabling diseases there are not enough prevalence or epidemiological studies to support this claim with data in India. This means a large number of patients are not being identified, screened, or managed despite early red flags and warning signs being present while visiting their primary care physician. Suicide in medical illness is a public health and hospital safety concern. There is an urgent need to understand suicidal trends in medical illness and the prevention and treatment strategies for various healthcare settings in India which will be further discussed in subsequent sections.

Concept of Chronic Illness/ Critical/Life-Threatening/ Debilitating Illness/Terminal Illness

Medical illnesses that pose high suicide risk can be examined in the perspective of spectrum of medical illness on the basis of severity and chronicity. *Chronic illnesses* which last for more than a year and require continued medical attention and affect activities of daily living. *Life-threatening diseases* which usually are long-lasting and incurable diseases and lower the life expectancy of people, while *critical illness* covers serious medical conditions referring to specific injury, illness, or medical episode. *Debilitating conditions* are medically diagnosable conditions which cause serious impairment in the patient's strength and ability to function in their daily lives. *Terminal illness* is an illness wherein it has a predictably fatal outcome and there is no known cure (in which death is expected within 6 months).

Epidemiology: Pattern and Prevalence Across Medical Illness

The population-based studies on chronic and life-threatening diseases have shown that the rate of suicide for cancer is 28.2 per 100,000 and suicide mortality ratio for suicide is 4.44,[37] for HIV the completed suicides are at 9.4%,[14] for chronic kidney disease (CKD) 22% of patients going through hemodialysis were reported to have suicidal ideations,[20] the rate of suicide among people with neurological conditions according to a retrospective Danish study was 44 per 100,000.[7] Of these neurological conditions, studies have shown that the rate of suicide for "multiple sclerosis" is 30.1 per 100,000[2] and 12% of people with epilepsy are under the risk of suicide. Historically, neurological conditions have reported the highest number of suicides among all medical illnesses. According to a Finnish study, the rate of death by suicide in hospital treated cardiovascular disease was 11% same as the general population but for patients with coronary artery disease the risk was two times more as compared to general population.[22] Another study showed that congestive heart failure (CHF) had the highest suicide mortality rate (SMR) of all cardiovascular diseases at 2.10 and peaked at year 2 and 10 of diagnosis.[35] Swedish study comparing death by suicide in traumatic brain injury (TBI) and healthy controls among 200,000 population found that death by suicide is three times more likely in TBI than in healthy controls.[8] A cross-sectional study on chronic pain patients (42% back pain) found that 19% had current passive suicide ideation, 13% had active thoughts of committing suicide, 5% had a current suicide plan, and 5% had a previous suicide attempt.

A study on 12 case series on 286 completed suicides carried out in general medical settings across America from 1947 to 2002 has shown that medical diagnoses that most often saw death by suicides were neoplasms at 25.2%, cardiovascular diseases at 16.1%, pulmonary diseases at 15.4%, neurological conditions at 13.3%, gastrointestinal diseases at 5.6%, injuries at 5.2%, orthopedic and rheumatological conditions at 4.2% allergies, and infectious disease at 4.9%, genitourinary at 4.2%, and others were at 5.9%.[1]

In India, one in every five suicides in India is because of identified illness. According to the data given by the National Crime Records Bureau (NCRB) out of 139,123 suicides in 2019, 17.1% died by suicide because of the fear, stress, and anxiety caused by their illness. According to these numbers, 23,830 people suffering from various ailments including cancer, paralysis, and HIV/AIDS chose to end their lives in 2019.[36] An analysis of NCRB data on suicides between 2001 and 2015 has shown 21% (385,000) of 1.84 million suicides were due to their ailments. 237,000 died by suicide because of their chronic illnesses. People suffering from cancer (11,099), paralysis (9,036), and HIV (9,419) died by suicide within the 15-year period. Maharashtra, Andhra Pradesh, Tamil Nadu, Karnataka, and Kerala are the states with the highest number of suicides reported.[17]

Psychopathology of Suicidality and Pathway of Suicidal Behavior in a Medically Ill Person

The interpersonal theory by Joiner and the stress (triggering)—diathesis (distal risk factors) model can be used to explain the suicidality in medical ill person **(Flowchart 1)**.[23]

In the stress-diathesis model, the contributing factors to suicidality and death by suicide can be categorized into state- and trait-dependent factors, or "proximal (triggering factors) and distal risk factors (predisposing factors)". Some of the proximal risk factors are psychiatric illness or its exacerbation, substance abuse, adverse life events, marital or financial issues, availability of lethal means to kill oneself and emotional pain. Distal risk factors are comprised of impulsive-aggressive personality traits, TBI, cognitive inflexibility, sensitivity to social stress, pessimism/hopelessness, childhood abuse, and family history of suicide.

In the interpersonal theory of suicide in context to medically ill person can be conceptualized as follows. Cognitive distortions induced by severe or critical injury or medical illness led to suicidal behavior. Cognitive distortions, mainly are of perceived burdensomeness (*"I am a burden/hopelessness"*) and/or thwarted belongingness (*"I am alone/feeling of loneliness"*). Both of these cognitive distortions, when present together, may lead to "readiness to die" or passive suicidal ideation. Transformation of suicidal desire into suicidal intent occurs only when an individual's fear for death is lowered. "Readiness to kill" may develop with repeated exposure to pain (emotional or physical) leading to a higher threshold for tolerating pain and decreased fear of death. Impulsivity and aggression, endophenotypes of suicidal behavior, may also elevate readiness to kill. In the presence of both "readiness to kill" and "readiness to die", probability of engaging in suicidal behavior increases substantially. Also, with each subsequent act of attempted suicide, one's "readiness to kill" increases due to habituation of the fear of death and dying, as well as there is increase in tolerance for pain.

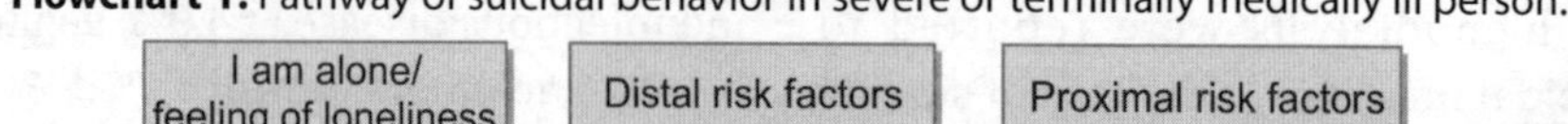

Flowchart 1: Pathway of suicidal behavior in severe or terminally medically ill person.

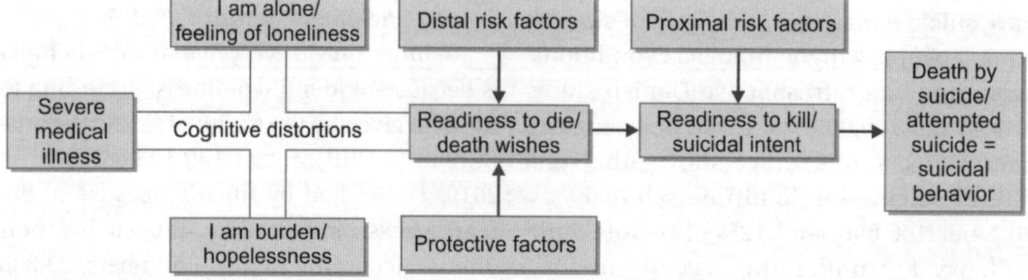

Source: Adapted from Joiner Interpersonal model and diathesis Model of Suicide by Mann et al, 1999.

FACTORS ASSOCIATED WITH SUICIDE IN MEDICAL ILLNESS

Majority of medical illnesses with increased risk of suicide are mostly associated with psychosocial construct that might be a gateway to syndromal psychiatric illness, substance use disorder, and drug-related side effects (**Box 1:** Risk factors). For example, in parkinsonism suicidality is associated with side effects of antiparkinsonian medications and the presence of neuropsychiatric manifestation.[21]

Table 1 below illustrates internal and external protective factors that hinder a patient's suicidal behaviors.

Depression as a Risk Factor for Suicide in the Medically Ill Person

Major depression in elders hospitalized with severe medical illness has been found to be over 10 times that reported in the community. Serious medical illness leads to an increased rate of depression, and further leads to an increased risk of suicide. Most importantly, physicians often fail to detect depression in the medically ill, or they view it as "appropriate" to the patient's condition. Therefore, depression, an important risk factor for suicide, is missed frequently or goes untreated. These patients often present with medically unexplained somatic symptoms and may be diagnosed incorrectly as being "somatizers" in primary care setting. Even other psychiatric illnesses and substance use disorders associated with high suicide risk, often go undetected and are not perceived as high risk in a medical setting.[31]

BOX 1: Risk factors for suicidality in medically ill person.

Individual factors:	*Treatment/Illness-related risk factors:*
• Previous psychiatric disorders or comorbidity • Family history of suicide • Problem-solving deficits • Advancing age • Male gender • Type A personality	• Poor outcomes • Pain • *Poor physician-patient relationship*: This includes failure to monitor the patient's emotional state. • Functional disability • Cognitive impairment • Burden of healthcare and expenditure
Psychological factors: • Loss of dignity • Dependency on others • Losing control of one's life • Burden to family • fear of abandonment • Seizing control by determining how and when to die	
Spiritual factors: • Receiving a deserved punishment • Uniting with others who died	
Social/Environmental factors: • Absence of family support • Earlier experiences with family members • Nonavailability of a competent doctor	

TABLE 1: Illustrating internal and external protective factors.

Internal	*External*
Increased threshold for frustration tolerance	Positive relationship with healthcare provider
Spiritual/Religious beliefs	Family responsibility
Coping skill	Social support
Capacity for reality testing	Illness information and adherence

SPECIFIC MEDICAL ILLNESSES AND SUICIDAL BEHAVIOR

HIV/AIDS

Suicide and HIV/AIDS continue to be major health problems. Global HIV/AIDS trends show that the number of people living with HIV/AIDS rose from around 8 million in 1990 to 34 million by the end of 2010.[10]

Fear of having AIDS could be a risk factor for suicidal ideation or behavior in young individuals diagnosed with HIV. It mostly affects younger people with less chance of comorbid medical illnesses, which generally affects the research finding of cause-effect relationship. The suicide rate in individuals infected with HIV/AIDS weas substantially higher in the earlier years of the epidemic. The rate began to fall in 90s. This decline was due to the improved treatments and emerging therapies. However, recent research studies still find a significantly increased rate of suicide in HIV/AIDS patients. It is not clear what factors (e.g., hopelessness, depression, and neuropsychiatric manifestation secondary to the disease) contribute to the pathways to suicide among HIV/AIDS patients.

Studies have found that during the first week of HIV testing, some asymptomatic HIV-infected people have a higher incidence of suicidal behavior than AIDS patients. The study also reported that a high level of suicidal ideation (27.5%) and suicidal plan in HIV-positive pregnant women. Gender is one of the important predictors of suicidal ideation. The risk of suicidal ideation in men is 1.8 times higher than in women. Others are lower levels of education and socioeconomic condition, who are vulnerable and succumbed to societal traditional belief or norms. It has been found that in certain beliefs, HIV/AIDS is sometimes conceptualized as a mysterious force, which leads to the negative social discourse and therefore the resistance to living with it is weakened, implying the experience of the "social death". Most seropositive patients with suicidal ideation belong to a younger age group (<30 years), which is consistent with the spread of age-related disease and the increase in suicidal behavior among young people.

It is well known that people living with HIV/AIDS experience stigma and discrimination in society. Stigma destroys a person's identity and ability to cope with illness, limits the possibility of disclosure, and leads to self-destructive behavior, despair, and depression.

Voluntary counseling and testing (VCT) gives patients the opportunity to understand their HIV status and, based on the test results, gives them the opportunity to receive immediate treatment and ultimately gives them the space to actively change their suicidal behavior. Suicide risk assessment and interventions in VCT clinics are important. Especially in the first 72 hours after transport in the diagnosis of HIV positive, these initial times can be considered as the best time to prevent suicide.[28]

Neurodegenerative Diseases

Suicide and neurodegenerative diseases share some common risk factors, such as depression, despair, and social isolation. The prevalence of suicidal ideation was 4.4% and 1.48%, respectively. These risk factors include men (single), aged 50–59 years or 70–89 years, financial problems, lack of social support, and lack of religious beliefs. Childhood mental disorders, despair, impulsivity, drug abuse, prior suicidal behaviors, and physical or sexual abuse play an important role. Neural structures that can be related to suicidal behavior are the tonsils, lateral septal nucleus, and the hippocampus which are involved in cognitive and behavioral control. Any neurological disease that involves these structures will increase the risk of suicide. Many known suicide risk factors, which have described earlier are common in Parkinson's disease (PD) patients (male gender, rural population, and history of psychiatric manifestation). Studies have shown that multiple sclerosis (MS) is closely related to depression; 25% of people find depression and it is related to the fatigue, anxiety, and pain associated with MS are associated with increased suicidal behavior. Most suicides occur within the first 5 years after diagnosis; younger patients, especially men, are at higher risk. These patients who committed suicide were more likely to be in a "chronic progressive" as opposed to an "exacerbating-remitting" pattern of symptoms at the time of death. They have more issues with mobility, vision as well as bladder and bowel function and severe depression. The suicide completers of MS were in the late stages of the disease at the time of death.[2] In TBI, neuropsychological deficits as mediators for increase in risk of suicidal behavior after moderate to severe injury. TBI usually results in injuries of focal and temporal lobes. Hence, behavioral, cognitive, and affective deficits are commonly present in these individuals. Also, personality changes, disinhibition, impulsivity, attention deficits, and lack of social awareness may contribute to suicidal behavior in these individuals. An increasing amount of evidence has linked inflammation and depressive symptomatology, which can be associated with suicidal behavior in TBI.[31] In Alzheimer's disease, studies have concluded that if there is suicidal ideation, it will occur in the early stages of the disease (within 6 months after the diagnosis with cognitive impairment). Depression is more prominent due to the loss of autonomy and the feeling of being a burden on others. In amyotrophic lateral sclerosis, the highest relative risk occurs in the first year after diagnosis. This peak responds to a strong emotional burden. In Huntington's disease, suicide is a serious problem, considering its high frequency. The period just before the diagnosis of the disease is the most turbulent phase because patients begin to realize that they have clearly lost their independence. Improved self-esteem, positive coping strategies, and strong social family support and religious belief, as well as adequate treatment for neuropsychiatric presentation are considered protective factors to prevent suicidal ideation in HD patients. For women, having children is considered as a protective factor.[5]

Cancer

Among nearly 4.6 million cancer patients, almost 1,600 died by suicide within a year of their diagnosis, which is thought to be twice as high as that of the general population. The risk of suicide in cancer patient persisted in almost all age and sex-specific subgroups. The risk is known to increase in first 5 years of follow-up. Suicide rate was increased in cancer involving multiple sites in compared with localized cancer. Among localized cancer, digestive organ (pancreatic and colon) cancer, lung cancer, and head and neck cancer have higher relative risk of suicide, but the risk did not seem to increase with breast and prostate cancer; may because of better treatment availability for these subtypes. Rates of death by suicide were nine times higher in persons with malignant neoplasms of the head and neck than in the general population, and about four times higher than in persons with other cancers, which might be due to cognitive inflexibility or nerve injury/inflammation which can cause affective symptoms.

Patients who underwent chemotherapy or no treatment had a higher risk of suicide than patients treated with surgery and/or radiation even when cancer is spread to multiple organs or sites. The risk of suicide in male compared with female was higher and the greater soon after diagnosis, which gradually decline with time.

Majority of the studies are epidemiological and provide little data on the psychopathology of those patients who committed suicide. Therefore, we do not know the mental status of the patient. Chemotherapy which increased risk of suicide either by inducing an affective symptoms/disorders or that the use of chemotherapy itself related to sense of hopelessness.

Vice versa, patient who suffers from illness of anxiety disorders and cancerphobia as psychopathology are correlated with high risk of suicidal behavior. It may be due to cancer which is considered as the most dreaded form of illness in our society. Hence, cognitive distortion of "going to die" might be hidden voice for suicidal behavior in cancer patients. Psychological care of cancer patient would be discussed in section 5.[21]

Cardiovascular Disease

Patients with cardiovascular disease are increased risk of suicide within 2 years after the diagnosis of congestive cardiac failure. A large proportion of patients with coronary heart disease (CHD) suffer from depression. Depression is related to several negative health outcomes of patients with heart disease and is an independent risk factor for death. The severity of depression and the anxiety are most significantly correlated with suicidal ideation in patients with heart disease. More than half of suicide patients with suicidal thoughts are more likely living alone, retired, having frequent chest pain and history of stroke. The physical functions of stroke patients are restricted, which explains the psychological distress. Even without a mental disorder, stroke is associated with an increased risk of suicide.[18]

In patient with CHD, clinicians must pay close attention to these psychological conditions that accompany suicidal ideation and quickly discover these variables and timely intervention is the golden rule. Even if the patient refuses to directly answer the questions about suicidal tendencies, doctors can obtain information about related vulnerabilities. With gradually acquired clinical skills, they can identify patients with a higher likelihood of suicidal ideation and immediately refer them to appropriate psychological care.[6]

Chronic Obstructive Pulmonary Disease

Chronic obstructive pulmonary disease (COPD) patients usually have various restrictions in daily activities. The high incidences of depression, anxiety, and low quality of life make this population a high-risk group of suicide, with an average prevalence of 27.1% in these patients. Studies confirmed a positive correlation between COPD and suicide. In addition, people with COPD are 90% more likely to commit suicide than people without COPD. A higher suicide rate is observed in the elderly. It has been observed that suicidal ideation is closely related to moderate restrictions in daily activities and severe pain. People with COPD are more likely to show suicidal behavior when there is previous history of suicidal thoughts or attempts.

Recognizing that the suicide and suicidal behavior in COPD patients indicates immediate intervention. It should be noted that COPD is a heterogeneous disease that will delay diagnosis and treatment. Furthermore, risk factors related to suicide in COPD, such as mental disorders, mostly have not been adequately diagnosed and treated. It is essential to implement suicide prevention measures in this group of patients, including psychological care and adaptation to activities of daily living, which must begin with the diagnosis of COPD. Patients with COPD should form a self-help group which requires the attention of the health team and decision makers to prevent the suicide and its consequences.[27]

End-stage Renal Disease

The nature of the disease, its treatment requirements, and its debilitating effects on health, function, autonomy, and overall outlook may trigger suicidal thoughts in patients. Depression, anxiety, and other forms of mental illness are common in this population. People with end-stage renal disease (ESRD) may have suicidal thoughts, attempt suicide, or die by suicide. It is irreversible and can cause major changes in lifestyle, affect mental health and well-being. It is estimated that 20–25% of patients with ESRD experience depression, and >45% experience anxiety. A source reported that the suicide death rate of patients with ESRD is 15 times than that of the general population. According to records, suicidal behaviors from conception to completion of suicide occur more frequently in this population than in non-ESRD populations. ESRD patients receiving multiple invasive treatments may have suicide risk factors.

This suggests that ESRD patients should be the target of suicide prevention. These measures can be implemented more easily and effectively in dialysis centers, where patients with ESRD need to spend a lot of time receiving treatment and providing and monitoring most of their care. Referrals and helpline numbers of counselors, psychologists, or mental health professionals (MHPs) must be provided to all ESRD individuals and their families.[26]

Diabetes

Diabetes is also one of the major health problems worldwide, and its global epidemic continues to increase. More than 400 million people worldwide suffer from diabetes, and its prevalence continues to rise every year. Mental illnesses are common in people with diabetes, such as depression and suicidal ideation. A study shows that the incidence and suicide rate of diabetic patients is 2.35 per 10,000 person-years, which indicates that approximately 94,000 diabetic patients commit suicide every year in the world. Depressive symptoms and suicidal ideation are often seen in diabetic patients. There are several reasons that contribute to suicidality in diabetic patients. In addition, diabetic patients usually have dysfunction and comorbidities. Due to these defects, poor quality of life will further increase the severity of depression and the risk of suicide.

There is a great need to identify high-risk patients, and effective psychological support is needed to reduce the risk of suicide in these patients. In clinical practice, we need to be more aware of the suicide risk associated with diabetes. In addition, more research is needed to develop effective strategies to reduce the risk of suicide in diabetic patients and improve mental health outcomes.[32]

Gastrointestinal Illness

Chronic abdominal pain syndrome due to peptic ulcer or duodenal ulcer increases the risk of suicidal behavior. There are numerous reasons for increase in risk of suicidal behaviors in patients with chronic abdominal pain. It might be due to faulty coping style, hypervigilance, and pain amplification which leads to visceral and somatic symptoms that may cause suicidal behaviors. This relationship can exist independently or can be coexisting with depression. Suicidal evaluation for these sufferers may need correction of faulty coping into positive coping (catastrophizing vs. lively coping skill) and to deal with interpersonal stressor especially in children and adolescents.[29]

RISK ASSESSMENT, MANAGEMENT, AND PREVENTION STRATEGIES

Risk Assessment

It is well known that people with physical illnesses are at an increased risk for suicide. Chronicity, severity, and disability all contribute to the risk of suicidality.

For these reasons suicide risk assessment has been identified as a fundamental safety issued by hospital settings. Primary healthcare providers are more likely to come in contact with the medical illness patients who are suicidal. They can plan a more comprehensive approach for suicide risk assessment and prevention. The suicide risk assessment allows the health provider to recognize specific factors that may contribute to risk of suicidal behaviors and provide targets for intervention. It also helps to address the patient's immediate safety and determine the most appropriate setting for treatment. The risk assessment for suicide includes the following:

Identifying Warning Signs

Strongest warning signs and symptoms:
- Threatening or talking about killing themselves

- Talking about being a burden to family
- Seeking access to lethal substances and devices.

Other warning signs:
- Anxiety, preoccupation with illness, agitation, and irritability
- Insomnia or sleep disturbance
- Purposelessness or hopelessness
- Rage about illness and limitations surrounding the illness or disability
- Withdrawing from everyone
- Dramatic mood changes
- Feeling trapped due to illness and the constraints.[34]

Suicide Inquiry

If any warning signs or risk factors are present then a suicide inquiry is warranted. The suicide inquiry needs to happen in collaboration with patient, family, primary healthcare physician for medical illness, paramedical staff, and law enforcement if they were involved. Suicide inquiry includes eliciting a patient's suicidal thoughts or ideation, past history of suicide attempts, any plans or rehearsals of suicide, the degree of suicidal intent including present self-harm behaviors and patient's mental status **(Table 2)**.

Psychometric Instruments

The psychometric tools can be used to quantitatively assess the level of suicidal behavior in a patient. It also gives a rationale while documenting the level of risk in a suicidal patient and the intervention that needs to be planned further for them. These various assessment formats include established assessments for suicidal behavior to be rated by a clinician, self-report questionnaires for patients or scales measuring severity of depression, and structured clinical interview

TABLE 2: Proposed suicide inquiry screening questions that can be asked by Gatekeepers based on (Karasouli E, et al 2014).[15]

Suicidal thoughts	Have you thought about stopping your medications or withdrawing from treatment?	Have you had any thoughts of harming yourself?	Do you often feel overwhelmed by your disease and think about escaping it through death?
Suicidal ideation	Do you ever feel like life is not worth living anymore?	Does the physical limitation of your illness (e.g., decreased mobility, decreased bladder/bowel function) make you feel suicidal?	Do you feel your illness makes you feel like you are a burden to everyone?
Suicidal intent/Aborted attempts	Have you tried to hurt yourself or end your life?	Do you have access to any lethal object or means?	What things about your illness make you want to end your life? What keeps you safe? (Reason to die vs. live)
Suicide plans	When you think about ending your life, what do you imagine?	What have you done to carry out your plan? For example, have you ever rehearsed your plan?	Have you made any preparations with personal belongings and finances?

assessing thought/ideation/intent/behavior/plan/past history **(Table 3)**.

Limitation and Assuming Professional Responsibility

The psychometric tools are not fully reliable in gauging suicide risk. The clinician has to rely on the clinical judgment based on structured and semi-structured interview along with the patient's history to identify the level of risk.

Suicide Management

The suicidal thoughts and behavior need to be identified as a modifiable target for management and intervention. Interventions usually target warning signs and dealing with motivational and skill deficits present in patients. In patients with medical illness, their illness-related thoughts and the management aspects include short term and brief strategies for crisis intervention as well as long-term strategies for inpatient and outpatient setting.

Safety Plan

Safety plans are lists of prioritized coping strategies used preceding or during a crisis by patient. It is made by patient and healthcare provider together and is said to be more effective than a no-harm contract. **Flowchart 2** illustrates the safety plan that can be followed for patients with medical illness.

Nonpharmacological Management Approaches

Nonpharmacological intervention is said to play a central role in suicide management. While there are no clear evidences on the reduction of mortality or morbidity in suicide

TABLE 3: Illustrating forms of suicidality and measuring tool.

Form of suicidality	Measurement tool	Author
Severity of depression (specifically focus on statements assessing suicide risk)	Hospital anxiety and depression scale (HADS)	Zigmond and Snaith (1983)
	Hamilton's scale for depression	Hamilton M (1988)
	Patient health questionnaire (PHQ)-9	Kroenke, Spitzer, Williams (1999)
Suicidal ideation	Beck's scale for suicidal ideation	Beck AT, Kovacs M, Weissman A (1979)
Suicidal ideation and suicidal behavior	Columbia suicide severity rating scale	The Columbia University, University of Pittsburgh and the University of Pennsylvania supported by National Institute of Mental Health of US (2008)
Deliberate self-harm	Self-harm inventory and semi-structured interview medical records	Sansone RA, Wiederman MW, Sansone LA (1998)
Planned suicide and arranged to end life	Composite international diagnostic interview (CIDI) 5.0	World Health Organization, World Mental Health (1990)
	Structured clinical interview	
Completed suicide	• Death reports • Interviewing family members • Hospital records	—

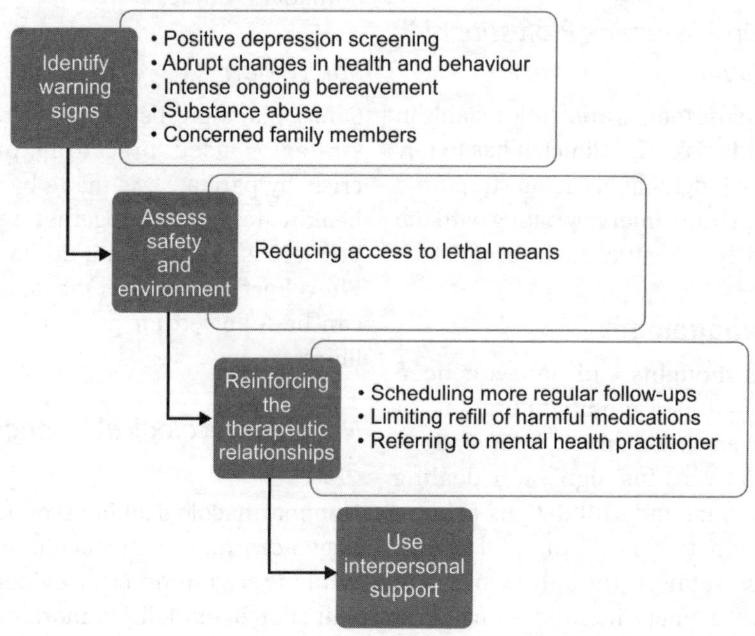

Flowchart 2: Illustrating safety plan for medically ill person.

with psychotherapy there are studies that prove the efficacy of these psychotherapies for depression and other mental disorders,[3] which are most often also associated with medical illness and suicidal behavior.

Nonpharmacological management toward suicide varies according to the settings and the level of healthcare facility available. **Figures 1 and 2** show psychosocial management in primary and secondary/tertiary care centers.

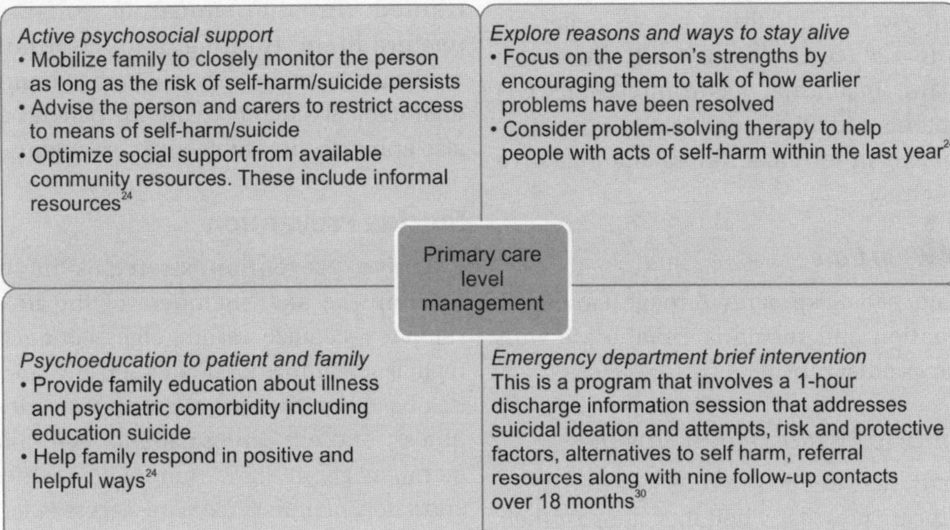

Fig. 1: Showing psychosocial management in primary care settings.

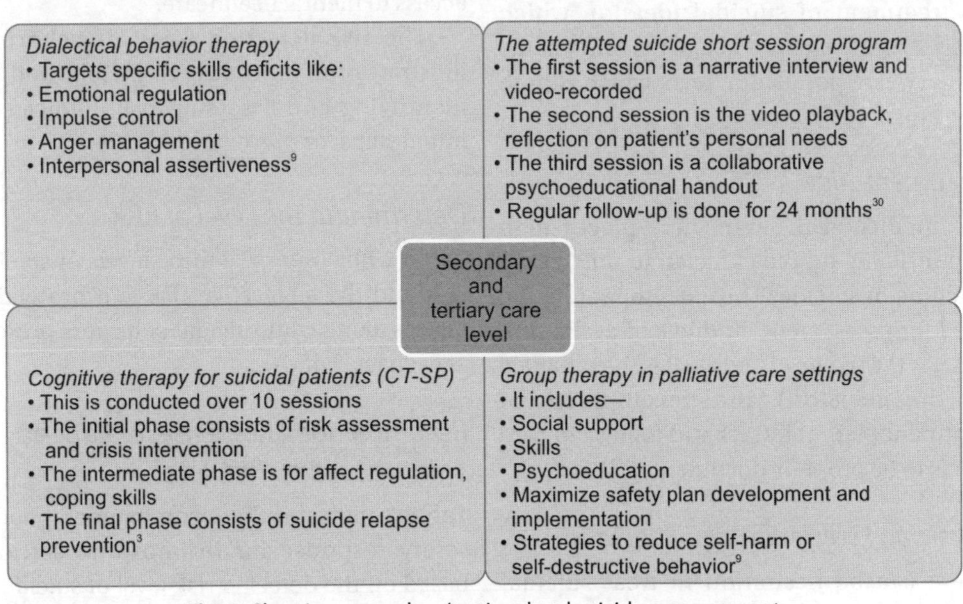

Fig. 2: Showing secondary/tertiary level suicide management.

Pharmacological Management

Identifying early sign of depression, anxiety, and other psychiatric morbidity and initiating appropriate pharmacological treatment is the significant way to mitigate the suicidal behavior in medically ill population. Off-label use of psychotropic drugs is a very effective way to reduce the distressing symptoms of pain, insomnia, gastrointestinal (GI) symptoms and other neurological symptoms especially in terminal illness and palliative care setting.

Follow-up Care

Monitor patient's progress through psychiatric evaluation and regularly collaborate with patient's other providers.[24]

Referral to Mental Health Provider

Physicians need to refer patients to healthcare provider when they are past their comfort level following failed trials to treat the psychiatric comorbidity. Establishing a primary care based collaborative approach for treatment of suicidal ideation which helps in reducing the suicidal tendency at the primary care population level which is both time and cost effective.[9]

Documentation

The medicolegal perspective places high responsibility on the clinician to predict the outcome of suicide. Thus, documenting the need for assessment, findings of evaluation (what is the risk level and what is the rationale for the decision), the development of treatment plan, referrals and follow-up care needs to be properly documented.[33]

Physician Evaluation and Education

There can be hesitation to treat suicidal patients due to lack of training. Physicians usually have a strong therapeutic alliance with patients having chronic physical illness as they have been treating them for a long time. This therapeutic alliance is a protective factor against suicide. To utilize this factor, it becomes essential that physicians are trained through education programs, postgraduate training and continuing medical education. This will help to improve their clinical outcomes with the patients and also enhance their subjective competency.[33]

Suicide Prevention

Effective prevention strategies include training the staff members of the health setup to recognize warning signs, conducting regular screenings for depression and suicide risk based on the chronicity and severity of illness, and educating patients and family members about the warning signs of suicide and safety planning/reducing access to lethal means. Suicide prevention also includes making effective strategies in hospitals and communities to improve public safety and access to mental healthcare.

The risk detection tree (**Flowchart 3**) illustrates the procedure to be followed for identifying and assessing risk followed by initial steps for preventing suicide.

Determining the Level of Risk

Table 4 illustrates the three levels of suicide risk and the suggestive risk and protective factors along with suicidal behaviors present at each level of risk.

Recommended Response for Patient Safety based on Risk level

Table 5 indicates the recommended patient safety response for the hospital settings based on the detected risk level of suicide in patient.

Flowchart 3: Suicide risk detection tree.

Identifying risk signs

- Current thoughts or plans of suicide/self-harm
- Worsening of medical illness/functional disability
- History of planning or attempts
- Lacks communication, agitated, hostile, distressed, etc.

Ask screening questions for detection of suicide risk → Document screening

At risk

No → Monitor changes in health and behavior in regular follow-ups

Yes → Do a comprehensive suicide assessment to detect the level of risk

- Psychosocial support
- Referral to mental health practitioners
- Regular follow-up for at least two months or until risk of suicide reduces

Source: Modified from Lewis DS et al (2014)[19] model for MS and mhGAP model for self-harm/suicide assessment by WHO (2016).[22]

TABLE 4: Illustration of characteristics of level of suicide.

Risk level	Risk factors	Protective factors	Suicidal evaluation
Risk of self-harm/suicide (Low risk)	Few risk factors, mild mood symptoms, evidence of self-control	Easily identified protective factors	Patient has thoughts of suicide but no plan or behavior during regular OPD visit for health checkup
Imminent risk (Moderate risk)	Baseline risk factors. Minimal mood symptoms, maintained self-control, rarely acute risk factors	Some identifiable protective factors	Patient might have suicidal ideation but no clear plan, previous suicide attempt might be present
Medically serious acts of self-harm (High risk)	Multiple risk factors, either at baseline or due to substances	Minimal protective factors	Patient has a plan with preparatory or rehearsal behavior

Source: Modified and based on Bryan and Rudd Model 2006[4] and pocket guide developed by WICHE Mental Health Program and Suicide Prevention Resource Centre.[34]

TABLE 5: Recommended Response for Patient Safety based on Risk level and common recommendations.

Risk level	Common recommendations	Recommended response for patient safety
Risk of self-harm/ suicide (Low risk)	• Do not leave the person alone and place them in a secure and supportive environment	• Further evaluate mood symptoms • Assess distress if worsening of illness is noticed
Imminent risk (Moderate risk)	• Manage pain related to illness or any concurrent mental health issues. • Offer and activate psychosocial support Offer caregivers support • Consult a mental health specialist, if available • Maintain regular contact and follow-up	• Repeated visits with increased duration • Involve family • Means restriction • Review the hospital protocols for crisis situation • If possible, offer a quiet room while waiting for treatment • Supervise and provide a named staff or family member to ensure safety • Attend to mental and emotional distress. • Provide psychoeducation to caregiver and patient
Medically serious acts of self-harm (High risk)		• Do not leave the person alone • Control mood symptoms with medications and psychotherapy • Reduce access to means • Frequent follow-up with phone calls • Hospitalize patient if suicide risk is increasing in each re-evaluation • Evaluation of patient on one-on-one basis • Care for person with self-harm behavior • Means restriction for acute period following hospitalization

Source: Modified and based on SAFE-T protocol developed through SAMSHA[33] and self-harm/ Behavior section of mhGAP Intervention Guide by WHO.[24]

Suicide Prevention at Community Level for Medical Illness

The following **Flowchart 4** illustrates the community level and public safety response for suicide prevention of people with medical illness.

PALLIATIVE CARE/END-OF-LIFE CARE, AND ASSISTED SUICIDE IN TERMINAL MEDICAL ILLNESS: EMERGING ROLE OF MENTAL HEALTH PROFESSIONALS

Individuals with terminal medical illnesses most likely to possess hopelessness, therefore, they frequently tend to commit suicides. However, it does not seem to be true for a fair proportion of individuals who have a terminal illness in current scenario because of improved medical facilities and better understanding of clinical condition. However, when there is loss of control of the final stages of life like irreversible brain damage, one should have autonomy of refusal of life-sustaining treatment. Decisions about the right to have dignified death should be made in advance in form of advance directive (Do not resuscitate or do not intubate; DNR/ DNI), which is not available in most of the time in our Indian culture, as our societal

Flowchart 4: Suicide prevention: At community level.

Step 1
- *Leading systematic and cultural changes in the attitude toward suicide*
- Community-based Suicide Awareness Programs along (Giving out brief pamphlates with information about suicide and mental health resources at hospitals and organizing awareness programs with local NGOs
- Holding mental health discussions on specific medical illness

Step 2
- *Crisis intervention plan*
- Telemedicine/Telecounseling
- National/state or NGO helpline numbers

Step 3
- *Train a competent and caring workforce*
- *Gatekeeper training:* Training community healthworkers, doctors, nurses, and paramedical staff to identify specific risk and protective factors for suicide in chronic illnesses
- Training for rural and lower income communities for identification, assessment, management, and referral of suicidal patients

Step 4
- *Identify individuals with suicide risk*
- Comprehensive screening and assessment for suicidal thoughts, behavior, and depression. Assess risk and protective factors in specific medical illnesses
- Assess people with physical illness on functional disability and associated severity of depression

Step 5
- *Engaging all patients at risk in suicide care management plan*
- Reducing access to lethal means most often used, e.g., in India having community storage of pesticides (most often used in rural India for lethal means suicide
- Community-based programs to reduce excessive alcohol and drugs use

Step 6
Treating suicidal thoughts using active psychosocial support at primary level and evidence-based treatments at secondary/tertiary level

Step 7
- *Transition individuals using warm handoffs and supportive contacts*
- Establish regular follow-up and checks on the patient and family

Step 8
Improve policies and procedures using continuous improvement

Source: Modified from Zero Suicide Model[30] and SPIRIT (Integrated Suicide Prevention Program, India).[25]

values and norms do not permit to talk about death. Hence, advance directive seems to be distant dream.

Role of MHPs is important in conditions such as neuronal injury, where deaths are prolonged due to medical advancement and sustaining life beyond certain point, when it is meaningless. MHPs should be able to assess capability to refuse treatment by patient with terminal medical illness. Mental competency can be assessed by patient's ability to make comparisons and manipulate pros and cons of continuing treatment. If mental competency assessment for withdrawal of life-sustaining treatment is not possible, then MHP has to look for advance directive, if that is also not available, then opt for surrogate decision makers (family members); when family members are also not available, then hospital ethics advisory committee have to decide and subsequently court have to be informed about the decision.[11]

Also, MHPs should know that life-sustaining treatments had a variation like one end, patients having multi-system failures are kept alive on a ventilator with very poor quality of life, while on the other end patients with ESRD who are maintained with dialysis treatments and may have very good quality of life. Therefore, withdrawal of life-sustaining treatment can be conceptualized in relation to the underlying condition and quality of life (whether it is administered just to delay the time of death).

Mental health professionals should be more focused and aware of rationale suicide. The concept of rationale suicide means withdrawal of life-sustaining treatment in background of the existence of a hopeless condition such as terminal illness along with chronic physical pain for which there are least possibilities of foreseeable improvement or relief. But, there are a number of caveats, which have to be addressed before accepting the rational suicide in the terminally ill. First, there can be increased rate of clinical depression among those with serious medical illness, which can be managed easily. Second, treating team decisions about ending life should be the last resort and as infrequent as

possible. Large time should be devoted to pain management and palliative care; recognize and treat underlying anxiety and depression; assist the patient in solving previously unresolved conflict with family members and friends; support the patient in grieving and saying good bye, therefore to bring good death with sense of ease and calmness. Lastly, in suicide-permissive society, elderly and terminally ill patients will be coerced into choosing suicide either by caregivers or family members, which has to be taken care by MHPs.[16] Role of MHPs in managing terminally ill patients is summarized in **Box 2**.

SUICIDALITY IN MEDICAL ILLNESSES IN INDIAN CONTEXT: GAPS IN RESEARCH AND WAY FORWARD

In a field of suicide research, the data from India in general is grossly inadequate in terms of availability, quality, and adequacy. The epidemiological studies regarding the prevalence and risk estimation of suicide behavior in medical illness is almost nonexistent. The official data source of National Crime Record Bureau (NCRB) is plagued by lack of clarity in systematic compilation of data, variable reporting methods and practices across states, underreporting and misreporting, and misplaced attribution of completed suicide to various factors. The legal ambiguity and stigma surrounding the suicide in Indian culture and society is also a significant limiting factor to conduct research in this field. The risk factors and good quality longitudinal cohort/case control design study in specific illness to estimate the relative risk/odds ratio and prediction of suicide behavior in Indian population with medical illness is glaringly abysmal. The experience of physical illness and its impact in terms of chronicity,

> **BOX 2:** Role of mental health professionals (MHPs) in managing terminally ill patients and in end-of-life care.
>
> - MHPs should use their therapeutic skills to bring about more-effective communication among patients, families, and hospital staff members. It will help them to talk about the emotional, legal, and ethical issues that generally complicate end-of-life decisions
> - Application of stress-management skills can promote a positive attitude and confidence about one's ability to function effectively
> - Providing compassion and support can help to patients who wish to continue living, and in those who are convinced to stop treatment
> - Helping patients and families getting in tune with dignified dying and the grief associated with it
> - Helping patients and families to resolve conflicts that was existing throughout, or at least they reach a level of expression and communication not previously possible. Such experiences can bring peace to the dying patient and to their family members
> - MHPs should work with the terminally ill to enhance the quality of their remaining life. They can educate different approaches for pain reduction and therapeutics to bear with difficult and invasive treatments. With such assistance, continued medical treatment may become tolerable
> - When end-of-life decisions need to be made, MHPs qualified by education and experience can evaluate patient's emotional and mental state and his/her mental capacity/competence to make treatment decisions
> - MHPs who are qualified by appropriate training can evaluate the decision-making capacity of patients who wish to refuse life-sustaining treatment or who wish to have their pain alleviation with increasing dose of medication even though it will accelerate death process
> - MHPs should be aware of state-mental-health laws (may expect them to prevent patients from committing suicide), when terminal ill patient is requesting assistance with suicide (voluntary euthanasia). MHPs should act as per law of land; however, they should voice for rational suicide in them

disability, healthcare, and economic burden is significantly influenced by the social, cultural, and economic factors which are quite different in low- and middle-income countries including India. Henceforth, it is imperative to do the good quality research (qualitative and quantitative) in Indian setting in order to understand the risk factors and interplay of biological, psychological, and social factors influencing the suicide behavior in medically ill population. The available global research data unequivocally supports the need to develop a prevention and management strategy for the suicidal behavior in such population. The suicide research should also be focused on developing culturally appropriate and locally acceptable models of suicide behavior management and prevention for different group of medically ill population as targeted intervention and primary prevention methods. The systematic and comprehensive approach for scientific and sustainable data collection of suicide behavior is the most fundamental and basic research gap in this field. A comprehensive data source which covers all possible sources of suicide-related information has to be developed to estimate and formulate a suicide prevention policy and program in India.

■ CONCLUSION

The medical illness is an important risk factor for suicide behavior and is associated with significant mortality and morbidity in our country. As the magnitudes of chronic physical illness are increasing in the population, the risk factors are compounding as the chronicity, multiplicity, and psychosocial impact of medical illness are multiplying. The noncommunicable diseases, terminal illnesses, and various types of neurological disorders are the important group of medical illness where the psychiatric assessment, assessment for suicide rate should be considered as an integral assessment protocol in the high-suicide-risk group of medically ill persons. The awareness, sensitization, and training of general healthcare staff are very important to identify and manage the high-suicide risk in the individuals at various levels of primary, secondary, and tertiary healthcare systems. The suicide research to evaluate and monitor the risk factors, suicide behavior pathways, and prevention and management strategy are significantly lacking in India. The integrated model of treatment and care of suicide behavior should be developed which is relevant for Indian social and cultural milieu. The bio-psycho-social approach is the most appropriate principle to decrease the magnitude and impact of suicide behavior in medical illnesses.

Conflict of interest: None.

Source of funding: None.

■ REFERENCES

1. Ballard ED, Pao M, Henderson D, Lee LM, Bostwick JM, Rosenstein DL. Suicide in the medical setting. Jt Comm J Qual Patient Saf. 2008;34(8):474-81.

2. Brenner P, Burkill S, Jokinen J, Hillert J, Bahmanyar S, Montgomery S. Multiple sclerosis and risk of attempted and completed suicide—a cohort study. Eur J Neurol. 2016;23(8):1329-36.

3. Brown GK, Karlin BE, Trockel M, Gordienko M, Yesavage J, Taylor CB. Effectiveness of cognitive behavioral therapy for veterans with depression and suicidal ideation. Arch Suicide Res. 2016;20(4):677-82.

4. Bryan CJ, Rudd MD. Advances in the assessment of suicide risk. J Clin Psychol. 2006;62(2):185-200.

5. Calero MG, Galiano AB. Neurodegenerative disease and suicide. Revista Científica de la Sociedad de Enfermería Neurológica (English edition). 2021.

6. Celano CM, Huffman JC. Heart failure and suicide: the role of depression. J cardiac failure. 2018;24(11):801.

7. Erlangsen A, Stenager E, Conwell Y, Andersen PK, Hawton K, Benros ME, et al Association Between Neurological Disorders and Death by Suicide in Denmark. JAMA. 2020;323(5):444-54.

8. Fazel S, Wolf A, Pillas D, Lichtenstein P, Langstrom N. Suicide, fatal injuries, and other causes of premature mortality in patients with traumatic brain injury: a 41-year Swedish population study. JAMA Psychiatry. 2014;326-333.

9. Jacobs DG, Baldessarini RJ, Conwell Y, Fawcett J A., Horton L, Meltzer H, et al. practice guideline for the Assessment and Treatment of Patients With Suicidal Behaviors. Am Psychiatr Assoc (APA). 2010.

10. Gizachew KD, Chekol YA, Basha EA, Mamuye SA, Wubetu AD. Suicidal ideation and attempt among people living with HIV/AIDS in selected public hospitals: Central Ethiopia. Ann general psychiatry. 2021;20(1):1-8.

11. Hendin H. Suicide, assisted suicide, and medical illness. J Clin Psychiatry. 1999;60(2):46-50.

12. Joiner T. Why people die by suicide. Cambridge, MA: Harvard University Press; 2005.

13. Jones JE, Hermann BP, Barry JJ, Gilliam FG, Kanner AM, Meador KJ. Rates and risk factors for suicide, suicidal ideation, and suicide attempts in chronic epilepsy. Editors' Bull. 2006;2(1):1-5.

14. Catalan J, Harding R, Sibley E, Clucas C, Croome N, Sherr L. HIV infection and mental health: Suicidal behaviour— Systematic review. Psychol Health Med. 2011;16(5):588-611.

15. Karasouli E, Latchford G, Owens D. The impact of chronic illness in suicidality: a qualitative exploration. Health Psychol Behav Med: an Open Access J. 2014;2(1):899-908.

16. Kleespies PM, Hughes DH, Gallacher FP. Suicide in the medically and terminally ill: psychological and ethical considerations. J clin psychol. 2000;56(9):1153-71.

17. Kumar Jain S. (2021). Troubled by illness, 385,000 people committed suicide between

2001 and 2015 [Internet]. Downtoearth.org. in. [online] Available from: https://www.downtoearth.org.in/news/health/troubled-by-illnesses-385-000-people-committed-suicide-between-2001-and-2015-56787 [Last accessed August, 2022].

18. Lehmann M, Kohlmann S, Gierk B, Murray AM, Löwe B. Suicidal ideation in patients with coronary heart disease and hypertension: Baseline results from the DEPSCREEN-INFO clinical trial. Clin psychol psychother. 2018;25(6):754-64.

19. Lewis DS, Anderson KH, Feuchtinger J. Suicide prevention in neurology patients: evidence to guide practice. J Neurosci Nurs. 2014;46(4):241-8.

20. Liu CH, Yeh MK, Weng SC, Bai MY, Chang JC. Suicide and chronic kidney disease: a case-control study. Nephrol Dial Transplant 2017;32(9):1524-9.

21. MacKenzie TB, Popkin MK. Suicide in the medical patient. Int J Psychiatry Med. 1988;17(1):3-22.

22. Mainio A, Hakko H, Räsänen P, Timonen M. Cardiovascular Diseases among Suiciders: a Population-Based Study in Northern Finland Population. Cardiovasc Psychiatry Neurol. 2010;2010:302102.

23. Mann JJ, Waternaux C, Haas GL, Malone KM. Toward a clinical model of suicidal behavior in psychiatric patients. *Am J Psychiatry.* 1999;156:181-9.

24. World Health Organization. (2016). mhGAP intervention guide for mental, neurological and substance use disorders in non-specialized health settings: mental health Gap Action Programme (mhGAP), version 2.0. World Health Organization. [online] Available from: https://apps.who.int/iris/handle/10665/250239 World Health Organization. [Last accessed August, 2022].

25. Pathare S, Shields-Zeeman L, Vijayakumar L, Pandit D, Nardodkar R, Chatterjee S, et al Evaluation of the SPIRIT Integrated Suicide Prevention Programme: study protocol for a cluster-randomised controlled trial in rural Gujarat, India. Trials. 2020;21:572.

26. Salvatore T, Dodson KD, Kivisalu TM, Harr D, Brown J. Suicide Risk and Suicide in End Stage Renal Disease Patients. Forensic Mental Health Practit. 2018;1(1):1-18.

27. Sampaio MS, Vieira WD, Bernardino ID, Herval AM, Flores-Mir C, Paranhos LR. Chronic obstructive pulmonary disease as a risk factor for suicide: a systematic review and meta-analysis. Respir med. 2019;151:11-8.

28. Schlebusch L, Govender RD. Elevated risk of suicidal ideation in HIV-positive persons. Depress Res Treat. 2015;2015:609172.

29. Spiegel B, Schoenfeld P, Naliboff B. Systematic review: the prevalence of suicidal behaviour in patients with chronic abdominal pain and irritable bowel syndrome. Aliment pharmacol therap. 2007;26(2):183-93.

30. Stone DM, Holland KM, Bartholow B, Crosby AE, Davis S, Wilkins N. Preventing Suicide: a Technical Package of Policies, Programs, and Practices. Atlanta, GA: National Center for Injury Prevention and Control, Centers for Disease Control and Prevention; 2017.

31. Wadhawan A, Stiller JW, Potocki E, Okusaga O, Dagdag A, Lowry CA, et al Traumatic brain injury and suicidal behavior: a review. J Alzheimer's dis. 2019;68(4):1339-70.9.

32. Wang B, An X, Shi X, Zhang JA. Management of endocrine disease: suicide risk in patients with diabetes: a systematic review and meta-analysis. Eur j endocrinol. 2017;177(4):R169-81.

33. Weber AN, Michail M, Thompson A, Fiedorowicz JG. Psychiatric Emergencies: Assessing and Managing Suicidal Ideation. Med Clin North Am. 2017;101(3):553-71.

34. WICHE Mental Health Program. Suicide Prevention and Primer-A guide for primary care physicians and medical practitioners., Final Tool Kit Version 2. Boulder: SPRC; 2018.

35. Wu V, Chang S, Kuo C, Liu J, Chen S, Yeh Y, et al Suicide death rates in patients with cardiovascular diseases: a 15-year nationwide cohort study in Taiwan. J Affect Disord. 2018;238:187-93.

36. Yasmeen A. 17.1% of suicides in 2019 linked to illnesses [Internet]. The Hindu. 2021 [online] Available from: https://www.thehindu.com/news/national/karnataka/171-of-suicides-in-2019-linked-to illnesses/article32564932.ece [Last accessed August, 2022].

37. Zaorsky NG, Zhang Y, Tuanquin L, Bluethmann SM, Park HS, Chinchilli VM. Suicide among cancer patients. Nat Commun. 2019;10(1):207.

Shubhangi R Parkar

ABSTRACT

The current chapter highlights the difference in suicidal behavior between the low- and middle-income countries and the western world. The various socio-cultural and biological factors leading to suicidal behavior and nonsuicidal self-injury are explored.

Keywords: Female suicide; Self-injury; Women.

◼ INTRODUCTION

Suicide is acknowledged as a major public health problem with wide-ranging social, economic, political, and psychological consequence. According to the World Health Organization (WHO), in 2015, about 800,000 suicides were recognized universally and 78% of all completed suicides occur in low- and middle-income countries. Southeast Asia accounts for roughly 40% of the estimated 800,000 annual suicide deaths globally. Generally, suicides account for 1.4% of premature deaths worldwide. Moreover, for every death by suicide, there are at least 8–20 more attempts. While it is important to understand the substantially heightened suicide risk for people with mental disorders, suicide is a multifaceted and highly stigmatized issue in India.[1] Though three times more men than women die by suicide worldwide, suicide attempts are higher in female gender. There is male–female disparity in completed suicides among various nations of the world. Female suicide completion rate is high in Sri Lanka, China, and also in India. However, the last decade has seen a sharp decrease in suicide rate of rural women. India has the highest number of suicides in the world. Indian men account for a quarter of global suicides, while Indian women despite making up less than 18% of the world's female population, account for more than 36% of all global suicides in the 15–39 age group.[2] Thus, making India as one of the countries with highest suicide rates among women, accounting for more than one-third of the total number suicides among women globally. According to the Global Health Data Exchange, India has the highest suicide rate among young and middle-aged women for countries with similar sociodemographics. In India, more girls below 14 years and young women than boys below 30 years are at a high risk of committing suicide. Suicide Death Rate (SDR) in India is higher than expected for its Socio-demographic Index level, especially for women, with substantial variations in the magnitude and men-to-women ratio between the states. Studies of female-only suicide are fairly sporadic. A comprehensive analysis and understanding of trends in SDRs over time for India and its states is nonetheless not readily available. The states of India have significant cultural, social, and economic variations, and various states have populations as large as mid-size or large countries. The escalating number of female suicides may be related to a conflict between women's increasing education and empowerment and the persistence of their subordinate status in Indian society. It is also speculated that these gender differences in SDR might be relatively less pronounced if suicide attempts were considered because women attempt more suicide attempts, but men are more likely to die in their attempts than women. Of women who committed suicides, the highest number was of house-wives followed by students and daily wage earners. The higher frequency of completed suicides among men and suicide attempts among women is called the gender paradox and has been reported in many different countries.[3] This paradox is absent in India and China where women and men present similar suicide rates. In addition, suicide among Indian and Chinese women may be preferred by the use of lethal methods such as self-burning in India and pesticides in China.

LIFE CYCLE AND SUICIDAL BEHAVIOR IN WOMEN

The literature revision revealed large cross-national differences in relation to life cycle and suicidal behavior in women.[4] Physical and sexual abuse, hormonal changes during the menstrual cycle and pregnancy, and the presence of psychiatric disorders are some of the known contributors to suicide in women. Some of the risk factors underline biological features, while others focus mainly on the feminine role and psychosocial aspects of gender.

Suicidal Behavior in Children and Adolescents

Infantile suicide is a rare incidence globally. Yet, the number of suicides among children and adolescents till 14 years of age appears to be increasing in several countries. In recent years, adolescent women from 13 years of age show an unpredicted upsurge of suicidal ideation, plans, and attempts together with a higher prevalence of mental disorders and substance abuse.[5] Additionally, young girls that committed suicide commonly had previous attempts and conflicts with their parents and left a note than male groups. The beginning of menarche is the moment when gender differences in the ratios of affective disorders and suicide behavior progress apart.

Women with Premenstrual Dysphoric Disorder (PMDD) and Premenstrual Syndrome (PMS) are at higher risk of suicidal thoughts, ideation, plans, and attempts compared with women without premenstrual disturbances. These findings were independent of other psychiatric comorbidities. Recent finding indicated that 30% of women with PMDD reported attempts to end their own life.[6] These inferences support regular suicidal risk assessments for women who suffer from moderate-to-severe premenstrual disturbance.[6]

Role of Reproductive Cycle and Maternity

Suicidal behaviors take place in 3–14% of the obstetric population. Depressed and anxious pregnant women have higher suicide risk compared to ones without these disorders. Younger age, unemployment, unplanned pregnancy, induced abortion, violence between intimate partners, low level of social support, sleep disturbances, drug abuse, and psychiatric disorders are important factors that increase suicidal behavior in women. In addition, these are independent predictors of suicidal ideations in women.[7] Suicidal ideations among the pregnant population are associated with several consequences that adversely affect maternal and infant outcomes including fetal growth restriction, premature labor, caesarean delivery, respiratory distress, and depression. There is a strong association between antenatal depressive symptoms and suicidal ideation in women. The presence of hormonal changes during pregnancy could be a risk factor for depression. Above and beyond that, depression decreases the level of the neurotransmitter serotonin, in which studies had shown an association between decreased level of serotonin and suicidal behavior.

Perinatal women who die by suicide are less likely than nonperinatal women who die by suicide to be receiving psychiatric treatment at the time of death. Pregnancy is a major common ground of discontinuing antidepressants. Several studies demonstrated that maternity plays a more significant role than marriage in the risk for completed suicide among middle-aged women when compared to men. Though the birth of a child is a protective factor against fatal and nonfatal self-harm, this protective function differs in pregnant women in presence of psychiatric disorders. The risk of suicide was calculated to be 70 times higher in women with psychiatric disorders during the first year after childbirth compared to the general female population. Approximately, 10–25% of pregnant and postpartum women experience depressive disorders or anxiety disorders. These women are more likely to complete suicide, especially within the first 2 months of the postpartum. Poor mental health, low socioeconomic status, and unmarried status are reported risk factors for suicide in the general population. Postnatal women who have a caesarean delivery, have a history of suicide, are unmarried, or have postpartum depressive disorder are at an increased risk of attempted suicide. Besides postnatal women with a low-birth-weight infant, lower education level, and a history of depression, anxiety and postpartum depressive disorder have an increased risk of completed suicide.[8] In addition, pregnant teens represent a high-risk group, with an estimated 16–44% prevalence rate of depression. Teen mothers are more likely to present suicidal thoughts or attempts, especially if it is the first pregnancy or if the pregnancy is unplanned. Suicide is the fourth cause of maternal deaths in the world and the leading cause of death in first-year postpartum women in the United Kingdom.

Suicide in Middle-aged Women, Marriage, and Divorce

In 2021, over 45,000 women died by suicide in India, 23,000 of them are housewives: [National Crime Records Bureau (NCRB) data 2021]. According to the accessible literature, married women are reduced risk to suicide than single, divorced, and widowed women. Marriage is known to be a protective measure worldwide. But in India, and other such low-income countries, marriage acts as an aggravating factor. Majority of suicides committed by housewives were reported in Tamil Nadu followed by Madhya Pradesh and Maharashtra which accounted for 13.9%, 13.2%, and 12.3% of total such suicides during 2021, respectively (NCRB Data 2021). Inability to adjust to a new environment and resolve interpersonal issues play a major role in pushing under-30 women to committing suicide. India being a progressive nation and gets more urban and rural women into the workforce, they are now facing double burden of traditional and modern workload that they are not fully equipped to cope up with. After marriage, the education and dreams of these housewives were put aside. Then, there are issues such as dowry, struggling to have a baby add up. All of this coupled with low coping skills and lack of economic independence and social support in patriarchy system leads to a lot of stress.[9] Quarrels with in-laws and problems in interpersonal relationships seem to be extremely common causes of attempted suicide in married women. Then despair and disappointment emerged into a suffering. Many women remain in violent situations but actively maintain their sanity simply because of the informal support they get. Additionally, there are other extreme problems that several women face, such as marital rape, emotional/physical abuse, or worse, that they often cannot remove themselves from. Even today it is not known the extent to which torture for dowry or other reasons resulting in death is passed off as suicide. Generally, housewives have poorer quality of life in comparison to working, married women who report higher self-esteem, and less hopelessness and insecurity than housewives, but further research is required in this area. During perimenopause, women have increased risk for suicidal ideation compared with pre- and postmenopausal women, as well as compared with men. Divorce touches in a singular way the risk of suicide among women. They present lower suicide rates after divorce than men, but the gender protection seems to decrease with advancing age.

Suicidal Behavior among the Oldest Women

Although suicide attempt rates reduce with age independently of gender, the rates of completed suicide augment with age in both men and women. In the group aged over 65 years, the male to female suicide ratio did not change in Eastern Europe or South America. There is greater risk of completing suicide in widowed, divorced, and never married old women. The death of the partner and loss of child is a prominent cause in the high rates of suicide in this age group.

■ CLINICAL PROFILE

The clinical risk factors are common in men and women. Depression the most known risk factor for serious suicidal behavior occurs twice as often in women as in men. The risk factors for men were a family history of suicide, comorbid substance abuse, and early separation. The risk factors for women identified are a previous suicide attempt, the lethality of the attempt, and lower number of reasons for living. Cougle et al. studied suicidal ideation and attempt in a national household probability sample of women.[10] The occurrence of merely post-traumatic stress disorder (PTSD) and a comorbid diagnosis of PTSD and Major Depressive Disorder (MDD) displayed the greater prevalence of suicide attempt than those with MDD only.[11] PTSD in general appears to be a particularly strong predictor of suicide attempt. People diagnosed with schizophrenia are significantly more likely to die from suicide than people in the general population. The risk of suicide is particularly increased in patients with prominent auditory hallucinations, paranoid delusions, and psychomotor agitation. It is also higher in patients with comorbid affective symptoms and substance use.

The researchers from National Institute on Alcohol Abuse and Alcoholism, USA reported that alcohol use may have been a core driver in the accelerated increase in suicide among US women. Kaplan and coauthors (2022) in their extensive study on 115,202 suicide decedents at the Center for Addiction and Mental Health, Institute for Mental Health Policy Research, in Toronto, found that while the prevalence of heavy alcohol use and the suicide mortality rate increased among men and women, women had experienced a notably higher increase in both. Borderline personality disorder has a strong relationship with self-harm and has been linked to childhood maltreatment and abuse.[12]

The death rate by suicide among people with eating disorders is not only higher than average, but higher than in those with depression, schizophrenia, or any other mental health disorder. Anorexia in women suicide is the second leading cause of death in those with anorexia and is projected to have a 50 fold increased risk of suicide. Both bulimia and anorexia are related to increased risk of suicide attempt. Furthermore, genetic factors, emotion dysregulation, trauma, stressful life events, and lack of body regard may have roles in the development of both eating disorders and suicidality.[13] In recent times, several studies have focused on attention-deficit hyperactivity disorder (ADHD) as a possible psychiatric disorder that may serve as a suicide risk factor in women as well. Impulsivity is a core symptom of ADHD that correlates to suicidal behavior.

Some studies have found that gynecologic cancer patients have a high risk of suicide than the general population. Women with gynecological malignancies (including ovarian, uterine cervical, vulvar, and vaginal cancers) have been found to have an increased risk of suicide compared with women in the general population.[14] Cluster headaches, which occur in cyclical patterns also called "suicide headaches" as the pain, aggravates suicidal thoughts, according to the Migraine Trust. Women with endometriosis had higher levels of depression leading to suicide compared with the control group.[15]

■ SOCIOCULTURAL ASPECT

Men and women vary in their roles, responsibilities, status and power, and these socially constructed differences intermingle with biological differences to contribute to divergence in their suicidal behavior. Despite evidence of intent, lethality, and hospitalization there has been a general tendency to identify suicidal behavior in women as manipulative and nonserious. One of the explanations for the lack of speculation in female suicidal behavior may be that of recognizing their suicidal attempts as "unsuccessful," "failed," or "attention-seeking" and generally inept or incompetent. Global focus being on the mortality of suicidal behavior (dominated by male deaths in all countries except China), the attempts of women are not taken critically. If both mortality and morbidity are considered collectively then it is apparent that the weight of disease burden in suicidal behavior is clearly female. Also, there has been increasing concern concerning the comparative significance of social determinants such as poverty and gender disadvantage related to oppressive attitudes toward women in many countries as being major contributors to the risk for attempted and completed suicide.

Data from a number of societies point out that wife abuse remains one of the most significant precipitants of female suicide and suicide attempts. The preference for the male child and the ill-treatment of the mother who gives birth to a female child is also seen in India. Dowry disputes is an additional distinctive form of abuse in Indian society is associated with suicide in women. In Indian study the most common reasons for suicidal attempts were marital and interpersonal problems with in-laws followed by psychiatric and physical illnesses, respectively.[16] A recent systematic review also found that women who experienced childhood maltreatment, particularly sexual abuse, were more at risk of engaging in "self-injurious" thoughts and behaviors.[17] The probability of death due to suicide jumps from 0.013 to 2.74% (>200 hundred-fold) for an Indian woman solely by virtue of being a housewife.[10] There is some evidence to suggest that having children or dependents can be a protective factor for women; this does not appear to extend to men. Social support has been found to be a protective factor against suicide for both men and women.

Domestic violence, in fact, is one of the most significant precipitants of suicide amongst women, with one-third of Indian women who take their lives having a history of suffering domestic violence. In India highest suicide rates in women are associated with the situation of extensive domestic violence. When they do not die from this cause, women may have physical and psychological squeal related to suicide attempts. These can be avoided through the prior recognition of warning signs of suicidal behavior, namely: rigidity of thought, impulsivity, and ambivalence. The recognition of violence as a major risk factor for women's ill-health must be fully included into mental health policy. Resources must be allocated to prevent violence against women and mitigating its consequences in order for the mental health needs of women to be effectively addressed. Many studies had found a strong and consistent association between intimate partner abuse and both suicidal ideation and attempts. The preference for the male child and the ill-treatment of the mother who gives birth to a female child is also seen in all socioeconomic sections of India. There is social evidence of an association between female suicidal behavior and childlessness in developing countries including India. Besides more married women reported marital violence, husbands with alcohol abuse, and extramarital affairs by husband as triggering factors for their self-destructive behaviors and suicide.

GENDER DIFFERENCES IN SUICIDE METHODS

Women who commit suicide use less violent methods, such as drugs and carbon monoxide poisoning, than do men, who more often use violent methods such as guns and hanging. Theories that enlightened this finding focus on gender differences in suicidal intent, socialization, emotions, interpersonal relationships, orientation and access to methods, and neurobiological factors. One assumption is that men tend to drift down toward more lethal methods than females because they have higher suicide intent. Men tend to choose violent (more lethal) suicide methods, such as firearms, hanging, and asphyxiation, whereas women are more likely to overdose on medications or drugs, drowning, and exsanguinations. It is proposed that women and men use different suicide methods as a result of the sex roles in their culture.[3] Suicide by burning or self-immolation amongst women is a major apprehension in India as it has become pervasive throughout all social strata and geographical areas.[16] The easy accessibility and familiarity of kerosene at home contribute to self-immolation being common method of suicide in general and even for women of

Indian origin even after migrating to UK. The use of lethal pesticides in suicide attempts by young women in Asia may contribute in higher suicide rate even if the intent was low. Women are more prone than men to make multiple suicide attempts, but this does not mean the attempts are not serious. In fact the likelihood of a critical outcome increase with further unsuccessful attempts—so it is essential that intervention is possible.

NONSUICIDAL SELF-INJURY

Nonsuicidal self-injury (NSSI) behavior is a rising clinical as well as public health problem. NSSI is defined as the direct and deliberate destruction of one's own bodily tissue in the absence of lethal intent and for reasons not socially sanctioned. Research on NSSI has focused on young women and girls, underpinning conventions of self-injury as a "feminine" behavior. More levels of NSSI in young women are moderately explained by their greater levels of psychological distress. Women are more possibly than men to experience depression and anxiety and this gender difference is the largest in mid-adolescence. Self-injury has been described as "impulsive" and impulsivity has been fundamental to academic explanations of women's explanations for self-harming.[18] Higher levels of depressive and anxious symptoms—which can be measured as psychological distress—may therefore contribute to women's greater prevalence of NSSI.[17]

PREVENTION OF SUICIDE IN WOMEN

Universally, there is an increasing emphasis on the need to identify suicide risk and prevention among women toward modification of prevention approaches by incorporating women's experiences. Certain factors communicate greater risk for suicide among women than among men, and which reasons may cluster together to rise risk among women. Women's needs in recovering from a nonfatal suicide attempt—increasing a sense of self-worth and developing stronger relationships with others. In India younger age, marital status, interpersonal conflicts, poverty, mental health concerns, undergoing violence, and medical comorbidities may altogether contribute to suicide risk among women. Hence, along with universal gender neutral model of suicide prevention, special attention is desirable to engage in identification of social determinants of suicide to develop suicide prevention strategies for women. Addressing stigma related to psychiatric disorders is another very critical area to be considered. The common issues of sexual discrimination, interpersonal violence, and economical difficulties require to be focused in the prevention strategies. Multipronged strategies to decrease domestic violence, endow with poverty relief, and improve treatment of mental and physical disorders are needed to reduce the population burden of attempted suicide.[19]

REFERENCES

1. Armstrong G, Vijayakumar L. Suicide in India: a complex public health tragedy in need of a plan. Lancet Public Health. 2018;3(10):e459-60.
2. R Dandona, G Anil Kumar, RS Dhaliwal, M Naghavi, T Vos, DK Shukla, et al. India Has a Female Suicide Crisis. Scientific American. 2016;319(6):20-1.
3. Canetto SS, Sakinofsky I. The gender paradox in suicide. Suicide Life Threat Behav. 1998 Spring;28(1):1-23.
4. Mendez-Bustos P, Lopez-Castroman L, Baca-García E, Ceverino A. Life cycle and suicidal behavior among women. ScientificWorldJournal 2013;2013:485851.

5. Eaton DK, Kann L, Kinchen S, Shanklin S, Ross J, Hawkins J, et al. Youth risk behavior surveillance—United States, 2007. MMWR Surveill Summ. 2008;57(4):1-131.

6. Khalifeh H, Hunt IM, Appleby L, Howard LM. Suicide in perinatal and non-perinatal women in contact with psychiatric services: 15-year findings from a UK national inquiry. Lancet Psychiatry. 2016;3(3):233-42.

7. Prasad D, Wollenhaupt-Aguiar B, Kidd KN, de Azevedo Cardoso T, Frey BN. Suicidal Risk in Women with Premenstrual Syndrome and Premenstrual Dysphoric Disorder: A Systematic Review and Meta-Analysis. J Womens Health (Larchmt). 2021;30(12):1693-707.

8. Reck C, Struben K, Backenstrass M, Stefenelli U, Reinig K, Fuchs T, et al. Prevalence, onset and comorbidity of postpartum anxiety and depressive disorders. Acta Psychiatr Scand. 2008;118(6):459-68.

9. Mayer P. Thinking Clearly about Suicide in India: Desperate Housewives, Despairing Farmers. Economic and Political Weekly. 2016;51(14):44-54.

10. Zadey S. Suicide and Indian housewives. Think Global Health; 2014.

11. Cougle JR, Resnick H, Kilpatrick DG. PTSD, depression, and their comorbidity in relation to suicidality: Cross-sectional and prospective analyses of a national probability sample of women. Depress Anxiety. 2009;26:1151-7.

12. Lange S, Kaplan MS, Tran A, Rehm, J. Growing alcohol use preceding death by suicide among women compared with men: Age-specific temporal trends, 2003–18. Addiction. 2022;117(9):2530-6.

13. Brezo J, Paris J, Turecki G. Personality traits as correlates of suicidal ideation, suicide attempts, and suicide completions: a systematic review. Acta Psychiatr Scand. 2006;113:180-206.

14. Smith AR, Ortiz SN, Forrest LN, Velkoff EA, Dodd DR. Which Comes First? An Examination of Associations and Shared Risk Factors for Eating Disorders and Suicidality. Curr Psychiatry Rep. 2018;20(9):77.

15. Mahdi H, Swensen RE, Munkarah AR, Chiang S, Luhrs K, Lockhart D, et al. Suicide in women with gynecologic cancer. Gynecol Oncol. 2011;122:344-9.

16. Lakshmi L. Suicide in women. Indian J Psychiatr. 2015;57(Suppl 2):S233-8.

17. Serafini G, Canepa G, Adavastro G, Nebbia J, Murri MB, Erbuto D, Pocai B, et al. The Relationship between Childhood Maltreatment and Non-Suicidal Self-Injury: A Systematic Review. Front Psychiatry. 2017;8:149.

18. Chandler A, Myers F, Platt S. The construction of self-injury in the clinical literature: A sociological exploration. Suicide Life Threat Behav. 2011;41(1):98-109.

19. Maselko J, Patel V. Why women attempt suicide: the role of mental illness and social disadvantage in a community cohort study in India. J Epidemiol Community Health. 2008;62(9):817-22.

Suicide in Young

Vivek Agarwal, Chhitij Srivastava

ABSTRACT

Suicide is a severe global public health issue. In the Indian population, it is the second leading cause of death in both genders in the 15–29 years age group. While suicide is more common in males, the rates in females are significantly higher in India as compared to global rates. Suicidal behaviors are multifactorial and result from a complex interaction between biological and psychosocial factors. A proper understanding of these factors transcends various boundaries that define and differentiate between various genetic, biological, psychological, psychiatric, and sociocultural domains. However, the natural history of suicidal behavior among children and adolescents is not well studied making any risk prediction very difficult. Studies from India have shown that the most common contributors to suicide are a combination of psychiatric disorders and social problems. Impulse control disorders are stronger predictors of suicidal behavior than affective disorders in the Indian population. Assessment of any person who has attempted or is contemplating suicide or self-harm should be holistic and should itself be therapeutic. Treatment should address not only the psychiatric disorder but also the accompanying psychosocial issues. We discussed differences in suicide rates, its methods, and the risk factors between India and the developed world as well as the various challenges in assessing and managing this group of patients along with some suicide prevention programs that are helpful.

Keywords: Suicide; Children and adolescents; Risk factors; Prevention.

■ INTRODUCTION

Suicide has existed in various cultures from ancient times. While most societies have generally condemned suicide, they have also glorified it at times. Given the rising rates of both suicidal attempts and completed suicide globally, it is an area of huge public health concern. In 2019, suicide accounted for 1.3% of all deaths globally thereby making it the 17th leading cause of death.[1] 77% of the global suicides take place in low- and middle-income countries. These numbers assume even more significance for the younger population in the 15–19-year age group in whom suicide is the fourth leading cause of death worldwide.[2] As per the WHO report of 2016, the suicide rate in India was 16.5/100,000 population which is significantly higher than the global rates of 10.5/100,000.[3] India has one of the world's highest suicide rates for youth aged 15–29 years despite for the fact that official statistics are likely to be an underestimate. Based on a nationally representative survey in India, suicide was the second leading cause of death at ages 15–29 years in both males and females.[4]

Suicidal behaviors are multifactorial and result from a complex interaction between biological and psychosocial factors. Mental health care is an area of huge gap in India especially in the young population. It is well known that mental health problems begin early in life with nearly half by 14 years of age and three-fourths by 24 years.[5] The prevalence of mental disorders in the 13–17 years age group is around 7.3% based on the National Mental Health Survey of India.[6] Addressing these mental health concerns in a timely manner is important for suicide prevention.[7]

ROLE OF AGE AND GENDER

Rates of suicidal behaviors are low in young pre-pubertal children. A population-based cohort study on the natural history of self-harm from adolescence to adulthood showed that self-harm is relatively common among teenagers and the rates were higher among girls, especially with regards to self-cutting.[8] Self-harming behaviors appeared to be related to puberty and somewhat independent of age.[9] The rates of self-harm among girls in late puberty are more than four times the rates in early puberty. The activating effects of changing hormones and changes in brain development during puberty may have a profound effect on emotional regulation. This resolves with the eventual maturation of the prefrontal cortex and most adolescents subsequently stop hurting themselves. However, persistent and more frequent self-harm may be a sign of anxiety and depression.

While girls self-harm more than boys in teenage years, the gender ratios tend to equalize by the mid-twenties and rates of self-harm drop generally. However, completed suicides have a general male preponderance. As per WHO, the rates of completed suicide in India are higher in males (18.5/100,000) as compared to females (14.5/100,000).[10]

This is significantly less than the male-to-female ratios of around 3:1 in high-income countries. The higher rates of female suicide in India as compared to the developed world are probably multifactorial but at least partly reflect the gender disadvantage experienced by females in India.

METHODS OF ATTEMPTING SUICIDE

Indian studies have reported that the most common methods of suicide are self-poisoning (mainly pesticides) and hanging.[4,11] In females, self-immolation accounts for one-sixths of all suicides.[4] Other common means for suicide in India include firearms, jumping off bridges and in front of trains.[2] The methods employed depend on the motives behind the act and expectedly highlight the multifactorial nature of suicidal behaviors. Those who have a strong desire to end their lives utilize more drastic measures in a planned manner such as hanging, self-immolation, and firearms. However, a number of unplanned, impulsive attempts in India end up in completed suicides because of the easy availability of pesticides. The death rates get further elevated because of inadequate health services in many parts of India. This impulsive group that more often says that their behavior was related to tension reduction or self-punishment[12] does not have a high completion rate when using other means such as self-cutting because of lack of planning and more likelihood of rescue. However, the boundaries between planned and impulsive attempts often get blurred in clinical settings.

RISK FACTORS

Suicide is a complex phenomenon with a multitude of factors that play a role **(Table 1)**. A proper understanding of these factors

TABLE 1: Risk factors for suicidal behavior.

Biological factors	Temperament and character	Adverse life events	Psychiatric factors
• Family history of suicide • Abnormalities in serotonin transmission	• Neuroticism • Perfectionism • Pessimism • Poor self-esteem • Maladaptive coping styles • Interpersonal dependency • Novelty-seeking • Impulsivity	• Childhood sexual abuse • Interpersonal problems within the family • Academic pressure and ragging in schools • Exposure to suicidal behavior • Cyber victimization • Homosexual/bisexual orientation	• Depression • Bipolar disorder • Anxiety disorders • Psychosis • ADHD • Substance use disorders • Eating disorders • Antisocial and borderline personality disorders • Previous suicide attempt

(ADHD: attention-deficit/hyperactivity disorder)

transcends various boundaries that define and differentiate between various genetic, biological, psychological, psychiatric, and sociocultural domains. Indian studies have shown that the most common contributors to suicide are a combination of psychiatric disorders and social problems.[4] Self-harm and suicidal behaviors exist on a continuum. They range from occasional mild nonsuicidal self-harm to frequent self-harm to severe attempts that result in completed suicide. While occasional self-harm is often due to social stressors, frequent self-harm more often than not is a sign of a serious psychiatric or personality disorders. Repetitive self-harm and recent serious suicidal attempt are a significant factor for predicting future risk of suicide.[13]

Accurately predicting suicidal risk especially in adolescents is still an area that needs further development, as the natural history of suicidal behavior among children and adolescents is not well studied.[14] A recent review discussed the limitations of any suicide risk assessment and concluded that much of the uncertainty about suicide is due to chance factors rather than from lack of knowledge.[15] This means that despite improving our knowledge about the risk factors of suicide, we may still not be able to accurately predict it. Nevertheless, we discuss some of the important factors that can positively or negatively impact the risk of suicide in the young population.

Genetics

Studies have consistently shown that family history of suicidal behavior is a risk factor for suicide.[9] The increased risk of suicide may be transmitted through social learning where suicide is seen as an acceptable means to escape the troubles of life. However, research has shown that the rates of suicide are higher in monozygotic as compared to dizygotic twins thereby implicating the role of genetics. Moreover, adoption studies show a higher rate of suicides in adopted children who were born to high-risk parents. It is quite likely that the actual traits that are transmitted are impulsivity, irritability, aggression, and increased rates of psychiatric disorders while suicide is a behavioral manifestation of these.

Summary of Biological Correlates

Various neurotransmitters have been implicated as relevant to the neurobiology of suicide, although studies are mainly in the adult population. The most consistently reported one is serotonin.[9,16] The reported abnormalities may be secondary to the psychiatric disorders present in this group of patients, although serotonin may also be related directly with suicide. Low serotonin levels in CSF have been found in people engaging in suicidal behavior in different psychiatric diagnoses including depression and psychotic disorders, both with and without depression.[17] There has also been a lot of interest in genes involved in serotonin, with most studies focusing on serotonin transporter (SERT), tryptophan hydroxylase (TPH), and serotonin receptor genes. Polymorphism at the SERT gene, particularly the short allele of the promoter variant 5-HTTLPR, is associated with a higher risk of suicide in adults.[9] Other areas of interest have involved the cannabinoid system, hypothalamic pituitary adrenal (HPA) axis, dopamine, acetylcholine, noradrenaline, opioid, gamma-aminobutyric acid (GABA), and glutamate systems, although results are inconsistent.

Early Temperament and Personality Factors

An individual's resilience or vulnerability has roots in the early temperamental traits that a child exhibit. Based on their temperament, 65% of children can be classified into one of the following—easy, difficult, and slow to warm up.[18] During early development, a number of environmental factors interact with the child's temperament to promote resilience or make the child more vulnerable.[19] If given a nourishing environment during the formative years, it promotes the development of resilience, which is a multidimensional construct that includes characteristics of tenacity, self-efficacy, optimism, emotional and cognitive control under pressure, adaptability, tolerance of negative effect, goal orientation, good stress coping mechanisms, and problem-solving skills.[20] On the other hand, neuroticism, perfectionism, interpersonal dependency, novelty seeking, impulsivity, pessimism, poor self-esteem, and maladaptive coping styles have been implicated as risk factors for suicide in adolescents.[14]

Adverse Life Events

In the clinical population, there is a high rate of adverse life events that precede both suicidal and nonsuicidal self-harming behaviors.[16] Although the immediately preceding event is often blamed by the person attempting suicide, it is the accumulation of many stressful life events that appear to be related to later suicidal behaviors. Also, these adverse events contribute to the prevalence of psychiatric disorders in the long run, which increases the suicidal risk. Studies have also shown that social factors account for a significant number of suicides in India without necessarily causing psychiatric morbidity.[4]

Early Childhood Adversity

Studies have shown that cumulative early childhood adversity increases the risk of suicide. While early and prolonged maternal separation, physical and childhood sexual abuse are associated with increased vulnerability,[14] stimulating environment and close relationship with a caring adult promotes resilience. Other relevant factors include physical abuse, child neglect, parental loss, and severe family discord.[21] Studies undertaken to understand the extent and magnitude of child abuse report a higher incidence of self-harm, suicidal ideations, and an elevated risk of committing suicide.[22-24]

Family and Parenting

Family environment and parenting are perhaps the most important modifiable influences on a child's development and behavior.[22] A supportive family set-up is seen as preventive. Marital conflicts, domestic violence, low socio-economic status and deprivation, parental psychiatric illness, drug use, suicidal behaviors in family, early parental death can all lead to various stressors that can increase the rate of psychiatric disorders and of suicide. At times, apparently minor events such as being scolded by family members, critical comments by a sibling, and demands not being met by caregivers can trigger an impulsive act of self-harm.

School Environment

Harsh discipline, physical punishment, and ragging are still quite prevalent in Indian schools. A recent review found that school-related factors such as academic difficulties, school absenteeism, pressure to achieve, control by teacher, and poor peer acceptance were important risk factors for emotional and behavioral disorders in adolescents in India.[25] These stressors can also lead to a higher risk of suicidal behaviors.

Peer Group

Peer group and siblings influence each other's behavior in various ways. Bullying in peer group is a major risk to the wellbeing of children and is quite prevalent in Indian schools. Recurrent bullying leads to behavioral and emotional problems, school refusal, and increases the chances of self-harm and suicide.[26] Sexual relationships during adolescence can also be a source of significant stressors. Premarital sex has a lot of stigma in the Indian society and can lead to significant guilt and anxiety. Break-ups can sometimes trigger an act of impulsive self-harm or suicide attempt. Peer influence can also lead to copycat behavior. There is evidence to show that nonsuicidal self-harm may be more common among teenagers when they know someone who self harms.[27] Such copycat behaviors have become more common in the era of internet and social media and sometimes extend beyond non-suicidal self-harm.

Role of Social Media and Internet

The easy accessibility of internet has a lot of advantages but the drawbacks especially in an unsupervised and unsupported home environment can have negative consequences. Social media sites place constant pressure on youngsters to portray themselves positively, which can be source of significant stress. People can take revenge by posting things about others on these sites. The stressors are amplified manifold given the wide audience on social media sites and this cybervictimization can lead to suicide attempts.[28] Moreover, there are some suicide websites and chat rooms where other participants support one another to commit suicide. Certain types of media coverage can also influence and increase the risk of suicide. This was recently witnessed when the media coverage of a Bollywood celebrity suicide was portrayed in a dramatic manner and details were repeatedly shown on popular TV channels. That was a time when India had imposed a nationwide lockdown because of the coronavirus disease (COVID) pandemic and it probably pushed vulnerable young people into further despair. Celebrity suicides can also give a sense of validation to suicide. All these factors put together consequently led to a spate of copycat suicides among the young Indian population.

Sexual Orientation

Studies have shown increased rates of suicidal behavior among youth who identify themselves as gay, lesbian, or bisexual.[9] The increase in risk is probably multifactorial. In the Indian society, there continues to exist considerable stigma against this population. This leads to an increased risk of adverse life events, poor social standing, and discrimination in the society. The increase in suicidal risk is both direct and indirect by increasing the rates of psychiatric disorders in this population.

Psychiatric Disorders

Studies have consistently demonstrated high rates of psychiatric disorders in young people who engage in suicidal behaviors—both fatal and nonfatal.[9] A systematic review of studies in adolescents and young adults found that 47–74% of suicides were due to a psychiatric disorder of which mood disorders were the most common.[29] Comorbid substance use disorders increased the risk. While depression was the most common associated disorder, other reported disorders were bipolar, anxiety, psychosis, attention-deficit/hyperactivity disorder (ADHD), substance use disorders, eating disorders, and personality disorders including antisocial and borderline.

A recent study that recruited adolescents from The Millennium Cohort Study (a longitudinal developmental study of young people throughout the United Kingdom) identified two distinct pathways to self-harm.[30] The "psychopathology" pathway was associated with emotional and behavioral difficulties as early as age 5 years, which was persistent over time. This group self-reported poor mental health and self-harming behavior at the age of 14 years. The other "adolescent risky behavior" group was much larger, did not have significant psychopathology, and showed risk-taking behavior and self-harm later into adolescence. It appears that this second group is similar to the majority of adolescents who self-harm in India although a smaller psychopathology group also exists.

A recent review of studies done in the Indian population indicated that impulse control disorders are stronger predictors of suicidal behavior than affective disorders.[11] Alcohol use disorders are also important risk factors but not to the extent reported in developed counties.

Chronic physical illness has also been associated with suicidal behavior. It is possible that this may be due to the increased risk of psychiatric disorders especially depression in chronic physical illnesses, which may lead to suicidal behavior.[31]

ASSESSMENT

Any child presenting with self-harm should be assessed thoroughly for behaviors related to suicide such as method, circumstances, intent, motive, reasons, previous attempts, planning, and influence of social media. They should also be assessed for psychiatric disorders, substance use, family environment, problems in psychosocial environment such as bullying, abuse, or interpersonal issues, and any physical problem. Risk and protective factors should be assessed keeping in mind the possibility of future self-harm. The challenges with the assessment of adolescents are that often these acts are impulsive without much planning. Also, adolescents are usually not very forthcoming about their problems and avoid help seeking from adults. It is, therefore, important that the initial assessment is more than just an information gathering process. Therapeutic assessment is an assessment model based on the cognitive-analytic model and there is evidence to show that it improves engagement in the young population.[32] For details of assessment and prevention, please refer to the specific chapters.

■ TREATMENT

Treatment of youth involved in self-harm should involve treatment of underlying psychiatric disorder, for example, depression along with interventions to address any specific psychosocial situations, for example, bullying at school. Often, there are significant issues within the family network, which need to be addressed sensitively. Specific therapies such as cognitive behavior therapy, cognitive analytic therapy, dialectical behavior therapy, and mentalization-based therapy have been found effective in reducing recurrences of self-harm in adolescents and young adults.[33] Pharmacotherapy has been studied largely in context of depression. There is no clear evidence of use of pharmacotherapy leading to reduction of self-harm in long term.

Hospitalization may be required depending upon the risk of further suicide, severity of psychiatric disorder, and safety issues in psychosocial environment. Otherwise, hospitalization does not lead to reduction in suicidal attempt in future.

■ PREVENTION

Suicide is primarily preventable public health problem. As it is associated with multiple factors, preventive interventions should work at multiple points in the complex pathways leading to suicide **(Table 2)**. The most common preventive approach has been to identify and treat individuals in crisis.

■ CHALLENGES IN SUICIDE PREVENTION

There are challenges related to record-keeping such as proper reporting of suicide attempt as well as of fatal suicide. Also, there is no national level registry to record suicide-related events. As suicide is a rare outcome, so it is difficult to assess the outcome of any

TABLE 2: Suicide prevention strategies.

Primary prevention	Secondary prevention	Tertiary prevention
• The good behavior game • Youth aware of mental health program • Life skill education	• Gatekeeper training • Sources of strength • Signs of suicide • Screening of social media uses • Screening in pediatric medical settings	• Psycho-therapy • Pharmaco-therapy

intervention. Besides, any suicide that is potentially prevented becomes a nonevent making it difficult to measure the efficacy of intervention at an individual level. These intervention programs are also very expensive making it difficult to sustain them.

Given the limitations of any suicide risk assessment, prevention efforts should focus more on promoting positive mental health and health promotion. Another way can be the increasing awareness about mental health problems, suicide, and early detection of adolescent at risk. There are programs for primary and secondary prevention, which have generally targeted at schools because children spend large part of the day at school.

Primary Prevention

There are many ways of primary prevention at community level like means restriction, for example, restrictions on pesticides sales, construction of barriers at jumping sites, changing packaging of medications to blister packs, restricting sales of medicines, and responsible media reporting. Similarly, there are programs to enhance resilience in children at community level. Here, only few specific programs are discussed.

The Good Behavior Game

The PAX Good Behavior Game (GBG) was designed to train the students in the first and second grades by trained teachers at the school.[34] The main focus of GBGs was developing self-regulation. Better self-regulation is important for development of overall good behavior, interpersonal relationships, and impulse control. These students were reassessed at the age of 19 and 21 years. They reported almost 50% drop in lifetime rates of suicide ideation and attempts compared with controls. The GBG also reduced the incidence of other disorders such as substance use, antisocial personality disorder, and violent and criminal behavior.[35]

Youth Aware of Mental Health Program

It is a primary prevention program with aims to enhance mental health awareness including especially depression and anxiety. It uses role-plays in a workshop format. It also focuses on developing skills to cope with stress. This program has been successful in reducing suicide attempts over 1 year in a European trial.[36]

Life Skill Education

It is a very good program, which should be implemented in all the schools. It helps in developing critical thinking and creative thinking, decision-making and problem-solving, communication skills, and interpersonal relations skills, coping with emotions and stress and self-awareness and empathy. Developing such skills will help a lot in prevention of suicide and other psychological problems in youth.[37]

Secondary Prevention

Sources of Strength

Sources of Strength has been developed for 10th to 12th grade students. It trains peer group leaders to help spread healthy practices among the students and also aimed to enhance student and adult connectedness and help seeking.

Sources of Strength is delivered in high schools and it has three phases namely school and community preparation, peer leader recruitment and training, and school-wide messaging. The training aimed to increase students' ability to use "sources of strength" so as to cope with psychosocial problems, for example, conflict with parents, relationship breakups. Also, it prepares them to cope effectively with emotions such as anger, depression, and anxiety. Program is intended to strengthen connectedness with adults, family, and school, and social integration with competent peers.

A controlled trial in 18 schools with 465 peer leaders and 2,700 students reported that the intervention-enhanced protective factors along with reducing suicide at a school.[38]

Signs of Suicide Program

This program was developed to increase awareness of youth about symptoms of depression and signs of suicide. They were educated through short videos of case vignettes followed by discussion. They were educated about screening for depression in themselves and friends and whom to seek help. Similarly, teachers and parents were also educated about depression and how to provide supportive environment. This program has been found very helpful in increasing awareness about depression and suicide as well as enhanced help seeking.[35]

Gatekeeper Training Program

This program is developed for the people who are likely to see children at risk of suicide, for example, school teachers and staff, school counselors, juvenile justice staff, parents, and health care professionals. The program aimed to increase awareness and skills to identify children at risk and make referrals when necessary. The focus of the program was to increase awareness and improve attitudes about suicide. Also, decrease reluctance to ask about suicide and help suicidal individuals to get help. However, this program alone was not found very effective without additional measures.[35]

Social Media/Online Platforms

As youth are using internet and are comfortable seeking help on social platforms or with online services. It is possible to reach large number of and diverse population through online platforms who otherwise hesitate to seek help for example LGBTQ community. There are some preliminary researches available on the use of social media or web-based messaging in suicide prevention. Studies have shown that it is possible to predict suicide risk by machine analysis of sociodemographic and psychological variables of students in Korea.[39] Studies have examined the use of text messaging as extension of Sources of Strength program, which students found useful. Similarly, studies have evaluated the use of websites developed for helping suicidal individuals, social media for expression of suicidal intent, and social support provided by the online community to such persons. Although initial findings are encouraging but the problems with social media are related to identity of such persons and controlling their behavior, actual risk assessment, and situation going out of control. It requires large methodologically sound studies to reach any firm conclusion about usefulness of social media/online programs.[40]

Education Reforms

Reforming the way children are educated in our schools will help a lot in suicide prevention. The environment of school should be made friendly so that the child looks forward to going to school. Efforts should also be made to reduce corporal punishment and bullying at schools. The teaching–learning methods should change from rote learning to more understanding based. There should be flexibility in choosing the subjects. Allowing the child to mix and match subjects from art and science streams with reduction in content of course. The focus should be on holistic development of the child, and strengthening his/her other aspects of personality rather than academics only. Hopefully new education policy will help with this aspect.

Parenting

Parental/family support plays a major role in suicide prevention. There is a significant need to educate Indian parents about the psychological needs of children including good communication between parent and children and psychological availability of parent for the child. More autonomy should be provided to children while choosing a career and decision-making related to the life of children. Need to learn good parenting practices and effect of parenting styles on children's psychology should be taught in colleges and to the prospective parents.

There are children and young adults who are not in any formal system of the country, for example, child laborers, street children, and children in juvenile homes, etc. There is a need of NGOs, which may reach out to them and work with this vulnerable population for suicide prevention.

■ CONCLUSION

The suicidal behavior among young in our country is not completely delineated. Although many risk factors have been identified, still it is difficult to predict which adolescents are likely to repeat their suicidal behavior. More research is required to understand the complex relationship among different risk factors for suicidality. Only few psychological treatments have been found effective in treatment of suicide. Role of pharmacological interventions is not clear. There are many effective suicide prevention programs available in the Western countries, which may be used with modification in our country to help the younger population.

There is need to reduce stigma and increase awareness about suicide in younger population. There should be a national program specifically for addressing the suicide in India. It should systematically address the risk factors specific to our country and develop strategies to prevent suicide, which will be effective and acceptable in our culture along with focus on positive mental health especially in younger population.

■ REFERENCES

1. World Health Organization. (2021). Suicide data [Internet]. [online] Available from: https://www.who.int/teams/mental-health-and-substance-use/data-research/suicide-data. [Last accessed July 2022].
2. World Health Organization. (2021). Suicide [Internet]. [online] Available from: https://www.who.int/news-room/fact-sheets/detail/suicide. [Last accessed July, 2022].
3. World Health Organization. (2021). Suicide - India [Internet]. [online] Available from: https://www.who.int/india/health-topics/suicide. [Last accessed July 2022].
4. Patel V, Ramasundarahettige C, Vijayakumar L, Thakur JS, Gajalakshmi V, Gururaj G, et al. Suicide mortality in India: A nationally representative survey. Lancet. 2012;379(9834):2343-51.
5. Kessler RC, Amminger GP, Aguilar-Gaxiola S, Alonso J, Lee S, Ustün TB, et al. Age of onset of mental disorders: A review of recent literature. Curr Opin Psychiatry. 2007;20:359-64.
6. Gururaj G, Varghese M, Benegal V, Rao GN, Pathak K, Singh LK, et al. National mental health survey of India, 2015-16: Prevalence, patterns and outcomes. NIMHANS Publication No. 129. Bengaluru: National Institute of Mental Health and Neuro Sciences; 2016.
7. Organization W. (2021). Preventing suicide: A global imperative [Internet]. [online] Available from: https://apps.who.int/iris/handle/10665/131056. [Last accessed July 2022].
8. Moran P, Coffey C, Romaniuk H, Olsson C, Borschmann R, Carlin JB, et al. The natural history of self-harm from adolescence to young adulthood: A population-based cohort study. Lancet. 2012;379(9812):236-43.
9. Hawton K, O'Connor RC, Saunders KEA. Suicidal behavior and self-harm. In: Thapar A, Pine DS, Leckman JF, Scott S, Snowling MJ, Taylor E (Eds). Rutter's Child and adolescent Psychiatry. West Sussex: John Wiley & Sons; 2015. pp. 893-910.
10. WHO. (2021). Suicide rate estimates, age-standardized - Estimates by country [Internet]. [online] Available from: http://apps.who.int/gho/data/node.main.MHSUICIDEASDR?lang=en. [Last accessed July 2022].
11. Rane A, Nadkarni A. Suicide in India: A systematic review. Shanghai Arch Psychiatry. 2014;26(2):69-80.
12. Rodham K, Hawton K, Evans E. Reasons for deliberate self-harm: Comparison of self-poisoners and self-cutters in a community sample of adolescents. J Am Acad Child Adolesc Psychiatry. 2004;43(1):80-7.
13. Castellví P, Lucas-Romero E, Miranda-Mendizábal A, Parés-Badell O, Almenara J, Alonso I, et al. Longitudinal association between self-injurious thoughts and behaviors and suicidal behavior in adolescents and young adults: A systematic review with meta-analysis. J Affect Disord. 2017;215:37-48.
14. Carballo JJ, Llorente C, Kehrmann L, Flamarique I, Zuddas A, Purper-Ouakil D, et al. Psychosocial risk factors for suicidality in children and adolescents. Eur Child Adolesc Psychiatry. 2019;25:1-8.

15. Large M, Galletly C, Myles N, Ryan CJ, Myles H. Known unknowns and unknown unknowns in suicide risk assessment: Evidence from meta-analyses of aleatory and epistemic uncertainty. BJPsych Bull. 2017;41:160-3.

16. Radhakrishnan R, Andrade C. Suicide: An Indian perspective. Indian J Psychiatry. 2012;54:304-19.

17. Trivedi JK. Serotonin and its metabolites as biological markers of suicidal behaviour. Indian J Psychiatry. 1992;34:174-97.

18. Thomas A, Chess S. The Temperament Trap: Recognizing and Accommodating Children's Personalities. New York: Brunner/Mazel; 1977.

19. Feder A, Nestler EJ, Charney DS. Psycho-biology and molecular genetics of resilience. Nat Rev Neurosci. 2009;10(6): 446-57.

20. Connor KM, Davidson JR. Development of a new resilience scale: The Connor-Davidson resilience scale (CD-RISC). Depress Anxiety. 2003;18(2):76-82.

21. Vargas-Medrano J, Diaz-Pacheco V, Castaneda C, Miranda-Arango M, Longhurst MO, Martin SL, et al., Psychological and neurobiological aspects of suicide in adolescents: Current outlooks. Brain Behav Immun Health. 2020;7:100124.

22. Agarwal V, Srivastava C. Social Dimensions of Childhood and Adolescent Psychiatric Disorders. In: Chadda RK, Kumar V, Sarkar S (Eds). Social Psychiatry: Principles & Clinical Perspectives. New Delhi: Jaypee Brothers Medical Publishers (P) Ltd; 2019. Pp. 284-93.

23. Danese A, McCrory E. Child Maltreatment. In: Thapar A, Pine DS, Leckman JF, Scott S, Snowling MJ, Taylor E (Eds). Rutter's Child and Adolescent Psychiatry. West Sussex: John Wiley & Sons; 2015. pp. 364-75.

24. Glaser D. Child sexual abuse. In: Thapar A, Pine DS, Leckman JF, Scott S, Snowling MJ, Taylor E (Eds). Rutter's Child and Adolescent Psychiatry. West Sussex: John Wiley & Sons; 2015. pp. 376-88.

25. Aggarwal S, Berk M. Evolution of adolescent mental health in a rapidly changing socioeconomic environment: A review of mental health studies in adolescents in India over last 10 years. Asian J Psychiatr. 2015; 13:3-12.

26. Klomek AB, Sourander A, Niemelä S, Kumpulainen K, Piha J, Tamminen T, et al. Childhood bullying behaviors as a risk for suicide attempts and completed suicides: A population-based birth cohort study. J Am Acad Child Adolesc Psychiatry. 2009; 48(3):254-61.

27. Syed S, Kingsbury M, Bennett K, Manion I, Colman I. Adolescents' knowledge of a peer's non-suicidal self-injury and own non-suicidal self-injury and suicidality. Acta Psychiatr Scand. 2020;142(5):366-73.

28. Sedgwick R, Epstein S, Dutta R, Ougrin D. Social media, internet use and suicide attempts in adolescents. Curr Opin Psychiatry. 2019;32:534-41.

29. Cavanagh JT, Carson AJ, Sharpe M, Lawrie SM. Psychological autopsy studies of suicide: A systematic review. Psychol Med. 2003;33(3):395-405.

30. Uh S, Dalmaijer ES, Siugzdaite R, Ford TJ, Astle DE. Two pathways to self-harm in adolescence. J Am Acad Child Adolesc Psychiatry. 2021;60(12):1491-500.

31. Greydanus D, Patel D, Pratt H. Suicide risk in adolescents with chronic illness: Implications for primary care and specialty paediatric practice: a review. Dev Med Child Neurol. 2010;52(12):1083-7.

32. English O, Wellings C, Banerjea B, Ougrin D. Specialized therapeutic assessment-based recovery-focused treatment for young people with self-harm: Pilot Study. Front Psychiatry. 2019;10:895.

33. Ougrin D, Tranah T, Stahl D, Moran P, Asarnow JR. Therapeutic interventions for suicide attempts and self-harm in adolescents: Systematic review and meta-analysis. J Am Acad Child Adolesc Psychiatry. 2015;54(2):97-107.

34. Kellam SG, Brown CH, Poduska JM, Ialongo NS, Wang W, Toyinbo P, et al. Effects of a universal classroom behavior management program in first and second grades on

young adult behavioural, psychiatric, and social outcomes. Drug Alcohol Depend. 2008;95:S5-28.

35. Wilcox HC, Wyman PA. Suicide prevention strategies for improving population health. Child Adolesc Psychiatric Clin N Am. 2016; 25(2):219-33.

36. Wasserman D, Hoven CW, Wasserman C, Wall M, Eisenberg R, Hadlaczky G, et al. School-based suicide prevention programmes: The SEYLE cluster-randomised, controlled trial. Lancet. 2015;385:1536-44.

37. Srikala B, Kishore KK. Empowering adolescents with life skills education in schools - School mental health program: Does it work? Indian J Psychiatry. 2010;52(4): 344-9.

38. Wyman PA, Brown CH, LoMurray M, Schmeelk-Cone K, Petrova M, Yu Q, et al. An outcome evaluation of the Sources of Strength suicide prevention program delivered by adolescent peer leaders in high schools. Am J Public Health. 2010;100: 1653-61.

39. Bae SM, Lee SA, Lee SH. Prediction by data mining, of suicide attempts in Korean adolescents: A national study. Neuropsychiatr Dis Treat. 2015;11:2367-75.

40. Robinson J, Cox G, Bailey E, Hetrick S, Rodrigues M, Fisher S, Herrman H. Social media and suicide prevention: A systematic review. Early Interv Psychiatry. 2016;10(2):103-21.

14

Farmer's Suicide in India

Manik C Bhise, Anuradha Patil

ABSTRACT

Suicide by farmers in India is a protracted issue over last 3 decades. Despite repeated demands there is no systemic prevention policy in the country. There is scarcity of literature in India about risk factors, especially about mental health of farmers. Objective of this chapter is to take a systematic review of available literature from India and suggest some prevention strategies taking cues from available literature from other countries. Analysis of government data on farmers' suicide and its limitations will also be covered in brief. This chapter will also discuss about similarities and differences in prevalence, risk factors and prevention strategies among farmers' suicides, and suicides in general population.

Keywords: Farmer suicide; Suicide.

◼ INTRODUCTION

Farming had been primary base of human existence on this earth since thousands of years. Historically, human civilizations have flourished alongside the river beds across globe. Farming is one of the oldest professions learnt by human beings which helped us to thrive over thousands of years. Over last century, industrialization gradually took over the farming as profession in majority of the globe. Middle- and low-income countries such as India however continue to be predominantly agriculture-based economies with gradual shift toward industrialization. Apart from farming as occupation, it is a major economic base for many industries which supply seeds, fertilizers and implements to farmers. Also there is another large group of industries that thrives on agricultural produce as raw material.

Over last few decades, farmer as an occupation and farming as an industry has been persistently under distress across globe. This has resulted in high number of suicides by farmers. Most farms are owned by families since years together. Farmers are exposed to volatility of markets, the variability of weather patterns and influence of respective government regulations.[1] This exposes farmers to a high level of stress and difficulties in life. Farmers experience high level of physical stressors and hazards of farm environment which are compounded by regulatory framework and economic dynamics of managing farm business. Over decades farmers are witnessing declining trends of trade for agricultural produce; volatile markets; limited availability of off-farm employment on one hand; and growing cost of machinery and production; and loss of farm or livelihood due to repeated crop failures.[2] Multiple studies from countries such as Canada, Australia, the United Kingdom, and Sri Lanka have reported high level of distress and high suicide rate among farmers.[3-6]

GLOBAL SCENARIO OF SUICIDE AMONG FARMERS

Way back in 1984, an estimated 220,000 pesticide-related suicides worldwide annually. Most of these victims are engaged in agricultural activities with easy access to pesticides. Approximately 3 decades later, review of data from a few countries in Asia suggested that there may be 300,000 suicides by deliberate ingestion of pesticides annually in Asia alone.[7] This goes in line with the World Health Organization (WHO) reporting pesticides as the most common method of suicide worldwide. High rate of suicide deaths by intentional ingestion of pesticides in Asian countries, most of which are developing countries, is the high-case fatality associated with pesticide ingestion compared to the relatively low-case fatality of many of the substances commonly taken in acts of self-poisoning in the western countries.[8] The proportion of all suicides using pesticides varies from 4% in the European region to over 50% in the western Pacific region, but this proportion is not concordant with the volume of pesticides sold in each region; it is the pattern of pesticide use and the toxicity of the products, not the quantity used, that influences the likelihood they will be used in acts of fatal self-harm.[9] Following is discussion on literature from few countries where suicide in farmers had been a concern.

United Kingdom

England and Wales have identified farming as one of the high-risk occupations for suicide. Based on proportional mortality ratios farmers were among the 10 occupational groups with the highest proportional mortality rate in the United Kingdom. Upland farmers and farmers keeping livestock were particularly at high risk for suicide. Hawton et al. found that over a period of 1981–1993, there was significant decline in farmers' suicides in England but not in the Wales region. Among different counties in England the largest number of farmers' suicides was in southwest region, but rest of the counties varied greatly. These authors have also found that farmers' suicide rates were higher in the regions where rates of suicide among general population were also high, focusing influence of local factors such as local density of farmers, financial deprivation, and unemployment levels on suicides.[5] An important observation which has high implication in designing prevention strategies was that farmers who commit suicide tend to use methods to which they have easy access. This applied particularly to the firearms. After Firearms Act 1988, it was noticed that there was a marked decline in the number of firearm-related suicides in farmers; also rates of suicides by other means did not change significantly. This is a good example of prevention of suicides by restriction of access to lethal methods. A later study found that despite of preventive measures taken so far, agricultural workers still have second highest proportional mortality rates (PMR) in the United Kingdom.[10]

Australia

Australia is another developed nation facing problem of farmers' suicides. Here, suicide accounts for one-fifth of the all the deaths in age group of 20–34 years. Age standardized suicide rate is 8.7 per 100,000 general population. By the start of 21st century, one farmer was taking his life every 4 days, and farmers' suicide rate was twice the national average in the country. Male farm managers and agricultural laborer suicide rates are higher than male national suicide rates and rates in the wider rural population.[4] Firearms figure as the most common method of suicide. In Australia, suicide by farmers is linked with drought. Most of the Australia experiences frequent and wide spread droughts. Farmers experience crop loss, and loss of jobs in agriculture leads to distress. In the year 2006, Australia was faced its 5th year of continuous drought. Due to this farms which were irrigated by rivers, were not provided water for irrigation.[11] In that year livestock prices were down by 80% as farmers preferred to sell off their animals rather than watch them to die in the fields. With this situation, a wave of farmers' suicides had struck the country. The emotional stress from the lingering drought had impacted not only farmers, but also their families, communities, and even the drought support services themselves. While the drought may have a limited life span, its ramifications continue for many years.[12] Even in times outside of drought, farmers' stress levels in Australia are rising due to the changing nature of farming (e.g., globalization, restructuring, and the aging farmer population) and the prevalence of increasingly restrictive legislation affecting day-to-day farming activities (particularly native vegetation and occupational health and safety). Literature from the country shows that elevated rate of suicide among Australian farmers does not seem to be simply explained by an elevated rate of mental health problems. This again has significance in devising suicide prevention strategies for farmers. Individual personality, gender, and community attitudes that limit a person's ability to acknowledge or express mental health problems and seek help for these may be significant risk factors

for suicide in Australian farmers.[13] Deaths from suicide of male farmers and farm workers are approximately double that of the Australian male population. There are also a significantly higher number of accidents (e.g., death by firearm and car accidents) occurring in the bush, particularly in remote areas. Despite the disproportionately high levels of depression and other mental illnesses in rural and remote areas, communities in these areas continue to have poorer access to mental health support, a problem that must be addressed as a matter of urgency.

Sri Lanka

In the early 1990s, Sri Lanka had one of the highest suicide rates in the world. Between 1950 and 1995 rates increased eightfold to a peak of 47 per 100,000 in 1995. However, after 10 years in the year 1995, Sri Lanka's suicide rates declined by 50%, a very significant decline in a decade.[9] Understanding suicides and prevention strategies in Sri Lanka will be beneficial for devising suicide prevention strategies for low-income countries. In Sri Lanka, pesticide self-poisoning accounts for about two-thirds of suicides. The marked decline in Sri Lanka's suicide rates in the mid-1990s coincided with the culmination of a series of legislative activities that systematically banned the most highly toxic pesticides that had been responsible for the majority of pesticide deaths in the preceding 2 decades. Apart from restricting or withdrawing a number of pesticides, Sri Lanka has also actively pursued a number of other initiatives to reduce use and increase the safety of pesticide use by farmers. Few examples include integrated pest management, use of lockable boxes to restrict access to pesticides.[6] Furthermore, there has been considerable research interest in Sri Lanka in the medical management of self-poisoning and so it is possible that the improved management of pesticide self-poisoning has also contributed to the favorable trends observed in deaths due to suicide.

INDIAN SCENARIO OF SUICIDE BY FARMERS

Historical Review of Suicide by Farmers in India

Suicides by farmers in India were first reported by print media around early 1990s. By that time globalization of Indian markets had started leading to flooding of agro-based industries in country. This started putting rising pressure on Indian farmers. Till early 1990s farming was done in season-wise pattern using home grown seeds and live-stock dung-based fertilizers. This needed minimal financial input from farmers as everything needed was available in own farms. Gradually, seeds, chemical fertilizers, and pesticides were promoted and introduced at subsidized rates. This started destroying prior indigenous traditional methods of farming. This was coupled with flooding of entertainment and daily needs goods from global markets, leading to rising expenditure by farmers for living daily life. Over years subsidies were reduced and concept of crop loans introduced by the governments, putting farmers in a vicious cycle of debt (will be discussed later in this chapter). Over next few years, signs of distress started appearing in farmers. Now youngsters perceive farming as less profitable business and opt for work in cities as industrial workers. By year 2006–2010 suicide by farmers became a major political issue in country with relief packages announced by the Central Government of India. What started as mere media hype now was at forefront of debates on news channels

and was a major concern for ruling parties. Within next few years farmers' suicides were reported by police to National Crime Records Bureau (NCRB) of India as a separated category, posthumous help was announced and later in next decade separate report was yearly published by the NCRB for few years.

Analysis of Government Data

National Crime Records Bureau of India has centralized suicide reporting system. These events are reported to the NCRB, an authority under Ministry of Home Affairs by police departments across nation. Same data with statistical analysis is published every year on the NCRB as an open for public document under title "Accidental Deaths and Suicides in India" which can be downloaded from their website: https://ncrb.gov.in/en/accidental-deaths-suicides-india-adsi. The NCRB did not have separate category for farmers' suicide till mid of 2nd decade of this century. However, inferences can be drawn from category—"self-employed (farming/agriculture)" under heading of "Professional status of suicide victims". Though there is variation in writing style of reports over years (for few years only percentage of total suicide is available, while for other years only number of suicides is available), we have calculated and collected required data from this source. We have done descriptive analysis of the data and same is presented below in **Figure 1**. During this 20-year timeframe, 294,806 farmers have committed suicide. During initial 12 years period between 2000 and 2011 itself, there were total of 201,013 suicides by farmers and agriculture workers. This makes an alarming average of 16,751 suicides by farmers every year! This is an official figure but actual suicides may be double or more than this official figure for two reasons, as many large states have reported "nil" or minimal

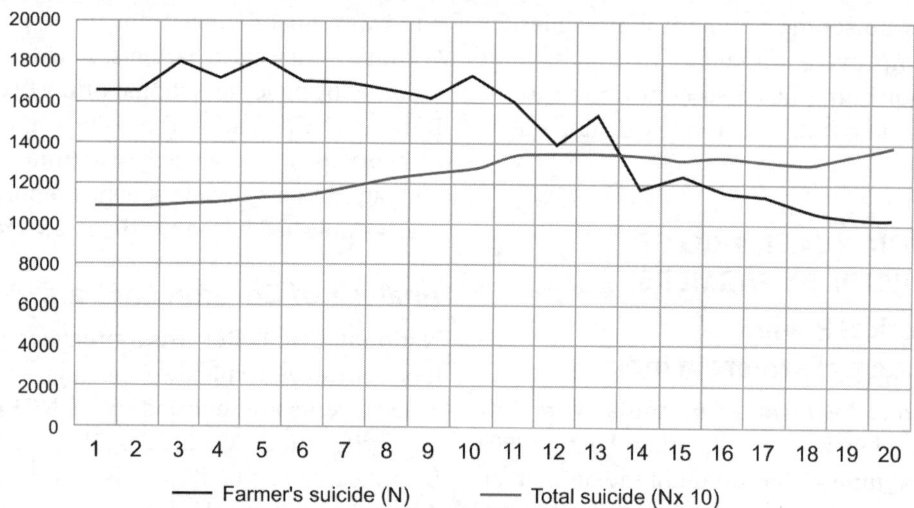

Fig. 1: Relative Trend of general suicides and farmers' suicide over 20 years. (Analysis of 20 years of NCRB data from year 2000 to 2019).

suicide figures in this category and studies across country have found that there is high under reporting of suicide in India. This trend has continued with little ups and downs over next 5 years. It was only after year 2016 that reported farmers' suicides have come below 12,000 per year. It is a bit of relief that between years 2016 and 2019 (latest available NCRB report) we can see steady decline in number of suicide by farmers in the country, though there is rise in number of suicides in general population.

Reliable number of farmers in India can be obtained from two census of India performed in year 2001 and 2011 during past 2 decades. Due to coronavirus disease 2019 (COVID-19) pandemic scheduled census of 2021 appears to be cancelled. Based on farmers population in year 2001 census, suicide rate among farmers in the country was 12.9 per lakh farmers, which was about one-fifth higher than the general suicide rate, which was 10.6 in that year. It is disheartening to note the marginal rise in farmers' suicide rate to 13.2 per lakh farmers in year 2011.[14]

We will be discussing the suicides by farmers in India in details in this chapter hence discussion here is limited. Considering the farming as a sector it is clear that farmers face unique challenges than other industries or general population. Also they face uncertainties and have to adapt rapidly to losses in business to sustain over generations. Suicide rate in farmers is substantially higher than general population. All these warrant study of suicides by farmers as a special category which will help in devising targeted prevention strategies for farmers.

Regional Patterns in Farmers' Suicides in India

Based on analysis of data provided by the NCRB over years, few inferences can be made as mentioned below. There is a high degree of variation in terms of number, as well as rate of farmer's suicides across different states in the country. A similar variation also exists for suicides in general population as well. In fact there seems to be a strong relationship between suicides in general population and suicides by farmers in terms of these variations across different states. The correlation coefficient between the number of general suicides and farm suicides is high and positive (+0.85, $N = 21$ in 2001; and +0.78, $N = 21$ in 2011), thus objectively establishing strong relationship.[14] States with high number of suicides in a general are also the ones with high number of farmers' suicides. The top five states in terms of the number of farm suicides in 2001 and 2011—Maharashtra, Karnataka, Andhra Pradesh, Chhattisgarh, and Madhya Pradesh—also accounted for nearly two-thirds (63 and 67%, respectively) of the general suicides in the country.

There is a large continuous region consisting of 8 states in North India has least number of farmer's suicides in country. Large part of this region falls in the Plains of Ganga and its tributaries. The number of farm suicides in this region is just around 1,400 per year on an average. This seems to be not very alarming, at least in comparison with some other parts of the country, and considering that this is a very large region both in terms of area and population. The rate of farm suicides in this region, at 2.6, is much lower than the all-India average. This is also the region where the suicide rate in general population is low. And lastly, the number of farm suicides, after showing an initial spurt in the years 1998 and 1999, has in fact shown a declining tendency after that. All in all, at least from NCRB data this is not the zone where problems of farm suicides are not very acute.

Shifting Patterns within and Among States

Discussion above gives picture that few states are consistently dealing with issue of suicide by farmers over past 3 decades in India. However, on close look, there is shifting trend and pattern within a state also. For example, in Maharashtra, in first decade of 21st century Vidarbha region was hotspot for suicides by farmers. While in 2nd decade, Marathwada region was hot spot. Similar variations can be observed in other states also. This shifting of trends among different geographical regions is closely associated with risk factors that impact lives of famers. From year 2011 to 2015, there was continuous drought in Marathwada region with severe water crisis. At districts like Latur and Osmanabad, drinking water was transported by trains! Successive crop failures led to severe distress among farmers leading to increased suicides by them. This was evident from media reports and few scientific studies conducted in the region.[15] This was the time when NAAM foundation and Paani Foundation were formed and started working to help farmers. On our request, information was provided by the District Collector Office of Aurangabad for a number of farmers' suicides in past 2.5 years in June 2017. As per their record, there were 144 (year 2015), 151 (year 2016), and 60 (first 6 months of year 2017) suicides by farmers. Of these suicides majority were in age group of 30–50 years and had used pesticide consumption as method of suicide. Compared to our research in Wardha district there were around 111–120 suicides by farmers every year in the district. In that comparison, number of 140–151 is quite high in Aurangabad district. This clearly indicates shifting pattern of suicide by farmers in response to draught situation. This is in line with shifting patterns and trends of suicides by farmers in as per draught situation observed in Australia.[12]

RISK FACTORS FOR SUICIDE BY FARMERS

Despite grave picture of farmers' suicides in India, there are very few studies by mental health professionals that have assessed the risk factors comprehensively. Literature search on the topics is highly biased toward findings of studies from field of social science and economics. Here for comprehensive discussion, we have included the studies from rural India as in rural areas farming is the predominant occupation and source of living. Bhalla et al. conducted a study on suicides in rural Punjab. This was the beginning of in depth studies to assess sociodemographic and mental health issues in farming population. They reported that those who committed suicide were more likely to be single, separated, and staying in nuclear families. Factors such as indebtedness, crop failures, and acute financial loss or financial responsibility (e.g., marriage in family) were significantly associated with farmers' suicides in rural Punjab.[17] Similar findings were also noticed among farmers' suicide victims in Vidarbha, Maharashtra.[16] Suicide victim's families reported a very low average annual income (₹ 20,000/- to ₹ 45,000/-). Irony of the situation is that these families do not have sufficient resources to rise above certain barrier of income. Loss of male farmer made things worse for these families. There was a complete lack of other allied sources of income for these victim farmers such as dairy, fishery, etc. To meet the ends in face of inadequate income, farmers have to obtain loans from private money lenders who extort them with high interest rates. In Karnataka state, trends in farm economy revealed that there is an increase in lease system of land due to inability of marginal and small scale farmers to do farming on their own. In a study from Vidarbha region of central India, it was found that recent deterioration in financial status, indebtedness, crop failures, and marriage of sister or daughter were closely associated with farmers' suicide.[18] Literature

available so far on the farmers' suicide in India reveals that it has been studied from different viewpoints with wide variation of risk factors. As stated before, Indian literature is dominated by articles from social science and economics field with minimal from mental health perspective of farmers. Its etiology is multifactorial and study involves complex interactions between social, economic, administrative, and psychiatric risk factors acting together. In following section we will be discussing findings from few psychological autopsy studies in India. We have included studies exclusively focusing on farmers as much as possible, but due to scarcity of data, we have compared these findings with studies done on rural population and some references from abroad are also compared.

Sex

In India, farms are primarily managed by males in family. This also puts male farmers at very high-risk of suicide with male to female ratio of 8.8:1 which is very high.[18] This ratio is much higher than the ratio of 2.33:1 for suicides in general population globally as per the latest estimates of the World Health Organization for 2019 (WHO, 2019), and as reported in India 2.35:1 by the NCRB 2019 in Indian population.[19,20] Analysis of NCRB Data over last 2 decades reveals that 85% of farmers' suicide victims were male. It can be seen that the number of suicides among male farmers has been increasing quite rapidly, while the number of suicides by female farmers in sharp contrast has remained almost static.[14] Apart from farm business being predominantly run by males in India there may be some bias in reporting also. Usually to categorize suicide as a farmers' suicide, criteria commonly considered is title of agriculture land in name of suicide victim. In India, traditionally male members in family have title of farm land, hence female suicides in farming families may be categorized under either housewives or other category.

Age

Majority of the farmers' suicide victims were in middle-age group, 3rd to 6th decade of their life. Similar age distribution is also reported in other studies on farmers' suicides.[18] This implies that most of the victims of farmers' suicides were in the economically productive age group and were the breadearners for the family. This puts survivors of farmers' suicides in a very distressing situation as is reported from Vidarbha and Marathwada regions in Maharashtra State.[15,21]

Education and Living Status of Farmers

Farmers who committed suicide usually had similar education and literacy status as reported by district administrators on official website for suicide victims in general population. This indicates that literacy plays little role as risk factor for farmers' suicide. Most farmers who died of suicide in India were married, and were living with their families.[15,17,18,23] Most of the Indian farmers who committed suicide were living in their homes with families intact, apparently had a good family support prior to committing suicide. This is in contrast to findings reported in western studies where a significant number of farmers who committed suicide were living alone (18%) and lacked close friend (31%) giving a picture of social isolation as a significant risk factor there.[24]

Caste and Religion

India is known for diversity of population and variety of faiths and religions across country. Above-mentioned studies from India also state that if ethnic (religious) composition of local population under study area is considered as base, there is no significant difference in proportion of suicides among different religions or castes. For example, study by author in Wardha district of Maharashtra showed that >50% farmers suicide victim belonged to other backward class (OBC) as category.[18] When one looks at religious composition of the farmers in district, its OBCs (Kunabi, Teli, etc.) who are doing farming there in large numbers than other categories. This implies that caste or religion is not a significant risk factor for suicide by farmers.

Farming Characteristics

As stated earlier, farming in India is a family-owned business run over generations. With every next generation, there is division of farm land holding happening. Usually this generation span is of 20–30 years. Over years, there is constant decline in size of farm land owned by a farmer. This has significant impact on running farming as business. Most farmers suicide victims owned marginal (<1 hectare) and small (1–4 hectares) farms. Small scale farmers are more likely to be exposed to financial stressors due to market fluctuations, small capital and risk of crop failures as there is less scope for mixed crop or multiple crop patterns. Due to less earning from marginal farms they own, to meet their needs they need to work on other's farms as laborers. This puts them in disadvantaged position as they need to balance their time for own farm and that of the other farmer. These small-size farms are less likely to have irrigation facilities. Irrigation in India is either supply of water from small dams or irrigation by well water (well and tube well). Small-scale farmers usually cannot afford either. So most of these marginal farmers lease out their farms or sell it under economic distress. Most of the suicide victims lacked the basic implements like plough, thresher, or live stocks. Leasing out farms, selling bullocks, and absence of livestock have significant association with suicides by farmers in India.[18]

Economic Distress

Over last 20 years, farmers' suicides in India have occupied prominent place in media. With this happening in public domain, social science and economic institutes started their research from social science and economic views. Unfortunately, till the 2nd decade of 21st century, most of the psychiatry institutions and psychiatrists or other mental health professionals were not actively involved in research on this issue. This has been reflected in economic factors being projected as *"the"* cause for farmers' suicides. Though not enough in themselves, compared to general suicides, economic distress is an important risk factor for farmers' suicides in India. Hence, it is pertinent to discuss this here. Case control studies from central India revealed that both farmers who committed suicide and their age, sex, and socioeconomically matched controls had procured debt similarly.[18,23] Similarly there was no difference in total amount of debt procured and irregular repayment of debt among suicide cases and their controls. However among debt characteristics, suicide victims differed significantly from controls in terms of sources of debt, reason for procuring debt, and amount of debt pending to be repaid. Significantly more proportion of suicide victims had sought debt from private moneylenders, who are known to take higher interest rates and also to threaten for repayment. Significant number of farmers suicide households had gone through recent financial deterioration

and about one-fourth of the suicide victims were reportedly pressurized to repay debt by moneylenders in these studies.[18,22,23] Farm business is heavily reliant upon a small labor force (usually within the family) and often has volatile and/or slim profit margins, resulting in limited flexibility to procure additional laborers from outside family. For the farming business to survive, it is crucial for members of the farming family unit to fulfill their roles, creating a clear imperative for a person to suppress negative feelings, or leave the profession. This creates stress and burden on farmers to contribute to the family business.[13] Author based on his own research on this subject and after considering corroborating findings from other studies proposes a *"Viscous Cycle of Indebtedness"* **(Fig. 2)** an important risk factor for suicide by farmers. Considering the fact that larger proportions (82% of all farmers interviewed) of suicide and nonsuicide households had debt, and that cost of living and cost of doing farming have both increased significantly in recent years, we can say that seeking debt is a common practice among farmers. Also most common source of debt is commercial or public sector banks, which issue "crop loan" to farmers, intended to be utilized for agriculture expenses only. Like any other business, it is hoped that providing money to spend on agriculture will help in better inputs and ultimately good yields from crops so that these debts are paid back to banks with good profit to farmers. This seeking of loans and repaying back goes on for years together. This cycle of debt (shown in dark grey color) should goes on for years, without causing much distress to farmers. But, in real life of a farmer, scenario is different. There are so many additional expenses that a farmer is experiencing with rapidly changing lifestyle. A farmer gets trapped into this cycle

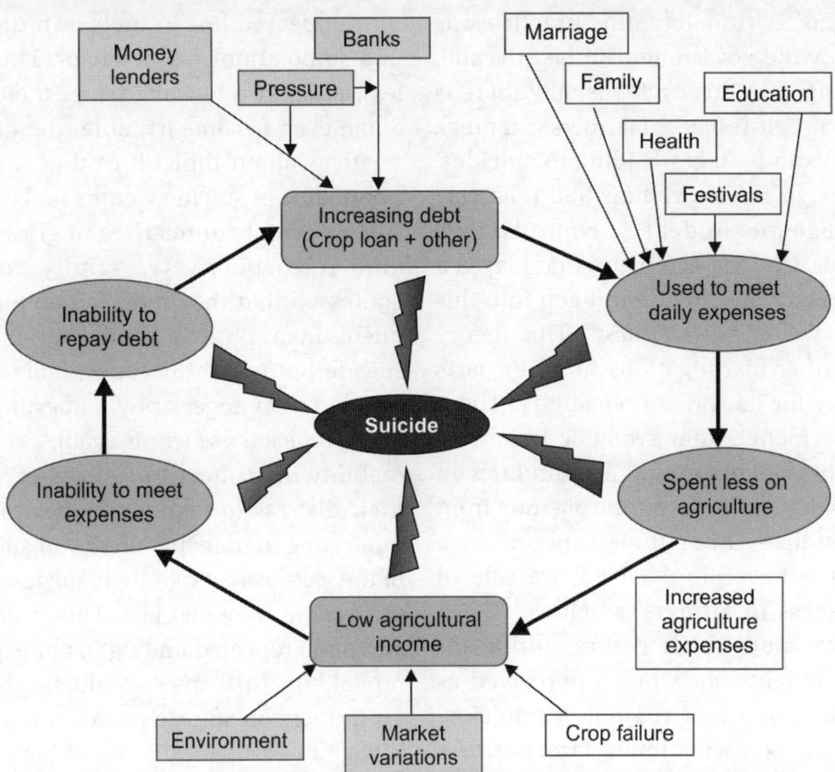

Fig. 2: Vicious cycle of indebtedness as risk factor for farmers' suicides.

with mounting amounts of debt when these additional or unexpected expenses come in his way (few are shown by white color).

Most common reasons for these additional expenses that were present in suicide victims in our study were expenses for events in family (e.g., health, education, and festivals), marriage of sister or daughter, etc. When these expenses come in the way, either crop loans are diverted or additional loans are procured by farmers to meet these financial burdens. This, in turn, leads to shortage of finances to run agriculture, which may lead to compromised spending on crops. This in association with rising costs of seeds, pesticides, and agricultural labor, etc. ultimately lead to low agricultural income. This is compounded by frequent draughts or excess rains, crop failures, and fluctuating market prices for agricultural produce. This leads to inability to repay existing debt as was evident among suicide victims in above study. Current banking policy is that unless previous debts are cleared off, fresh loans cannot be obtained. This leads to feeling of helplessness to run farming business. This along with additional expenses that cannot be met with by only crop loans propels farmers toward private moneylenders who charge very high interests. All these factors lead to severe distress among the farmers. Pressures from moneylenders and banks (showed in light grey color) further add to the distress among farmers. Till the 10-years back, banks used to send their people to demand repaying of loans, just like moneylenders send goons. Fortunately, this practice was banned by the government in last decade. Once trapped in this cycle, usually there is no way out. Self-respect of farmers can break down at various stages leading to suicides. Thus, though suicide victims had relatively similar amounts of debt as controls, they have other debt characteristics that played a crucial role in pushing them deep into this *"vicious cycle of indebtedness"*. This theory needs further investigations in other parts of country for its wide applicability. There is some evidence from available literature. Srijit Mishra had reported similar findings on indebtedness in his case control study from central India.[23] Other Indian quantitative studies too have emphasized the role of indebtedness in farmers' suicides.[17,18,25] A qualitative study from central India has reported indebtedness being perceived as one of the important reasons for suicide, along with high cost of running farm business and low market price for farm produces.[22] In the United Kingdom also farmers were found to be more concerned about their financial problems and indebtedness.[24] However, a study on suicide in rural Tamil Nadu reported relatively lower contribution of financial problems as significant stressor and risk factor for suicides.[26]

Psychiatric Illnesses in Farmers

Mental health status of farmers had been assessed in depth in developed countries. However, there is paucity of such studies in India. From few studies published so far, family members had noticed a recent change in behavior of suicide victims before suicide. Most commonly victims appeared "tensed" or under some "stress" without apparent reason. They became withdrawn and had problems with sleep and appetite. In local language they described as "bhram" meaning

they appeared lost in their own thought or had some abnormal behavior. They talked less, and were reluctant to share their distress. Some even became irritable when asked by relatives about difficulties they are facing. About 20% of suicide victims had expressed suicide intents to relatives or close friends, and retrospectively, family members confessed that they have felt about suicide intents many times in few days prior to actual suicide. But, most of the times family members responded in anger or by requesting person not to repeat these words again.[18] This shows inability of farmers to express or ventilate their distress to family members also. It is interesting to note that on day of suicide, 5% of the victims had told their suicide intent to the person they met last. This is important and often repeated finding in our experience on field. In 2018, after conducting a session for farmers on suicide prevention in Manoli Village in Parbhani district of Maharashtra, a young farmer met us. He stated that his friend who committed suicide had expressed suicide ideas to him in morning, for next 3–4 hours he accompanied his friend and repeated "counseled" about why he should not commit suicide. However, in noon, when he went for lunch in his own home, his friend committed suicide by pesticide ingestion. When we conduct sessions about suicide prevention, it is important to emphasize about allowing person to express distress and to insist on immediate actions to seek mental health support which is easily available now. Similar findings were reported from Punjab State where 15% of the victims expressed suicide ideas prior to actual suicide to the relatives.[17] These are significant findings with implications in suicide prevention. We mental health professionals need to spread awareness among general population to take "any" suicide threat as serious and consider immediate consultation of a psychiatrist which can save a life. Most of the farmers who expressed suicide ideas had a diagnosable psychiatric illness on psychological autopsy.

Mental illness has been associated with suicide since long. In our psychological autopsy study, there was some diagnosable psychiatric illness in 60% of the farmers who committed suicide. Psychiatric epidemiological research emphasizes central role of current psychiatric status in determining suicide risk with estimates suggesting that up to 90% of suicides can be attributed to a series of common mental disorders. These studies have consistently shown that the relative contributions of social and economic factors, at the individual level, to the suicide risk of individuals are smaller than the overall contribution of mental illness.[27] Psychological autopsy studies from different parts of India have reported varied prevalence of mental health problems in suicide victims. Findings of these studies need to be interpreted in the light of difference in methodology adopted in conducting these studies. Also a note should be taken that these are not studies in farmers. These rates varied and may be depending upon method of diagnosis. In Chennai where structured instruments were used, 88% had diagnosable mental illness compared to 43% in Bengaluru, where structured interview tool was not used.[28,29] Most common psychiatric diagnosis was depression followed by alcohol dependence in these studies which is also reported from psychological autopsy studies in farmers' suicides. There are studies in farmers' suicides from west as well which emphasize role of mental illness in farmers' suicides. Study on farmers' suicides in the United Kingdom reported that 46% definitely and another 23% probably had mental illness. Depressive disorders and substance abuse were most common diagnosis.[24] In studies from central India, mental illness was recognized as major contributor to farmers' suicides.[18,23] In a study from Punjab, 63% suicide victims had alcohol dependence while 90% were reported to have mental stress.[17] Most significantly associated predictors for having a diagnosable psychiatric illness were noticeable change in behavior and expression of suicide ideas by farmers. Study on suicides in young, rural Tamil Nadu population reported mental illness were important contributors to suicide.[30]

Stressful Life Events

Psychological autopsy study by us in central India reported the most common stressful life event as "crop failure", accounting for 60% of all stressful events. This was followed by interpersonal problems (17%) and any physical illness or disability (10%). About 40% suicide victims had more than one stressful life event. Most common additional stressful; life event was marriage of a female family member, usually daughter or sister. Studies from India have reported occurrence of significant stressors prior to suicide event.[18] Other studies on farmers' suicide had described the role of stressful life events prior to suicide by farmers in India.[22,23,25] Study from Tamil Nadu also reported that acute stressors such as family conflicts, domestic violence, academic failures, unfulfilled romantic ideas were important risk factors associated with suicide in young.[30] Studies from abroad show importance of life stressors on the farmers. Here, occupational stressors were the most common, followed by relationship problems and then physical problems.[24]

Perceived Cause of Suicide

It is important to note the perspective of family members on probable reason behind suicide by their loved one. This gives idea about perception of society and farmers in particular as to what are etiological factor for suicide. With this background we had asked all suicide households and nonsuicide controls about what led the person to commit suicide.[18] On field during our psychological autopsy when relatives were directly asked about their opinion regarding reason behind suicide by victim, most common explanation offered by them was indebtedness (43%). Another 12% were not sure about reason of suicide but felt it is "probably related to debt". Thus, about 55% of farmers themselves perceived indebtedness as directly or indirectly as cause of suicide. Looking from another view, 45% of the farmers interviewed did not perceive indebtedness as direct cause of suicide. Thus, though important in itself, apart from indebtedness, there are other factors that are playing important role in the farmers' suicides. Relationship problems (15%) and mental illness (11%) were next most common attributes of suicide as per them. Though mental illness was perceived as one of the important causes for suicide, only 5% of the victims had consulted psychiatrist. We also asked relatives whether psychiatrist should be consulted in case of attempted/ threatened suicide. Sixty-one percent of the family members of suicide victims felt that one should consult psychiatrist in case of attempted suicide as compared to 75% of the controls. This is important for us as mental health professionals. We need to be proactive in community to propagate importance of seeking mental healthcare if someone expresses suicide ideas or attempts suicide. This needs to start from medical colleges itself where budding doctors should be emphasized about the need of psychiatric evaluation and intervention of every patient with attempted suicide before discharge. This will save many lives as these budding doctors will be working as medical officers and specialists who will later be treating persons with suicide attempts in community.

PREVENTION OF SUICIDES BY FARMERS

To prevent deaths of farmers by suicide, we need to accept and understand that "farmer's suicides are preventable". Most of the risk factors discussed above are modifiable to large extent. All mental health professionals should take pride in saving lives by preventing suicides. Active involvement is suicide prevention programs at various levels, and is a direct contribution to saving lives by preventing suicides. Same applies to prevention of suicides by farmers. Preventive strategies can be devised to work at various levels and can modify risk factors. There are examples from across the globe for devising and implementing these strategies effectively. Same will be discussed at relevant places below.

Over last decade, the government had taken few initiatives to reduce distress in farming sector. Most preventive measures taken so far reflect dominance of social scientists on preventive strategies devised. Most of the special financial packages announced have been diverted to the agriculture and allied industries rather than direct benefit to farmers. Less than 60% households who lost a farmer by suicide got full ex-gratia financial help from government. Most were provided few implements etc. as ex-gratia help. Few states like Maharashtra had implemented "Prerna Prakalp (Policy)" and appointed part time psychiatrists in few districts affected with high number of suicides by farmers to run some mental health awareness programs. Proactive screening of distressed farmers was expected but never actually started. Andhra Pradesh and Karnataka government had formed state level commission and devised policy to prevent suicides by farmers, but implementation at ground level was not satisfactory.

Based on our personal work experience and backing of knowledge gained from available literature here we will discuss few suggestions for what should be part of strategies to prevent suicide by farmers in India. These are just few suggestions and strategies may go far beyond what we have discussed below. Farmers' suicide prevention can be viewed from principles of primary, secondary, and tertiary prevention as discussed below.

Primary Prevention

Here, identification of high-risk farmers and training community gatekeepers to identify and guide them is key strategy. Early detection of at-risk groups is very important in suicide prevention.

Early Identification and Treatment of Mental Health Problems

Farmers with mental health issues are at high-risk for suicide. Indentifying of farmers in community suffering with depression, alcoholism, previous suicide attempts, etc. by using simple screening tools at village level and their prompt guidance to seek mental health care can be a good initial starting point.[25] A significant association exists between crop failures, marriage of sister or daughter in home and suicide by farmers. A more humane and scientific approach needs to be evolved to deal with loan defaulters. Bank personnel need to be trained in this approach. Psychological help may be provided when dealing with defaulters in distress. Alcoholism is another

important contributor to farmers' suicides. Alcoholism should not be projected only as a moral problem of individual. Availability of medical facilities at primary health center level to treat withdrawal and prompt referral to psychiatrists appointed at almost all district hospitals under the National Rural Health Mission (NRHM) program can play a vital role in reducing this menace. Training should be imparted to all medical and paramedical professionals for early detection and treatment of mental illnesses. This is being done to some extent for Community Health Officers being recruited by current central Government. Rigorous monitoring of this training should be done to make it more effective. Depression as an illness often goes undiagnosed. Simple self-administered tools available and validated in local dialects such as self-reporting questionnaire-20 (SRQ-20) may be useful in detecting those suffering from psychological distress.[31] Awareness programs for general public and high-risk individuals should focus on promotion of better mental health, stress management and coping skills, proper financial planning, life-skills development, and early identification and treatment of mental illnesses. Community gatekeepers such as representatives of local bodies, teachers, spiritual leaders, aanganwadi, and ASHA workers can be trained in these simple suicide prevention strategies. Apart from these, some of the specific primary prevention measures for farmers' as a group could be:

Restriction of access to pesticides (includes herbicides): Suicide by ingestion of pesticide is the most common method of suicide among farmers in the country. Like there is a list of essential medicines and restricted medicines in India, similarly there should be lists of essential pesticide list and restricted pesticides. Restricted pesticides should include extremely lethal compounds. Strict regulation of their formulation, packaging and sale, and storage should be implemented urgently. A simple intervention like providing a lockable storage box to keep pesticides safe and out of reach is also effective. Study in Sri Lanka on Introduction of *lockable boxes* for storing pesticides to farming households was found to be acceptable. Most households used the boxes responsibly, although there was some decline in the proper usage over time. Most informants regarded the box as useful with convenience for storage, security, avoiding wastage, and protection of children being major factors.[6] A message on the box about how to deal with bad feelings and the importance of safer storage can be very effective in guiding farmers about keeping composed. We, in India, need to start this initiative as pesticide market highly nonregulated and is corrupted by giant MNCs who do marketing of their products at village level with blind eye to hazards of these chemicals.

Farmer friendly economic policies: Economic distress is an important risk factor for suicides by farmers. This should be viewed from a farmers' perspective. Provision of seeds, fertilizers, and farm implements at subsidized rates will reduce input cost for farming. Group farming and farming via co-operative societies will help marginal and small farmers to share crops and incomes from small pieces of land. This will ensure economic well-being by reducing input cost as a group of farmers can bargain for less cost for seeds, fertilizers, etc. as quantity required will be large. Also shared labor and farming implements can reduce cost of crop maintenance. When yield comes in bulk quantity, transport at larger scale can be arranged by group of farmers or co-operative society to a distant market offering better price for their produce.

This can be promoted by government via announcing special packages for a small/large group of farmers. At individual level, "state" should ensure fresh crop loans to every farmer at the beginning of each season. Loans should carry a minimal interest and for nonirrigated farmers, this may be interest free. Crop insurance needs to be covered well. Current practice of leaving farmers at mercy of private insurance companies should be shunned. Insurance companies should be made accountable for any losses without discretion. There should be fast grievance redress system for farmers so that they are not harassed by private insurance firms. This will ensure that when a yield failure occurs, finances of poor farmers do not collapse all of a sudden. Suicide prevention campaign in Sri Lanka had slogan "agricultural loans only for agricultural purpose" which very well suits Indian scenario as well. So that crop loans will be utilized to maximize yield and farmers do not get trapped in vicious cycle of indebtedness.

Coping skills: As we have seen above the farmers are exposed to various stressors and farming is highly uncertain industry when it comes to yielding results. Indian farmers heavily rely on things beyond their control such as poor rain, attacks by pests, fluctuation in market price for their produce, lack of storage facilities, etc. increasing this uncertainty many folded. Farmers need to be trained in coping skills so that they can adapt to favorable defense mechanisms in face of adversities. Improving communication with neighbors, utilization of social contacts, and supports when in difficulty is important. Co-operation with neighbors for farming and social support also play an important role. Creation of small groups to help each other in distress will go long way in their sustainability in volatile times. Spirituality is another important way to cope with adverse events in life. Another important aspect is avoiding competition within village. At present many farmers get trapped in expenditure to "show off" their superiority in village. Excessive intrusion of politics within villages and families is also destabilizing healthy bond within these social units. In times of adversity, it is important to learn from mistakes and minimize costs rather than falling into addictions as is visible in current farming community. It is important to make farmers aware of availability if mental health services nearby so that they can seek round the clock help when in distress.

Training farmers in new agricultural practices: Most of the farms in India are family run businesses that adopt the farming practices prevalent over generations. Newer technologies in this field should be made available to farmers at low cost. There should be proper information portals that will provide information in villages rather than in cities. When it comes to new technology cost is often a barrier. Poor farmers will need subsidies on these so that it is affordable to them.

Secondary Prevention

This involves early intervention and treatment of high-risk farmers and suicide attempters. For this we can use existing three-tier system of healthcare infrastructure in India. At primary health center (PHC) and sub-center level, healthcare workers and other voluntary workers can screen for mental illness with simple questionnaires. Those with distress or some suspected illness or who harbor suicide ideas should be treated at PHC by medical officer who should have received some training in mental health. If healthcare workers at PHC feel that urgent referral is needed in view of high suicide risk or they are not confident in treating case, this should be done immediately to District Hospital where Class-I psychiatrist with his team is appointed. At this level option should be given to patient to visit any other psychiatrist in private practice immediately. A team should be formed under the leadership of a psychiatrist at district hospitals which serves as level-2 in current public health infrastructure. Those found to have mental illness and also all those who attempt suicide or threaten to do so should be evaluated and treated here with all mental healthcare facilities, including electroconvulsive therapy (ECTs). Proper follow-up and monitoring of treatment of suicide attempters should be ensured in the community. Psychiatrists in private sector and nursing homes and local associations of psychiatrists may also be involved in providing help at this level with appropriate incentives to them. If patients require further management they may be referred to psychiatry departments in medical colleges, mental hospitals which serve as level-3 institutes in current healthcare structure. These institutes can also be utilized efficiently as training centers for health professionals at PHC and grass-root workers.

Apart from strengthening mental healthcare services, there is an urgent need to train healthcare workers including doctors at PHC in treatment of pesticide poisoning, drug over dosages, attempted hanging, traumatic injuries, basic life support (BLS), etc. This will ensure prompt and early treatment of a farmer with a suicide attempt, increasing chances of saving his life many folds. At PHC level itself, medical officer should start antidotes such as atropine, pralidoxime (PAM), do intubation and ventilation if needed, perform gastric wash to remove ingested poison, etc. can save many lives. Also prompt primary care of burns with immediate infusion of IV fluids can help victim to survive till he reaches higher center. Splinting of traumatic injuries, provision of neck fixations and spine support will save lives of many who adopt traumatic methods of suicide. All these should be systematically devised and training imparted frequently.

Tertiary Prevention

This involves rehabilitation of rescued attempters and helping the survivors of the suicide. A psychological autopsy should be performed on all farmers' suicides as this objectively brings out relationship between suicides and sociodemographic, psychological factors, stressful life events, etc. This is particularly important in case of farmers' suicides as there are many unscientific speculative reports in the media which misleads the policy makers and public as well. For any preventive strategy to be effective, it should be based on sound research and should have frequent evaluations for its success. Families of suicide victims (suicide survivors) should be offered psychological support via professionals. This is important and urgent need in India as studies have found very high level of psychological distress in survivors of farmers' suicide in the country.[15,21] Those families affected by farmers' suicides should receive economic support to restart their distressed business, if need. But, only financial support is not enough in itself for the survivors. Long-term strategies are required to help the survivors cope with loss of a breadearner in family. Children of the victims are particularly at risk and should be offered support in education and other facilities. Any financial package should always be accompanied by mental health support to the survivors as above-quoted studies have clearly shown that mere financial help will not reduce psychological distress of suicide survivors.

■ CONCLUSION

Suicide by farmers is an ongoing pheno-menon since over 30 years now. Suicides by farmers need to be studied as a special category, as farming business operates in an environment of distinct risk factors unique to this sector. Literature on this issue is dominated from social science and economic sectors so have been the relief policies adopted by the government in India. There are very few scientific studies from mental health perspective of farmers who committed suicide in India. It is an appeal to all the mental healthcare workers in country to take up this issue as priority for research and community work so that policies of government can be mended accordingly. Psychological needs of farmers' suicide survivors need to be addressed urgently as nearly 80% of them are experiencing severe psychological distress. Preventive policies for farmers' suicide should have mental healthcare of farmers as a major component so that the best results can be obtained.

Acknowledgments

I am thankful to Prof Dr Prakash Behere and Prof Dr RS Murthy sir for their constant support and encouragement to me to continue work in this area of farmers' suicide.

■ REFERENCES

1. Behere PB, Bhise MC. Farmers' suicide: Across culture. Indian J Psychiatry. 2009;51:242-3.
2. Eklind PD, Carlson JE, Schanbel B. Agricultural hazards reduction through stress management. J Agromedicine. 1998;39(2): 159-65.
3. Pickett W, Hartling L, Brison RJ, Guernsey JR. Fatal work related farm injuries in Canada,

1991-1995. Canadian Agricultural Injury Surveillance Program. CMAJ. 1999;160: 1843-8.

4. Page AN, Fragar LJ. Suicide in Australian farming, 1988-1997. Aust N Z J Psychiatry. 2002;36:81-5.

5. Hawton K, Fagg J, Simkin S, Harriss L, Malmberg A, Smith D. The geographical distribution of suicides in farmers in England and Wales. Soc Psychiatry Psychiatr Epidemiol. 1999;34:122-7.

6. Hawton K, Ratnayeke L, Simkin S, Harriss L, Scott V. Evaluation of acceptability and use of lockable storage devices for pesticides in Sri Lanka that might assist in prevention of self-poisoning. BMC Public Health [Internet]. 2009;9:69.

7. Gunnell D, Eddleston M. Suicide by intentional ingestion of pesticides: A continuing tragedy in developing countries. Int J Epidemiol. 2003;32:902-9.

8. Bertolote JM, Fleischmann A, Butchart A, Besbelli N. Suicide, suicide attempts and pesticides: A major hidden public health problem. Bull World Health Organ. 2006; 84:260.

9. Gunnell D, Fernando R, Hewagama M, Priyangika WDD, Konradsen F, Eddleston M. The impact of pesticide regulations on suicide in Sri Lanka. Int J Epidemiol. 2007: 163-70.

10. Meltzer H, Griffins C, Brock A, Rooney C, Jenkins R. Patterns of suicide by occupation in England and Wales: 2001-2005. Br J Psychiatry. 2008;193:73-6.

11. Spiegel. Water Shut Off in Australia-wave of suicides follows drought down under [Internet] 2006. [Cited 2012 Aug 18]. [online] Available from: http://www.spiegel.de/ international/0,518,448677,00.html. [Last accessed July, 2022].

12. NSW Farmers Association. NSW Farmers' Mental Health Network, [Internet] 2006. [Cited 2014 July 15]. [online] Available from: http://www.nswfarmers.org.au/mental_ health_network. [Last accessed July, 2022].

13. Judd F, Jackson H, Fraser C, Murray G, Robins G, Komiti A. Understanding suicide in Australian farmers. Soc Psychiatry Psychiatr Epidemiol. 2006;41:1-10.

14. Nagaraj K, Sainath P, Gopinath R. Farmers' suicides in India: Magnitudes, trends and spatial patterns, 1997-2012. Rev Agrarian Studies [Internet]. 2014;4(2).

15. Bhise MC, Marwale AV, Mohide AC, Jadhav SS, Murambikar GP. Psychological distress in survivors of farmers' suicides in drought prone Aurangabad and Jalna Districts of Marathwada region in Maharashtra, India. Ann Indian Psychiatry. 2019;3:143-7.

16. Behere PB, Bhise MC. Farmers' suicides in central rural India: Where are we heading? Indian J Soc Psychiatry. 2010;26(1):1-3.

17. Bhalla GS, Sharma SL, Wig NN, Mehta S, Kumar P. Suicides in rural Punjab. By Institute for Development and Communication: Report submitted to Government of Punjab. Chandigarh: Himalaya Press; 1998.

18. Bhise MC, Behere PB. Risk factors for farmers' suicides in central rural India: Matched case–control psychological autopsy study. Indian J Psychol Med. 2016;38:560-6.

19. World Health Organization (WHO). (2021). Suicide worldwide in 2019: global health estimates. World Health Organization [Internet] 2021. [online] Available from: https://www.who.int/publications/i/ item/9789240026643 [Last accessed July, 2022].

20. National Crime Records Bureau of India. (2019). Accidental Deaths and Suicides in India 2019. National Crime Records Bureau of India, Ministry of Home affairs of India [Internet]. [online] Available from: https:// ncrb.gov.in/en/accidental-deaths-suicides-india-2019 [Last accessed July, 2022].

21. Bhise MC, Behere PB. A case–control study of psychological distress in survivors of farmers' suicides in Wardha District in central India. Indian J Psychiatry. 2016;58:147-51.

22. Dongre AR, Deshmukh PR. Farmers' suicides in the Vidarbha region of Maharashtra, India: A qualitative exploration of their causes. J Inj Violence Res. 2012;4:2-6.

23. Mishra S. (2006). Suicide of farmers in Maharashtra state: Report submitted to Govt of Maharashtra. [Internet]. 2006. [online] Available from: http://www.igidr.ac.in/pdf/

publication/PP-055.pdf [Last accessed July, 2022].

24. Malmberg A, Simkin S, Howton K. Suicide in farmers. Br J Psychiatry. 1999;175:103-5.

25. Xavier PV, Dinesh N, John AJ, Radhakrishnan VK, Suresh Kumar PN, Ali A. Position paper and action plan on farmers' suicide: Presentation to Chief Minister and Health Minister. Kerala J Psychiatry. 2007;22(1): 68-75.

26. Prasad J, Abraham VJ, Minz S, Abraham S, Joseph A, Muliyil JP, et al. Rates and Factors Associated with Suicide in Kaniyambadi Block, Tamil Nadu, South India, 2000–2002. Int J Soc Psychiatry. 2006;52(1):65-71.

27. Cavanagh JT, Carson AJ, Sharpe M, Lawrie SM. Psychological autopsy studies of suicide: A systematic review. Psychol Med. 2003;33:395-405.

28. Vijaykumar L, Rajkumar S. Are risk factors for suicide universal? A case control study in India. Acta Psychiatr Scand. 1999;99: 407-11.

29. Gururaj G, Isaac MK, Subbakrishna DK, Ranjani R. Risk factors for completed suicides: A case-control study from Bengaluru, India. Inj Control Saf Promot. 2004;11(3): 183-91.

30. Aron R, Joseph A, Abraham S, Muliyili J, George K, Prasad J, et al. Suicide in young people in southern India. Lancet. 2004;363: 1117-8.

31. World Health Organization (WHO). User's Guide to the Self Reporting Questionnaire. In: World Health Organization, Division of Mental Health Geneva: WHO/MNH/ PSF/94.8, Division of Mental Health; 1994.

Suicide and Indian Media

Vinay Kumar, KS Shubrata

ABSTRACT

This chapter deals with the role of media in influencing the suicide rates. The role of media in the Indian context has also been highlighted. The guidelines for proper media reporting have been discussed.

Keywords: Media and suicide; Suicide reporting guidelines.

■ INTRODUCTION

Suicides account for 1.3% of deaths globally. Out of 800,000 people dying by suicide worldwide every year, 135,000 (17%) are Indian residents. Suicide leaves a devastating and lasting impact on immediate family members. This negative effect is extended to other people in the community by media. The media portrayal of suicides can lead to several emotional complications in readers/viewers, rarely ending in suicides itself. At the same time, a sensible media report on suicide can help in "Suicide Prevention" too. Here, we discuss effect of "Media on Suicides", particularly in Indian context.

SUICIDE AND MEDIA: GLOBAL SCENARIO

David Philips, an American sociologist, was one of the first people who found the association between media and suicide. He observed that after stories about suicides had been published in the *New York Times*, their number rose significantly. He coined the term "Werther Effect" in 1974. Soon after the publication of a novel, *Die Leiden des jungen Werthers* (*The Sorrows of Young Werther*) by Goethe.[1] It was noted that many young men mimicked the main character by dressing in yellow pants and blue jackets. Werther, the lead character in the novel, when rejected by his lover, shoots himself with a pistol. During the immediate period after publication, there were reports of young men trying to kill themselves in similar method. This led to the book being banned at several places. Till date, the case of Werther is the most well-known, though other historical examples of spates of suicide following publicity about an index suicide have been described.[2-4] The "Werther effect" is now commonly used to describe the relationship between media portrayals of suicide and imitation acts, including completed suicides, attempted suicides, and suicidal thoughts.

"Social learning theory" or "identification theory" is being used to explain suicides which happen in subsequent days after suicide reporting in media. Human behaviors are learnt observationally through modeling. Already vulnerable persons (persons with depression, in crisis, etc.) tend to observe human behavior in media and come to a conclusion that personal problem may be solved by suicide and then may adopt suicidal behavior. While this is about social learning theory, the identification theory says that people tend to identify with persons who are similar to themselves. Persons who face similar emotional states or experience problems or crisis similar to those as suicidal victims presented in the media may develop a sort of attachment that encourages them to imitate suicidal behavior. This can be horizontal identification which is identifying oneself with persons of similar sociodemographic profile, or vertical identification, which is mimicking behaviors of persons whom they admire or perceive as socially superior/celebrities.[5]

But fortunately, it has been also suggested that under certain conditions, exposure to accounts of suicidal behavior in the media is associated with a lower risk of suicide attempts. It can have a more positive, i.e., educative or preventive, effect, especially when the media present constructive coping strategies with suicidal ideations or emphasize other solutions to adverse life circumstances. Niederkrotenthaler and his team studied this effect and have named it as "Papageno effect".[6] This is to indicate a positive preventive effect of media reporting on suicidal behaviors. Papageno, the main character in Mozart's opera *The Magic Flute* (1791), having lost his lover, tries to hang himself, when the three child-spirits appear and stop him. They advise him to play his magic bells to summon the lover. Then the problem gets solved and Papageno is happy. Hence, it is important to note the protective effects of media, if suicides are reported with constructive coping strategies.

SUICIDE AND MEDIA: INDIAN SCENARIO

The Indian media consists of several different types of communications of mass media: newspapers, magazines, television, radio, cinema, and internet-based websites/portals. Printing has been the basic tool of mass communication, storing, and dissemination of information and knowledge for about 600 years. From about the second half of the last century electronic media has somewhat taken over the mass media world by a storm but the print media has not lost its charm and its social relevance.[7] As of 2007, the country consumes 99 million newspaper copies, making it the world's second largest newspaper market. It is one of the world's oldest and largest media. India's media has been free and autonomous for most of its history, even before Ashoka the Great founded the Indian empire on the principles of justice, openness, morality, and spirituality.

The period of emergency (1975–1977) declared by the then Prime Minister was the brief period when India's media was faced with potential government retribution. According to the census of India, the average literacy rate of India is 74.4% in 2011 while National Statistical Commission surveyed literacy to be 77.7% in 2017–18* (Wikipedia). With approximately 551 million people being literate in India, more people—rural and urban—are reading newspapers and magazines. Print media now has a readership of approximately 316 million people.[7-9] There is tremendous pressure from the advertising agencies to make the news in papers, sensational, so that more copies are sold. There is a tough competition given by the numerous 24*7 news channels, which try to reconstruct the sensational events in the original manner.

In India, media portrayal of mental health issues has always been biased. A suicide report always makes it into front page with a sensationalized picture. Armstrong et al. conducted the first study in India to examine whether these media reports of suicides reflect the epidemiological data on suicide. They followed nine major newspapers (print versions) in Tamil Nadu over 7 months and collected a large sample of 1,631 media reports of suicides. They concluded that the suicide characteristics in the print media were not entirely representative of suicides in the broader Tamil Nadu population, which may lead the general public to develop misunderstandings about suicide in their state. In particular, overreporting compared to their occurrence in broader population was seen in cases of suicides involving females, those aged under 29 years, separated or widowed males, unmarried females, those using methods with a higher case fatality rate and those who were students or working in the agricultural sector. Under reporting was seen in suicides involving males, those aged over 30 years and above, those who were married and suicides by poisoning.[10]

A content analysis study of nine major newspapers in Tamil Nadu[10] was undertaken to assess the quality of newspaper reporting of suicide-related news in India against World Health Organization (WHO) suicide reporting guidelines. They reviewed 1.681 suicide articles in total. The mean number of suicide articles per day per newspaper was 0.9% and 54.5% of articles were 10 sentences or less. Nearly 95% of articles primarily focused on reporting specific suicide incidents. Harmful reporting practices were very common while helpful reporting practices were rare.

In a semi-structured qualitative interview study conducted with 28 print media and television media professionals with experience reporting on suicide-related news of north (New Delhi and Chandigarh) and south (Chennai) India, perspectives on the reason for regular reporting of suicides in mass media, a description of experiences and processes of covering suicide incidents on the crime beat and about the emergence of health reporter coverage of suicide were explored.[10] It was interesting to note that the socio-cultural factors such as profile of the suicidal person, presence of suicide notes, the social and political issues surrounding it, played a major role in determining the newsworthiness of a particular incident. Reporters believed that the suicide news was akin to crime report and hence they reported in a similar fashion. It was reassuring to note that many health reporters and editorial-level media professionals talked about the recent shift to introducing some coverage on suicide as a public health issue including social and psychological causes. On the 30th of January 2020, India recorded its first coronavirus disease (COVID) case,[11] and as the number of cases grew, the government of India progressively implemented a range of measures, beginning with the suspension of travel from certain countries, medical screening for international travelers, and finally a complete nationwide lock-down from March 24 to April 14, 2020. This study was done to understand whether media reporting of suicides and attempted suicides in India changed during these 40 days of lockdown from 24th March 2020 to 3rd May 2020. The study saw an increase in online news media reports of suicides and attempts during COVID-19 lockdown. They opined that this may be due to an increase in journalists' awareness about suicide or more sensational media reporting or may be a proxy indicator of a real community increase in suicidal behavior.[12]

■ ONLINE MEDIA

Growing digitalization efforts, paired with low data pricing, have enabled a large number of individuals in India to actively use the internet. The country's digital population amounts to approximately 624 million active users as of February 2021. Around 448 million of them were active social media users. As of January 2021, YouTube and Facebook have the highest penetration, with over 89% and 76%, respectively.[13]

Although more study is needed to demonstrate causal correlations, and it is yet unknown whether forms of online content are harmful and the degree of such an effect. Social Cognitive Theory supports one mechanism for such associations. According to the Social Cognitive Theory, conduct is taught through observation and interaction with others in a social context or social environment. Suicide-related behaviors are one such health behavior that is influenced by social learning from others. Indeed, social learning is especially crucial in adolescent populations, as research has shown that brain maturation at this age provides a greater sensitivity to social judgment and peer standards.[14] Suicide-related behaviors can unfortunately spread among youngsters, making it difficult for doctors and public health practitioners to notice them before they cause morbidity.[15]

It was discovered that teens with self-harming behavior and suicidal ideation use social networking websites to contact with and seek social support from other users. These users were more likely to be exposed to and engage in self-harm behavior as a result of factors such as reading negative messages supporting self-harm, replicating self-injurious behavior of others, and adopting self-harm practices through online social networking.[16]

Despite sharing risk factors with the world on social media sites like Facebook and Twitter, many teenagers and young people fail to mention them to physicians. Probably, the reason for this would be that they are able to reach nonjudgmental audience in an anonymous way. As professionals, we need to see an opportunity in this social media to reach a good number of hard to engage young individuals with "mental health promotion" and "suicide prevention strategies".

We see a limited number of studies from India on suicide and digital media.

Cyberbullying leading to cybervictimization which may end up in suicides are a raising matter of concern in adolescents and young people.

Every other day, a confusing array of games with novel components of fun and entertainment emerge to entice children. Games are designed to help youngsters and adults relax and strengthen their cognitive abilities. Teenagers are always interested in trying out new games, and e-gaming is one such platform that allows them convenient access and faster amusement. The perilous "Blue Whale Challenge", in which vulnerable teens are frequently involved, has taken the world by storm. The Blue Whale Challenge is neither an app nor an online game; instead, participants are given a link to enter this "deadly" challenge game through social media chat groups.

This is perhaps the only game in which the player must end his or her life in order to complete the game. To make matters worse, there is no way to exit the challenge. Narayan R and team describe a depressed boy who accepted the Blue Whale challenge and caution about the need for awareness in clinicians about the same.[17] From June to September 2019, an online contest called "Buddies for Suicide Prevention" was held with the topic "Action for Suicide Prevention". Instagram and Facebook were used to promote the campaign. Post-it: a poster-making competition, Inscribe 2.0: a slogan-writing competition, Script O: a script-writing competition, and Minute matter: short film contest were among the four categories of competitions. Following the promotions, the page reached a total of >10,000 users. They concluded that social media can be utilized to conduct mental health campaigns and it is an effective initiative as one can reach out to several people over a short-time period.[18]

MEDIA GUIDELINES FOR SUICIDE REPORTING

Experts have tried to find evidence-based therapies in their search for suicide prevention measures. Though there is inadequate proof, media techniques are one of the most important suicide prevention strategies used around the world.[19] In 2008, the WHO published "Media Guidelines" for reporting suicides. This was later updated in 2017 based on a systematic review of over 100 research studies on the impact of media reporting on suicide in collaboration with International Association of Suicide Prevention.[20]

The WHO guidelines for responsible reporting suggest practices which promote help-seeking behavior, increase awareness of suicide prevention, and provide alternative coping strategies for vulnerable readers.[21] More recently, the International Association for Suicide Prevention (IASP) highlighted the urgent need for the adoption of guidelines on responsible reporting of suicides during the COVID-19 pandemic and suggested additional tips to support and supplement existing guidelines during the pandemic.[22]

The WHO guidelines stresses on providing accurate information on help seeking, educating public without spreading myths, reporting stories of how to cope with life stressors or suicidal thoughts and to be cautious specifically in reporting celebrity suicides and when interviewing bereaved family members. The guidelines also talk about the things which should not be done while reporting suicides in media. It says not to place stories about suicide prominently, not to repeat such stories, avoid sensationalization or normalization and not to describe the method used and not to use photographs or video footage or social media links.

The Samaritans, a global organization, that spreads awareness on suicide prevention recommends "Suicide Reporting: 10 points to remember" based on WHO Guidelines.[23]

The growing popularity of social media, particularly among young people, has necessitated the development of additional standards to promote secure peer-to-peer contact. This has resulted in the #chatsafe project in Australia. It contains 173 items. These items were organized into the following five sections: (1) Before you post anything online about suicide; (2) Sharing your own thoughts, feelings, or experience with suicidal behavior online; (3) Communicating about someone you know who is affected by suicidal thoughts, feelings or behaviors; (4) Responding to someone who may be suicidal; (5) Memorial websites, pages and closed groups to honor the deceased.[24]

As a comment to the paper by Rakhi Dandona and colleagues, reported in *The Lancet Public Health, Armstrong and colleagues write that* suicide prevention is not solely or even primarily the domain of mental health practitioners providing interventions for suicidal individuals. They continue to say that with suicide being a complex and highly stigmatized issue in India, suicide prevention planning should be grounded in a broader public health approach framed around multisectoral collaboration. Population-level approaches such as responsible media reporting of suicides should be undertaken selectively targeting at-risk subpopulations.[25]

MEDIA GUIDELINES IN INDIA

No national guidelines were available on the subject of media reporting of suicide in India till 2015. The Indian Psychiatric Society (IPS) was the first body to take initiative in formulating guidelines for media reporting of Suicides[26] **(Box 1)**. These guidelines by IPS not only talk about what should not be done but also about the aspects related to positive reporting too.

The Press Council of India (PCI) issued a notification in 2019 endorsing the WHO guidelines for responsible reporting of suicide. The PCI cited the Mental Health Care Act 2017 which states that photographs or other information about a person undergoing mental health treatment should not be published without their consent.[27] Its key advantages are its conformance to the WHO guideline's international standards. The points such as lack of operationalization and a high level of subjectivity and ethical such as releasing personal information including possible triggers are the source of its methodological flaws. Because the recommendations are not operationalized, they are more subjective.[28]

India is yet to come up with guidelines specific to social media.

OUTCOME STUDIES

There have been few studies all over India to check if media coverage of suicides is accurate. Media reporting of suicide in Rajasthan, Puducherry, Kerala, Bangalore,

---

BOX 1: The Indian Psychiatric Society (IPS) guidelines for reporting of suicide in media.

News coverage should be neutral:
- Present facts in matter-of-fact language, without sensationalism; be objective rather than emotional
- Do not romanticize or glorify the event, or imply martyrdom
- Do not indicate blame unless clearly justified; instead, acknowledge that a combination of triggers and vulnerabilities were probably responsible

News coverage should be discreet:
- Avoid front-page reporting, presentation in boxes, large headlines, lengthy reports, and photographs of the deceased
- Do not provide detailed descriptions of the method of suicide
- Do not publish suicide notes

News coverage should be sensitive:
- Consider how the news coverage might occasion psychological and social harm to the survivors of the event
- Respect the privacy of the survivors

Other matters:
- Do not repeatedly play on the event or theme
- Do not allow readers to form the impression that suicide is a way of coping with a personal problem, or a way to teach others a lesson
- Exercise particular caution when reporting celebrity suicides

Suggestions for positive reporting:
- When reporting suicide, use the opportunity to improve public awareness about issues related to mental health and suicide, and sources of help. Possibilities include the provision of tips on early warning signs of suicidal behavior and assistance that can be provided to those at risk. List suicide helplines and counseling services
- Destigmatize the experience of stress, emotional difficulties, depression, and suicidal ideation so that help-seeking behavior is encouraged
- Promote the awareness that problems can be solved and depression and mental illness can be overcome. Describe how people have overcome suicidal thoughts and coped with stress

and Kashmir were assessed in different studies.[29-33] Unfortunately, they all found that the suicide reporting did not adhere to WHO guidelines. Most of the stories were sensationalized. Harmful reporting practices such as describing the location and method of suicide and the detailing of steps involved were common. No attempt was made to include any educational materials. Suicide reporting had a strong tendency toward sensationalism. On the plus side, most publications did not print the photograph of the deceased.[29] All studies concluded that there was an urgent need to improve the quality of media reporting. They suggested development of national guidelines as well as collaborative efforts in implementing the same. A cross-sectional study from India was undertaken to see whether online media adhered to the responsible suicide reporting guidelines. More than 80% of media reports departed from at least one of the suggestions, according to the findings. The news article's headlines, sensational reporting, and extensive descriptions of suicide techniques revealed a maximum breach.[34]

A team led by Lakshmi Vijaykumar has created a scorecard to examine and rate media accounts on suicide to encourage appropriate reporting. They came up with a scorecard that included 10 good and 10 negative parameters after speaking with a group of specialists. The scorecard can be a useful tool for evaluating and quantifying media reporting about suicide.[35]

■ CELEBRITY SUICIDES

In our country, celebrity suicide is one of the most widely reported events. Following the tragic death of a prominent Hindi actor by suicide in 2019, as expected, the media flew into frenzy, with pieces in newspapers, news channels, and social media detailing every aspect of the suicide attempt. Most of the news channels became so insensitive that they kept on showing the actor's lifeless body, evoking severe negative feelings in the audience. Different channels tried in myriad ways to reconstruct the whole scene, with making new assumptions and guesses about the unfortunate event. Numerous studies have happened following this celebrity suicide.

Quality of media reporting following a celebrity suicide was assessed by different teams.[36-39] One study analyzed 573 new articles on the topic. Several breaches of reporting were noted in relation to mentioning the word "celebrity" in the title of report, inclusion of the deceased's photograph, detailed descriptions of the method and location of suicide.[36]

Another study tried to assess the quality of online media reporting of a recent celebrity suicide in India and its impact on the online suicide related search behavior of the population. Nearly 85.5% of online reports violated at least one WHO media reporting guideline and only 13% articles provided information about where to seek help for suicidal thoughts or ideation. There was a significant increase in online suicide-seeking and help-seeking behavior after the reference event, when compared to baseline. However, the online peak search interest for suicide-seeking was greater than help-seeking.[37]

Recent cross-sectional study by Raj et al. (2020) explores the adherence of Indian media reporting of suicides for a month after the celebrity-death. It reveals that >80% of the news articles deviate from the prevalent Press Council of India (PCI) and the WHO guidelines for media-reporting of suicides.[40]

Vikas Menon and his colleagues have tried to offer some insights into mediators of suicide contagion following a celebrity suicide and propose suggestions from a preventive standpoint. Preexisting psychiatric morbidity or maladaptive cognitions, excessive identification and idealization, excessive discussion among peers amplifying the feeling of loss, greater emotional connectedness to the celebrity, and social and community factors were explained as mediating factors. Suggestions were given to mitigate the impact of celebrity suicide on Population Mental Health like increase public awareness about the negative impact of celebrity suicide (universal strategy), responsible media reporting of celebrity suicide (selective strategy), early identification and monitoring of vulnerable individuals (indicated strategy), positive thinking and promoting positive mental health approaches and postvention activities directed at family and close relatives of the deceased celebrity.[41]

CONCLUSION

Overall, the evidence till date suggests that suicide reporting in media can have substantial influence on the mindsets of the readers/viewers. While an insensitive and sensationalized report of suicide in media results in number of negative effects in the readers, a sensible, realistic report with educative material and information on help seeking can prevent further suicides. Now that there are specific guidelines in India regarding suicide reporting in media, it is vital that they are implemented. This implementation would mean active collaboration between different stakeholders such as mental health professionals, media personnel, police officials, and nongovernmental organizations. It is also important to have more long-term studies related to the beneficial effects of these implemented guidelines. We need to develop culture sensitive tools which can be used in social media for suicide prevention specific to India. There needs to be an inherent mechanism in all these digital media, which tries to screen for these suicide-related behavior.

REFERENCES

1. Thorson J, Oberg PA. Was there a suicide epidemic after Goethe's Werther? Arch Suicide Res. 2003;7(1):69-72.
2. Andriessen K. On the Werther effect: a reply to Krysinska and Lester. Crisis. 2007;28(1):48-9.
3. Krysinska K, Lester D. Comment on the Werther effect. Crisis. 2006;27(2):100.
4. Motto JA. Suicide and suggestibility: the role of the press. Am J Psychiatry. 1967;124(2):252-6.
5. Jan D. The Werther Effect, the Papageno Effect or No Effect? A Literature Review. Int J Environ Res Public Health. 2021;18:2396.
6. Niederkrotenthaler T, Voracek M, Herberth A, Till B, Strauss M, Etzersdorfer E, et al. Role of media reports in completed and prevented suicide: Werther vs. Papageno effects. Br J Psychiatry: J Mental Sci. 2010;197(3):234-43.
7. Press Council of India. (2017). Inaugural address by Mr. Justice GN Ray, Chairman, Press Council of India at the Seminar on "Future of Print Media" on 17th February, 2009 at Surendranath College for Women, Kolkata. [online] Available from: https://presscouncil.nic.in/OldWebsite/speechpdf/Future%20of%20Print%20Media%20February%2017,%202009%20Kolkata.pdf [Last accessed August, 2022].
8. WAN Report.
9. Lintas Media Guide 2008.
10. Armstrong G, Vijayakumar L, Niederkrotenthaler T, Jayaseelan M, Kannan R, Pirkis J, et al. Assessing the quality of media reporting of suicide news in India against World Health Organization guidelines: a content analysis stvudy of nine major newspapers in Tamil Nadu. Aust NZJ Psychiatry. 2018;52(9):856-63.
11. Rawat M. Coronavirus in India: tracking country's first 50 COVID-19 cases; what numbers tell. New Delhi: India Today Magazine; 2020. pp. 1-10.

12. Pathare S, Vijayakumar L, Fernandes TN, Shastri M, Kapoor A, Pandit D, et al. Analysis of news media reports of suicides and attempted suicides during the COVID-19 lockdown in India. Int J Ment Health Syst. 2020;14:88.

13. Statista. (2022). Penetration of leading social networks in India in 3rd quarter of 2021. [online] Available from: https://www.statista.com/statistics/284436/india-social-network-penetration/ [Last accessed August, 2022].

14. Somerville LH. The teenage brain: Sensitivity to social evaluation. Curr Dir Psychol Sci. 2013;22:121-7.

15. Lester D. Suicide as a learned behavior. Springfield, IL: Charles C Thomas; 1987.

16. Memon AM, Sharma SG, Mohite SS, Jain S. The role of online social networking on deliberate self-harm and suicidality in adolescents: a systematized review of literature. Indian J Psychiatry. 2018;60(4):384-92.

17. Narayan R, Das B, Das S, Bhandari SS. The depressed boy who accepted "Blue Whale Challenge". Indian J Psychiatry. 2019;61(1): 105-6.

18. Latha K, Meena KS, Pravitha MR, Dasgupta M, Chaturvedi SK. Effective use of social media platforms for promotion of mental health awareness. J Educ Health Promot. 2020;9:124.

19. Zalsman G, Hawton K, Wasserman D, van Heeringen K, Arensman E, Sarchiapone M, et al. Suicide prevention strategies revisited: 10-year systematic review. Lancet Psychiatry. 2016;3(7):646-59.

20. World Health Organization and International Association for Suicide Prevention (2017). Preventing suicide: a resource for media professionals, 2017 update. World Health Organization. [online] Available from: https://apps.who.int/iris/handle/10665/258814. [Last accessed August, 2022].

21. World Health Organization. Preventing Suicide: a Resource for Media Professionals. Geneva, Switzerland: World Health Organization; 2017.

22. IASP. (2021). Reporting on Suicide during COVID-19 Pandemic. [online] Available from: https://www.iasp.info/pdf/2020_Briefing_Statement_Reporting_on_Suicide_During_COVID19.pdf. [Last accessed August, 2022].

23. Samaritans Media. (2013). Guidelines for Reporting Suicide. Samaritans, 2013. [online] Available from: http://www.samaritans.org/sites/default/files/kcfinder/files/press/Samaritans%20Media%20Guidelines%202013%20UK.pdf [Last accessed August, 2022].

24. Robinson J, Hill NTM, Thorn P, Battersby R, Teh Z, Reavley NJ, et al. The #chatsafe project. Developing guidelines to help young people communicate safely about suicide on social media: A Delphi study. PLoS One. 2018;13(11):e0206584.

25. Armstrong G, Vijayakumar L. Suicide in India: a complex public health tragedy in need of a plan. Lancet Public Health. 2018;3(10):e459-60.

26. Ramadas S, Kuttichira P, John CJ, Isaac M, Kallivayalil RA, Sharma I, et al. Position statement and guideline on media coverage of suicide. Indian J Psychiatry. 2014;56(2): 107-10.

27. Press Council of India. (2020). Guidelines adopted by PCI on mental illness/reporting on suicide cases. [online] Available from: https://presscouncil.nic.in/WriteReadData/Pdf/PRtennineteentwenty.pdf. [Last accessed August, 2022].

28. Kar SK, Menon V, Padhy SK, Ransing R. Suicide Reporting Guideline by Press Council of India: Utility and Lacunae. Indian J Psychol Med. 2021.

29. Jain N, Kumar S. Is suicide reporting in Indian newspapers responsible? A study from Rajasthan. Asian J Psychiatr. 2016;24:135-8.

30. Menon V, Kaliamoorthy C, Sridhar VK, Varadharajan N, Joseph R, Kattimani S, et al. Do Tamil newspapers educate the public about suicide? Content analysis from a high suicide Union Territory in India. Int J Soc Psychiatry. 2020;66(8):785-91.

31. Menon V, Mani AM, Kurian N, Sahadevan S, Sreekumar S, Venu S, et al. Newspaper reporting of suicide news in a high suicide burden state in India: is it compliant with

international reporting guidelines? Asian J Psychiatr. 2021;60:102647.

32. Sheikh S, Arafat SM. Quality of Newspaper Reporting of Suicide in Kashmir: adherence to World Health Organization Guidelines. Psychiatry Interpersonal Biol Proc. 2021.

33. Chandra PS, Doraiswamy P, Padmanabh A, Philip M. Do newspaper reports of suicides comply with standard suicide reporting guidelines? A study from Bangalore, India. Int J Soc Psychiatry. 2014;60(7):687-94.

34. Raj S, Ghosh A, Sharma B, Goel S. Do online media adhere to the responsible suicide reporting guidelines? A cross sectional study from India. Int J Soc Psychiatry. 2020:20764020975797.

35. Vijayakumar L, Shastri M, Fernandes TN, Bagra Y, Pathare A, Patel A, et al. Application of a Scorecard Tool for Assessing and Engaging Media on Responsible Reporting of Suicide-Related News in India. Int J Environ Res Public Health. 2021;18(12):6206.

36. Menon V, Kar SK, Varadharajan N, Kaliamoorthy C, Pattnaik JI, Sharma G, et al. Quality of media reporting following a celebrity suicide in India. J Public Health (Oxf). 2020:fdaa161.

37. Ganesh R, Singh S, Mishra R, Sagar R. The quality of online media reporting of celebrity suicide in India and its association with subsequent online suicide-related search behaviour among general population: an infodemiology study. Asian J Psychiatr. 2020;53:102380.

38. Harshe D, Karia S, Harshe S, Shah N, Harshe G, De Sousa A. Celebrity suicide and its effect on further media reporting and portrayal of suicide: an exploratory study. Indian J Psychiatry. 2016;58(4):443-7.

39. Menon V, Arafat SMY, Akter H, Mukherjee S, Kar SK, Padhy SK. Cross-country comparison of media reporting of celebrity suicide in the immediate week: a pilot study. Asian J Psychiatr. 2020;54:102302.

40. Raj S, Ghosh A, Sharma B, Goel S. Do online media adhere to the responsible suicide reporting guidelines? A cross sectional study from India. Int J Soc Psychiatry. 2020.

41. Menon V, Padhy SK, Ransing R, Kar SK, Arafat SY. Impact of Celebrity Suicide on Population Mental Health: Mediators, Media, and Mitigation of Contagion. Indian J Psychol Med. 2020;42(6):588-90.

Survivors of Suicide

Rija Rappai, Priya Sreedaran, Anish V Cherian

ABSTRACT

The current chapter deals with various aspects of suicide survivors. Initially the concept of suicide survivors is delineated, followed by mental health issues and grief in survivors. The increased risk of suicide in the survivors is discussed. Finally, suggested interventions for this population has been discussed.

■ INTRODUCTION

"We do not know why she has done this; she was very small just 16 years old, all of us went in search of the answer for her death but we could not find anything. I wish if I were there in the house at that time, it was hardly 20–30 minutes, my mother gone out for something and she did wind up everything. Now we do not talk to each other at home, all are in their own world. My fiancé almost stopped talking to me as I am unable to continue the conversation with him, I know we will get married as decided but I will never able to be as earlier, I think he is worried that I will also commit suicide as my sister, he does not feel secure with me I guess, I cannot blame him, it is true that there is an uncertainty prevailing in our home, in all of us, I do not feel secure with myself, I find my own actions unpredictable, I think I lost myself. I could have been little more responsible and friendly with her as an elder sister, but I did not, and now I cannot too, is not it? Me, father, and mother are worried of each other to the extent that we keep an eye on each other even during night so that none of us commit suicide. We are planning to shift the house, this place (where they are residing for 20 years) is not good......"

This is a conversation that the first author of this chapter had with a suicide loss survivor. The conversation revolved around the subjective experience of a woman, who has been bereaved by the suicide of her younger sister. The concept of self, world and future, change for the survivor after the suicide, and the trauma has divided their life into two: before and after the suicide.

■ MAGNITUDE OF THE ISSUE

In 1970s Edwin Shneidman estimated that there were at least six survivors left grieving for every death by suicide. Studies in recent years give a bigger picture on the number of survivors. Studies estimate that the number of people "intimately and directly affected by" suicide death of their loved one, client, or colleague is around 45 and 80 (the estimate depends on the kinship relationship) with 14–30 of these individuals having been in weekly contact with the decedent prior to death. These include medians of 5.1 immediate family members, 14.5 extended

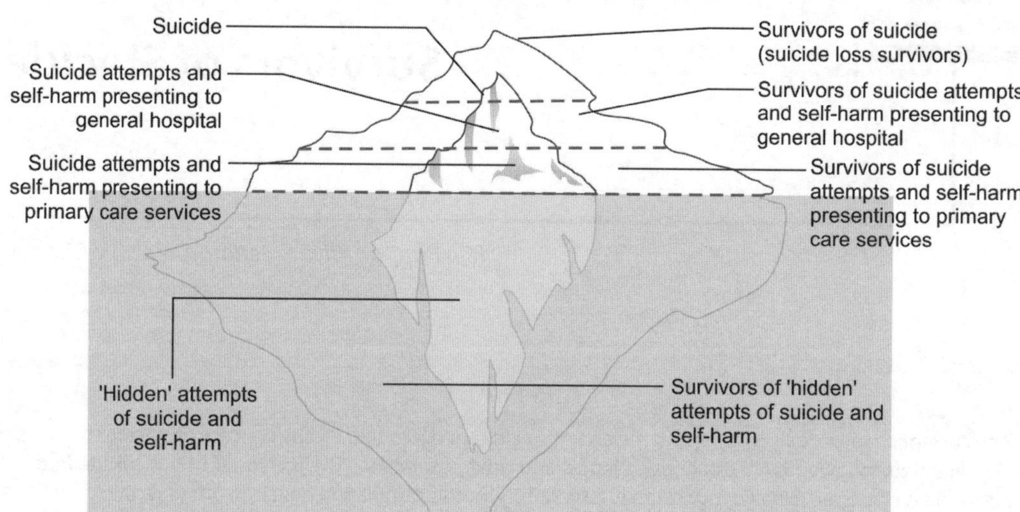

Fig. 1: Iceberg—survivors.

*Proportions illustrated in this diagram stem from international research findings; however, these proportions may vary between countries and regions, increased accuracy and uniformity of information is needed at all levels.

Source: Adapted from "The extent of suicidal behaviour'—WHO. (2016). Practice manual for establishing and maintaining surveillance systems for suicide attempts and self-harm. Geneva, Switzerland: WHO Document Production Services.

family members, and about 20 friends, coworkers, and classmates who survived and were significantly affected by each suicide. The number of survivors is based on the age, sex, marital status, personality traits, interpersonal relationship, etc. of the deceased individual. Thus, the prevalence of suicide survivors is nearly 80 times higher than the suicide rate; this is an invisible hidden population which needs immediate attention of the healthcare system **(Fig. 1)**.

■ DEFINITION

Though the term *"suicide survivor"* is used to describe individuals left behind to grieve, try to understand the reasons for the death and learn to carry on with their lives following a suicide death; there is no consensus on the definition of suicide survivor as different authors define the concept differently.

Globally, "bereaved by suicide" is the more widely used term in this context.

Jordan and McIntosh (2011) put forth a definition of a suicide survivor, as being "someone who experiences a high level of self-perceived psychological, physical, and/ or social distress for a considerable length of time after exposure to the suicide of another person".

Philip Seager (2004) defined contrary to common use, "suicide survivor" does not refer to those bereaved by suicide, but to a person who has made a nonlethal suicide attempt.

The chapter discusses about the survival journey of suicide loss survivors (suicide survivors), i.e., "someone who experiences a high level of self-perceived psychological, physical, and/ or social distress for a considerable length of time after exposure to the suicide of another person", as the phenomena is different for both suicide loss survivors and for suicide attempt survivors.

Who is a suicide survivor? How is each survivor's experience different?

A survivor could be anyone; family, friends, neighbors, classmates, patients, and coworkers could all be considered survivors. The self-identification as a survivor depends on the relationship the individual has with the deceased one.

"The experience of survival" of each category of survivors varies based on their age, the interaction and experience with the person who is no more, sociocultural background and other factors.

Family as survivor: The Family systems theory by *Bowen* states family members are interconnected, interdependent and operate as a group or as a family system. This connectedness makes the functioning of family members interdependent; hence, a change in one person's functioning will inevitably change the functioning of other family members. When there is a loss of a family member due to suicide, the functioning of each subsystem and the functioning of family as a system change.

Functional families are characterized by no evidence of preexisting family conflict or psychopathology; the suicide usually takes place in the context of chronic physical illness. In *encapsulated families*, psychopathology and conflict were generally observed only in the deceased, not in other family members. In *chaotic families*, clear evidence of psychopathology in multiple family members and/or turmoil prior to suicide is present.

Child suicide survivor: Child is more likely to be anxious, aggressive, or withdrawn immediately after the death. Internalizing symptoms and problems with school adjustment and symptoms of post-traumatic stress disorder will be present. Children tend to have following grief response: sadness, guilt, and withdrawn response, and an angry, hostile, and defiant response.

Peer group: Adolescents exposed to peer suicidal behavior were more likely to smoke cigarettes and marijuana, participate in high-risk drinking, and engage in aggressive behaviors resulting in injury. They are at greater risk for depression, post-traumatic stress, suicidal ideation, relationship conflict, and traumatic grief.

How the survival is different in "death" and "suicide"?

After the death of a loved one, anyone can identify themselves as a survivor. There is, however, a difference in the process of dying and suicide that itself makes the survival different in suicide. In suicide, the person appears to have chosen death and this makes a world of difference for those left to grieve. The suicide survivor faces all the same emotions as anyone who mourns a death, but they also face a unique set of painful feelings as follows:

- *Guilt:* People die because of diseases, accidents, and old age. Individuals know instinctively that they cannot cause or control these things. But, the suicide survivors—even if they were only on the periphery of the deceased's life—invariably feel that they might have, could have, or should have done something to prevent the suicide.
- *Anger:* It is not uncommon to feel some form of anger toward a lost loved one, but it is intensified for survivors of suicide. In suicide, the person lost is also the murderer of the person they lost,

bringing new meaning to the term "love-hate" relationship. The extension of this ambivalent relationship the survivor gradually develops with his/her self and the world.

- *Disconnection:* When we lose a loved one to disease or an accident, it is easier to retain happy memories of them. We know that, if they could choose, they would still be here with us. But it is not the same for the suicide survivor. As their loved one seems to have made a choice that is objectionable to them, they feel disconnected from their memory. They are in a state of conflict with themselves, and they are left to resolve that conflict alone.

- *Existential crisis:* For certain families the bread winner of the family would be the one whom they have lost to suicide so the whole grief and mourning process become an existential crisis in terms of physical and financial security. And this existential crisis can be layered with all the above-mentioned feelings, that is, guilt, anger, and disconnection.

MENTAL HEALTH ISSUES IN SURVIVORS

The mental health issues in suicide survivors range from immediate emotional response of anger or guilt to suicide.

- *Depression:* Survivors tend to experience depression as they undergo guilt and abandonment, they experience the negative triad of depression: worthlessness, helplessness, and hopelessness along with the cardinal symptoms such as sadness, loss of interest in pleasurable activities and fatigue and other symptoms of depression as well.

- *Post-traumatic stress disorder (PTSD):* Survivors of suicide are more likely than other bereaved individuals to develop symptoms of PTSD. The majority of suicide methods involve considerable bodily damage. Occasionally, survivors are witnesses to the final act, or the first to discover the dead body. Those left to find the deceased's body, struggle to get the gruesome images of out of their minds. In such circumstances, traumatic distress marked by fear, horror, vulnerability, and disintegration of cognitive assumptions arises. After a death by suicide, themes of violence, victimization, and volition (i.e., the choice of death over life, as in the case of suicide) are common and may be intermixed with other aspects of grief. Disbelief, despair, anxiety symptoms, preoccupation with the deceased and the circumstances of the death, withdrawal, hyperarousal, and dysphoria are more intense and more prolonged in suicide survivors.

- *Suicidality:* Individuals who have lost a loved one to suicide are themselves at heightened risk for suicidal ideation and behaviors. Survivors of suicide loss may wish to "join" their loved one; to understand or identify with the mental state of the deceased; to punish themselves for failing to prevent the suicide; or to end their own pain through death.

Survivors respond differently to the loss and studies have found some of the mental health issues in survivors as follows:

- Greater rates of bipolar disorder in persons exposed to the suicide of a parent.
- Greater depression across all kinship losses.
- Greater depression in parent survivors of a child's suicide, even when there was no evidence of premorbid depression before the death.
- Greater depression in bereaved mothers.

- Greater depression and complicated grief in adolescent siblings and young adult friends of the deceased.
- Greater depression and substance abuse in youth losing a parent.
- Greater psychiatric morbidity in elderly parents losing a child.
- Greater rates of complicated grief disorder.
- Greater mental health symptoms and social isolation in surviving spouses 10 years after a loss.
- Greater depression and suicidal ideation and poorer self-ratings of mental health in bereaved mothers and fathers 5 or more years after the death of a child when compared to a nonbereaved national sample. This pattern persisted for >10 years for the bereaved mothers. Similar patterns were also found for suicide loss survivors who were diagnosed with complicated grief.
- Greater social strain and stigmatization within the social networks of loss survivors.

■ GRIEF IN SURVIVORS

Concept of Grief

Grief is a natural and universal response to the loss of a loved one. The grief experience is not a state but a process. Most individuals recover adequately within a year after the loss; however, when individuals experience an extension of the grieving process, they are said to be experiencing complicated grief or prolonged grief disorder, which is thought to result from failure to transition from acute to integrated grief.

- *Acute grief* is the initial response to a loss, often intense and disruptive. Feelings of anguish and despair may initially seem ever present but soon they occur predominantly in waves or bursts—the so-called pangs of grief—brought on by concrete reminders of or discussions about the deceased. Once the reality of the loss begins to sink in, over time, the waves become less intense and less frequent. For most bereaved persons, these feelings gradually diminish in intensity, allowing the individual to accept the loss and re-establish emotional balance. The person knows what the loss has meant to them but they begin to shift attention to the world around them.
- *Integrated grief* is the permanent response after adaptation to the loss, in which satisfaction in ongoing life is renewed. For many, new capacities, wisdom, unrecognized strengths, new and meaningful relationships, and broader perspectives emerge in the aftermath of loss.

However, a small percentage of individuals are not able to come to such a resolution and go on to develop a "complicated grief" reaction.

- *Complicated grief* is a form of prolonged acute grief, where the term complicated is used in the medical sense of a superimposed process that impedes healing. Complicated grief is a distinct mental health disorder. It is a bereavement reaction in which acute grief is prolonged, causing distress and interfering with functioning. The bereaved may feel longing and yearning that does not substantially subside with time and may experience difficulty re-establishing a meaningful life without the person who died. The pain of the loss stays fresh and healing does not occur. The bereaved person feels stuck; time moves forward but the intense grief remains. Symptoms include recurrent and intense pangs of grief and a preoccupation with the person who died mixed with avoidance of reminders of the loss. The bereaved may have recurrent intrusive images of the death, while positive memories may be blocked or interpreted as sad, or experienced in prolonged states of reverie that interfere with daily activities.

Dynamics of Grief

Different authors have explained the dynamics of the grief differently:

- *Freud* proposed the original "grief work" theory, which involved the breaking of ties with the deceased, readjusting to new life circumstances, and building new relationships.
- *Kübler-Ross* proposed the "stage theory" where grief proceeded along a series of predictable stages including shock and denial, anger, resentment and guilt, depression, and finally acceptance.
- *Stroebe and Schut* proposed a "dual-process model" with grief being a process of oscillation between two modes, a "loss orientation" mode when the griever engages in emotion-focused coping, and a "restoration orientation" mode when the griever engages in problem-focused coping.
- *Bonanno* suggested chronic grief was associated with preloss dependency and resilience with preloss acceptance of death.
- *Neimeyer and Sands* suggested that the construction of meaning was the main issue in grief.
- *Hall* has proposed that loss provides the possibility of life-enhancing "post-traumatic" growth as the individual integrates the lessons of loss and resilience.

Grief in Survivors

Though there are different theories on bereavement and grief, the grief in suicide survivors is unique considering the process of dying in suicide. The suicide of a loved one frequently unleashes an emotional turmoil of guilt and self-reproach in survivors. Suicide can be understood as shattering the assumptive world of the survivor, meaning the foundational beliefs about one's world.

For example; "a mother whose 15-year-old daughter hanged herself in her bedroom after an argument with her parents was struggling with whether her daughter had intended to die or not. As she commented, "If the answer to that question is yes, then it means that I did not know my daughter."

In essence, her daughter's death had profoundly called into doubt who her daughter was, the nature of their relationship, and her own identity as a "good" mother. So, the world of reality of the mother is getting shattered with a single event, over the period of time her understanding about herself, others and future changes traumatically and end up uncertain.

The grief can involve complex, fluctuating emotional reactions unlike the five stages of grief by Kubler Ross. The grief in suicide survivors will be layered with shame, guilt, abandonment, self-blame, confusion, fear, uncertainty, etc. and the individual may or may not come to consensus with the reality that they have lost the loved one and they have to "normalize" the life with the loss. Survivors of suicide tend to grieve themselves; they tend to grieve the emotional and material security they experienced in the presence of the loved one. At times they realize the fact that they grieve their "previous self".

■ SUICIDALITY IN SURVIVORS

Survivors of suicide may be left to struggle with their own suicidal ideation, while seeing that the deceased escaped the anguish and put an end to their suffering. Despite the fact that the suicide bereaved intimately understand the intense pain and suffering experienced by all those who survive a suicide loss, survivors are at higher risk themselves for suicidal ideation and behavior as compared to other bereaved individuals. The pain of dealing with the loss of a loved one by suicide coupled with shame, rejection, anger, perceived responsibility, and other risk factors, can be too much to bear, and to some, suicide seems like the only way to end the pain. Some may feel closer to their loved one by taking their life in the same way. Finally, as with other types of losses, yearning for a loved one can be so intense, that the desire to join the loved one in death can be overwhelming. Evidence strongly supports the fact that suicide survivors are at an increased risk of developing physical ill health, poor mental health, psychiatric disorders, and suicidality.

Adolescent suicide survivors have a higher tendency than other survivor groups to engage in suicidal thinking and suicide attempts in the first year following a significant other's suicide. *A survivor: "I have thought about suicide a million times".*

It seems that survivors' exposure to suicide cases brings an acute awareness of suicide as a coping option for life's problems: Megan

A survivor: "One of my motivations (to attempt suicide) was that if he could do it, why can't I?... he could get out of his situation, why can't I?".

> **BOX 1:** The phenomena of "heightened stress".
>
> - Baumeister's theory provides an explanation of how being a suicide survivor could lead to a heightened state of stress because loss of a loved one to suicide is a significant negative life event. A suicide survivor's grief, stigma, shame, isolation, and self-blame could result in a state of heightened stress. This state of heightened stress may balloon into psych ache, a commonly identified trigger of suicide. Heightened stress leads to increased vulnerability
> - Often, the negative life event creates in the suicide survivor a need for social support, but prevailing attitudes toward suicide cause the suicide survivor to meet, at worst, animosity, and, at best, glib reassurance. Perversely, this type of social support engenders more stress and isolation. Increased stress and isolation may result in psych ache and suicide as an escape

Suicide thoughts are not uncommon among suicide survivors during the early months of bereavement. This may be as a result of the significant other's death that makes the very idea of suicide more real in the survivor's life. It reframes the previously unthinkable idea of suicide into a viable option in the event of great stress, difficulties or crises.

Risk of Suicide in Survivors-based— the Phenomena "Heightened Stress" (Box 1)

Recurrent themes in the existing literature include shame due to stigma, risk for developing depression and/or post-traumatic stress disorder (PTSD), feelings of abandonment and rejection by the deceased, and a need to answer the question "Why did he/she choose suicide?"

LIVED EXPERIENCE OF SURVIVORS

People with lived experience are individuals who are surviving the loss of suicide as their loved ones completed suicide.

Why it is important to know lived experience of survivors?

- People with lived experience can serve as models of hope for others at risk for suicide and who have lost someone to suicide.
- The insights of people with lived experience can be extremely valuable in prevention planning, treatment, and education, contributing to improved care, enhanced safety, reduced suicide attempts and deaths, and improved support for loss survivors.
- Involving people with lived experience in suicide prevention efforts can help you to better tailor approaches to meet the needs the needy **(Box 2)**.

BOX 2: Core values for supporting people with lived experience.

All activities designed to help suicide loss survivors should be consistent with one or more of the core values below:

- Foster hope and help people to find meaning and purpose in life
- Preserve dignity and counter stigma, shame, and discrimination
- Connect people to peer supports
- Promote community connectedness
- Engage and support family and friends
- Respect and support cultural, ethnic, and/or spiritual beliefs and traditions
- Promote choice and collaboration in care
- Provide timely access to care and support

Source: Adapted from National Action Alliance for Suicide Prevention: Suicide Attempt Survivors Task Force, 2014.

Themes Evolved in Studies on Lived Experience of Suicide Survivors

Several themes on lived experience have been evolved through various qualitative studies in the field:

- *Guilt:* Guilt feelings often follow the loss of relationships that were ambivalent and/or troubled. Such a pattern becomes a destructive process in which one is worthy and deserving of punishment. This guilt is often based in the imperfectness of human relationships. The suicide survivors tend to measure themselves against "perfect" relationship standards while ignoring the imperfect nature of relationships or failing to acknowledge their positive contributions to it. Feelings of having done something wrong are often based in social rules, religious beliefs, or the perception that a personal standard has been violated. Such feelings of guilt result in the expectancy that punishment and a need for compensation has to follow.

  "That was punishment; it was too much for me … at first I thought (my cousin) did it … because she did not even contact me to tell me anything … I felt I was not always in contact with her".

  The unfinished nature of guilt feelings often interferes with survivors' ability to accept and adapt to a changed life; it keeps them chained to the past. Part of what is so painful about survivors' guilt feelings is that they cannot confirm whether the guilt is justified or not; they can only speculate and continue to feel guilty.

- *Self-blame:* Self-blame is a common experience among suicide survivors. It refers to the sense that if only one had done more, loved more, listened more or been around more, then things might have turned out differently. Self-blame is closely related to guilt feelings. Guilt is primarily an emotional pattern based on actions that somehow contributed to the suicide ("acts of commission"), while self-blame is primarily a cognitive pattern based on the absence of efforts that seemingly could have prevented the suicide ("acts of omission").

- *Blaming others or God:* Blame refers to the attribution of personal responsibility, coupled with disapproval. The frequent ambiguity of causes and/or the specific context around a suicide seems to increase the need within the social network to assign blame. The act of blaming others or God is one way to release the deceased of blame and responsibility for the suicide. Survivors sometimes blame other significant persons for their perceived negative interpersonal relationship with the deceased that seemingly contributed to the suicide events.

  "(My cousin's) parents ... I am blaming them because they are the ones who made sure ... she was always restricted ... they did not want her to do anything ..."

- *Anger*: The emotional side of suicide is often a combination of blame, guilt, anger, and stigma. Suicide survivors sometimes focus their anger on the deceased's seemingly deliberate abandonment or avoidance of an interpersonal context where problems could have been sorted out. Instead of dealing with the problems within this context, the deceased apparently rather chose to betray trusted relationships that were not allowed an opportunity to help.

  "(My brother and I) were very close ... I would have thought if he had a problem, he would have told me ... I did not understand when he did something alone and I did not even know it ... that is why

I think I resented him ... if he could talk to me about anything else, why could not he talk to me about this?"

- *Loss or restriction of "self":* The death of a significant other often leaves survivors with a sense of loss/restriction of their past and future. It is not only as a result of the death of the other person, but also the loss of a part of the survivor's sense of "self".

  One significant loss of "self" suffered by suicide survivors is the socio-emotional support, care, and friendship.

  "A part of me died when my brother died ... a huge part of me ... I looked after him ... he is my big brother ... he (came to) pick me up after school ... it has (been) 3 years now; you (would) expect it (to be) better now ... but it seems as if it is getting worse because you think if he was here now, he will be doing this or we will be doing that ...."

  A second loss of "self" that survivors experience is the loss and/or restriction of significant personal emotions, thoughts, and self-regard. This experience can be thought of as an amputation that leaves survivors feeling as though a significant part of them is missing.

  "(when talking about a collage picture of a naked girl) '... she does not have any clothes on or have anything with her ... that is how I felt ... everything was taken from me ... I was absolutely naked ... my emotions were gone, my thoughts, my material worth, everything ..."

  A third, important loss of "self" is associated with a sense of restricted access to a meaningful future. Such an indifferent and fatalistic experience may originate from the survivors' sense of disillusionment in life. This often adversely affects relational commitments to significant others and to life events.

"I do not care about half the things that happen ... I have this "do not care" attitude now; I do not care ...' A last, salient loss of "self" is based in new role expectations from changed social and/or family interactions. These expectations are often experienced as something that restricts and overwhelms their personhood: Shirley: "Everybody just expects me to be this superhuman who can listen to (them) and not have problems of (my) own, and tell you what to do and what not to do ... I feel it is too much pressure for me at times and I cannot handle it ... I am expected to know how to deal with it, because (now) I am the big sister; I am the star of the family ... I think they are expecting way too much from me ... and I cannot ... now I feel like I have chains ...."

- *Depression*: It included feelings of apathy, fatigue, emptiness, despair, crying, sadness, and exhaustion. Depression plays an important role in survivors' tendencies to lose weight or overeat, as well in their tendency to not form new relationships due to low self-esteem.
- *Suboptimal behavioral coping patterns*: Bereaved individuals' lack of optimal coping skills can hamper their exploration of appropriate behavioral coping patterns for a life without a significant other. In the case of suicide survivors, the implicit motivation to engage in suboptimal behavioral coping patterns in the aftermath of a completed suicide is an attempt to escape or avoid direct engagement with intense emotions and thoughts. Some of the participants in our study resorted to two of the more common coping patterns, namely cigarette smoking and alcohol misuse. Cigarette smoking is frequently used to deal with life stressors:

"I started smoking, I just want something (to) take that away ... because I am thinking 'If I cannot take (it), I will smoke (it) away,' it does not help, but just smoke it away."

- *Changes in relationship dynamics*: The death of a significant other almost always results in altered relationship patterns and interpersonal dynamics due to its role in an individual's sense of meaning and purpose in life. Close relationships with significant others may become superficial in the aftermath of a significant other's suicide:

"(My dad and I) were very close, extremely close (before my mom's suicide) ... I think that I knew everything about my dad, he knew everything about me ... but now ... we are not as close as we were".

Survivors sometimes intentionally choose to avoid and/or distance themselves from close relationships in the aftermath of a completed suicide. The suicide is experienced as the ultimate rejection.

"I push people away ... I do not want anyone close to me ... because if they say they love you, like my brother did, they just leave you ... if people like that can put you through so much pain, what can stop a stranger? ... I find it very difficult to have somebody very close to me ... so I keep by myself".

The person who is no more's desertion of a significant relationship is interpreted by suicide survivors as an indication that their relationship was somehow not providing enough reason to choose life above death, or at least not providing a sufficiently safe and trusted context. As a result, survivors cannot find any reason why such a betrayal could not come from anyone else. This loss brings feelings of insecurity that deeply impacts on the survivor's sense of trust in relationships. Thus, to protect them from being rejected or abandoned again, the survivors now do the rejecting.

■ STIGMA AND SOCIAL ASPECTS

Social Process Around the Survivor

While mourners usually receive sympathy and compassion, the suicide survivor may encounter blame, judgment, or exclusion. Society starts to whisper about the cause of suicide and instead of consoling the bereaved one, the conversation after the suicide will revolve around the curiosity to know the cause of suicide and society might develop their own rationale for suicide as well. So, the bereaved one will be left out with lots of questions on morale and norms in the society.

Stigma: Stigmatization of suicide survivors can be traced back to early historic periods when family members of suicide were faced with being denied a proper burial of the deceased, property confiscation, and excommunication from the community. Although such cultural practices have ceased to exist, there is evidence that negative attitudes toward those bereaved by suicide prevail and that stigmatization has taken more subtle forms of isolation and shunning.

Negative attitudes within the public can be conveyed to the survivors through various pathways, such as attribution of blame by the survivor's social environment, gossip or negative media portrayal of the deceased. If suicide survivors internalize these negative attitudes, this could exacerbate existing feelings of shame, self-blame, and/or guilt. In order to avoid stigmatization, suicide survivors might also engage in maladaptive behaviors, such as concealment of the cause of death.

Reciprocal Relationship of Stigma, Suicide, and Suicide in Survivors

A negative perception is frequently held of suicidal people, labeling them as weak and unable to cope with their problems, or selfish. Individuals who have attempted suicide are subject to similar processes of stigmatization and "social distancing". Subjects with a direct personal experience of depression or suicide strongly endorse a feeling of self-stigma; those who have attempted suicide are often ashamed and embarrassed by their behavior and tend to hide the occurrence as much as possible. Similar processes are observed among family members of subjects who have committed suicide or made a suicide attempt, with a higher perceived stigma present in those bereaved by suicide. Perceived or internalized stigma produced by mental or physical disorders, or through belonging to a minority group, may represent a significant risk factor for suicide, being severely distressing, reducing self-esteem and acting as a barrier in help-seeking behaviors.

Psychological distress due to stigmatizing attitudes may be an exceedingly severe burden and at times result in extreme consequences. Exposure to suicide in someone close has been found to be associated with a series of negative health and social outcomes, including an increased rate of suicide among partners and mothers of people who died by suicide, a more pronounced recourse to psychiatric care by parents bereaved by the self-given death of an offspring, and a higher risk of depression in offspring of parents who had committed suicide.

Decriminalization of Suicide—A Milestone in the Antistigma Movement of Suicide—Mental Health Care Act (MHCA), 2017

"115. (1) Notwithstanding anything contained in section 309 of the Indian Penal Code any person who attempts to commit suicide shall be presumed, unless proved otherwise, to have severe stress and shall not be tried and punished under the said Code. (2) The appropriate government shall have a duty to provide care, treatment, and rehabilitation to a person, having severe stress and who attempted to commit suicide, to reduce the risk of recurrence of attempt to commit suicide."

Subsection 115, Chapter 16 of Mental Health Care Act, 2017 has discussed about the decriminalization of suicide and the need to focus intervention programs to reduce further suicide attempts. This would go a long way in reducing the stigma attached with suicide.

INTERVENTIONS FOR SUICIDE SURVIVORS

It has long been recognized that people bereaved by suicide have diverse psychosocial and health needs and effective postvention, i.e., suicide bereavement support, is seen as a major public and mental health challenge **(Table 1)**.

Postvention, a term first coined by *Shneidman* at the first conference of the American Association of Suicidology (AAS, 1972), is used to describe "appropriate and helpful acts that come after a dire event."

Andriessen (2009) defined postvention as: "those activities developed by, with, or for suicide survivors, in order to facilitate recovery after suicide, and to prevent adverse outcomes including suicidal behavior."

As per the United States National guidelines developed by the Survivors of Suicide Loss Task Force (2015): Postvention is an organized response in the aftermath of a suicide to accomplish any one or more of the following:

- To facilitate the healing of individuals from the grief and distress of suicide loss
- To mitigate other negative effects of exposure to suicide
- To prevent suicide among people who are at high risk after exposure to suicide.

Following factors influence the positive outcome of interventions—time: 8–10 weeks, active control group, psychoeducational, therapeutic group, and involvement of parents as per the existing literature.

CONCLUSION

Suicide survivors—an unnoticeable, hidden population, suffer significantly secondary to the loss of their loved one to suicide. The survivors undergo a wide range of response from immediate emotional response of shock to the extreme step of suicide. Including suicide survivors in the suicide prevention program is the need of the hour, for any country. The phenomena of "survival" is layered with the social process around the survivor, the process of dying in suicide, socio-cultural background, psychological factors of the survivor, etc. The complex phenomena of survival are yet to be understood completely. There is a need to incorporate the "postvention" programs to the general healthcare system of the country along with all the other healthcare needs to ensure the sustainability and better outcome.

TABLE 1: Summary of studies among survivors.

Author, year, location	Population	Time since bereavement, relationship to the deceased	Type of intervention, setting	Intervention	Duration/ frequency of intervention	Result
Zisook et al. (2018) USA	People bereaved by suicide—SB, accident, homicide— A/H, and natural causes—NC	Time—SB: M = 3.9 years A/H: 6.6 years, NC: 4.3 years Partner, parent, child, and other	Individual clinical setting	• Manual-based structured complicated grief therapy, therapists, including social workers, psychiatrists, psychologists • Antidepressant medication with individual follow-up • Facilitated by trained researcher	Therapy 16 sessions over 20 weeks Medication: 12-week with 2–4 weekly visits until week 20	• Lower improvement on clinician-rated CG-CGI-I in SB versus A/H and NC groups (p < 0.5) • Low rates of post-treatment active suicidal ideation in SB, A/H, and NC groups
Wittouck et al. (2014) Belgium	Suicide of a significant other	Intervention 9.8 months Partner, parent, sibling, and other	Group/family participant's home	Cognitive behavioral therapy-based psychoeducational intervention versus no treatment facilitated by clinical psychologist	2 h sessions, 4 sessions Frequency not reported	• Decrease in depression, hopelessness and grief in intervention versus control group • Decrease in intensity of grief, depression, passive coping style, social support seeking and behavioral expression of (negative) feelings in intervention group only (all p < 0.05)

Contd…

Contd...

Author, year, location	Population	Time since bereavement, relationship to the deceased	Type of intervention, setting	Intervention	Duration/ frequency of intervention	Result
De Groot et al. (2010) The Netherlands	First-degree relatives or spouses bereaved by suicide	3–6 months after suicide Spouse, parent, child, and in-laws	Group/family participant's home	Family-based cognitive behavior counseling program versus treatment as usual facilitated by trained psychiatric nurses	2 h, 2–3 weekly sessions, 4 sessions	• Decrease of complicated grief in suicide ideators • Reduction in maladaptive grief reactions (p = 0.03) and risk of suicidal ideation (p = 0.03) among ideators
De Groot et al. (2007) The Netherlands	First-degree relatives or spouses bereaved by suicide	3–6 months after suicide Spouse, parent, child, and in-laws	• Family-based cognitive behavior counseling program versus treatment as usual • Facilitated by trained psychiatric nurses	• Family-based cognitive behavior counseling program versus treatment as usual • Facilitated by trained psychiatric nurses	2 h, 2–3 weekly sessions, 4 sessions	A trend toward feeling less being to blame (p = 0.01) and fewer maladaptive grief reactions (p = 0.056)
Pfeffer et al. (2002) USA	Families where child's parent or sibling died by suicide disorders	Within a year after death Siblings, children, and parents	Group/family clinical setting	• Manual based bereavement group intervention for children grouped by age • Psychoeducational, support group for parents • No treatment control • Facilitated by trained psychologists	1.5 h weekly sessions 10 sessions	Children: Significantly greater reduction in anxiety and depressive symptoms in intervention versus control group (p ≤ 0.01)

Contd...

Contd…

Author, year, location	Population	Time since bereavement, relationship to the deceased	Type of intervention, setting	Intervention	Duration/ frequency of intervention	Result
Constantino et al. (2001) USA	Widows whose spouse died by suicide	1–27 months	Group setting not reported	Bereavement group postvention (BGP), i.e., group psychotherapy versus social group postvention (SGP), e.g., socialization, recreation Facilitated by trained mental health nurses	1.5 h weekly sessions, 8 sessions	Significant decrease in depression (p = 0.0001), total distress (p = 0.0001), grief symptoms (all p < 0.05), except for anger/ hostility and social isolation, and increase in total social adjustment (p = 0.0001)
Kovac and Range (2000) USA	Undergraduate students who had a close person die by suicide in the past 2 years and were upset by the death	Intervention M = 13.26 months	Individual experimental/ laboratory setting	Writing task: profound, death-related writing versus trivial writing Facilitated by researchers	15 min sessions, 4 sessions over 2 weeks	Reduction in impact of grief (p < 0.05), and general GRQ grief levels (p < 0.05) in intervention and control group. Suicide-specific grief GEQ more reduced in intervention than control group (p < 0.05)

(CG-CGI-I: complicated grief clinical global impressions scale—improvement; GEQ: grief experience questionnaire; GRQ: grief recovery questions)

Source: Adapted from Effectiveness of suicide bereavement interventions: Summary of studies—Karl Andriessen KK. Effectiveness of interventions for people bereaved through suicide: a systematic review of controlled studies of grief, psychosocial and suicide-related outcomes. BMC Psychiatry. 2019;19:49.

■ SUGGESTED READING

1. Aguirre RTP, Slater H. Suicide postvention as suicide prevention: Improvement and expansion in the United States. Death Stud. 2010;34(6):529-40.

2. Ali F. Exploring the complexities of suicide bereavement research. Procedia Soc Behav Sci. 2015;165:30-9.

3. Behere PB, Sathyanarayana Rao TS, Mulmule AN. Decriminalization of attempted suicide law: Journey of fifteen decades. Indian J Psychiatry. 2015;57(2):122-4.

4. Carpiniello B, Pinna F. The reciprocal relationship between suicidality and stigma. Front Psychiatry. 2017;8:35.

5. De fauw N, Andriessen K. Networking to support suicide survivors: Clinical insights. Crisis. 2003;24(1):29-31.

6. Farshid Shamsaeia SY. Exploring the lived experiences of the suicide attempt survivors: A phenomenological approach. Int J Qual Stud Health Well-being. 2020;15(1):1745478.

7. Feigelman B, Feigelman W. Suicide survivor support groups: Comings and goings, Part II. Illness Crisis Loss. 2011;19(2):165-85.

8. Force NA. The Way Forward: Pathways to hope, recovery, and wellness with insights from lived experience. Washington, DC: National Action Alliance for Suicide Prevention; 2014.

9. Hanschmidt F, Lehnig F, Riedel-Heller SG, Kersting A. The stigma of suicide survivorship and related consequences—a systematic review. PLoS One. 2016;11(9):e0162688.

10. Hoffmann WA, Myburgh C, Poggenpoel M. The lived experiences of late-adolescent female suicide: survivors: 'A part of me died'. Health SA Gesondheid. 2010;15(1):a493.

11. Ilanit Tal Young P, Alana Iglewicz M, Danielle Glorioso M, Nicole Lanouette M, Kathryn Seay B, Manjusha Ilapakurti M, et al. Suicide bereavement and complicated grief. Dialogues Clin Neurosci. 2012;14(2):177-86.

12. Jordan JR. Bereavement after suicide. Psychiatric Ann. 2008;38(10):679-85.

13. Lester D. Denial in suicide survivors. Crisis. 2004;25(2):78-9.

14. Ludwig J, Liebherz S, Dreier M, Härter M, von dem Knesebeck O. Public stigma toward persons with suicidal thoughts—Do age, sex, and medical condition of affected persons matter? Suicide and Life-Threatening Behavior. 2020;50(3):631-42.

15. Ministry of Law and Justice, New Delhi. (2017). The Mental Healthcare Act, 2017 (pp. 1-51). [online] Available from: https://egazette.nic.in/WriteReadData/2017/175248.pdf. [Last accessed July, 2022].

16. Mitchell AM, Kim Y, Prigerson HG, Mortimer-Stephens M. Complicated grief in survivors of suicide. Crisis. 2004;25(1):12-8.

17. Mughal S, Azhar Y, Mahon MM, Siddiqui WJ. Grief Reaction. Treasure Island (FL): StatPearls Publishing; 2022.

18. Pinna BC. The Reciprocal Relationship between suicidality and stigma. Front Psychiatry. 2017;8:35.

19. Pinto S, Soares J, Silva A, Curral R, Coelho R. COVID-19 suicide survivors—a hidden grieving population. Front Psychiatry. 2020;11:626807.

20. Pitman AL, Osborn DPJ, Rantell K, King MB. Bereavement by suicide as a risk factor for suicide attempt: A cross-sectional national UK-wide study of 3432 young bereaved adults. BMJ Open. 2016;6(1):e009948.

21. Shear MK, Ghesquiere A, Glickman K. Bereavement and complicated grief. Curr Psychiatry Rep. 2013;15(11):406.

22. Suicide Prevention Resource Center. (2014). Engaging People with Lived Experience. Retrieved from Suicide Prevention Resource Center. [online] Available from: https://www.sprc.org/keys-success/lived-experience [Last accessed July, 2022].

23. Wittouck C, Van Autreve S, Portzky G, van Heeringen K. A CBT-based psychoeducational intervention for suicide survivors: a cluster randomized controlled study. Crisis. 2014;35(3):193-201.

24. World Health Organization. Practice manual for establishing and maintaining surveillance systems for suicide attempts and self-harm. Geneva, Switzerland: WHO Document Production Services; 2016.

Suicide Helplines in India

Amrit Pattojoshi, Sai Krishna Tikka, Shobit Garg

ABSTRACT

The chapter deals with the evolution of the concept of suicide helplines. It discusses the need for such helplines, how to build resources, how to provide training and set up a proper helpline in the Indian context. The suicide helpline scenario across the world is also discussed.

Keywords: Suicide helpline; Befrienders; Helpline.

■ INTRODUCTION

Suicide prevention helplines are phone numbers that are set up to help people who are suicidal, specifically those contemplating dying by suicide and therefore help to prevent them from doing so. Such people can call this number and receive emergency counseling. Overtime, such helplines have also expanded on helping people to deal with emotional crisis emerging out of varied circumstances. Therefore, they are many times referred to as "crisis hotlines."

In this chapter, we discuss various aspects of suicide prevention helplines. We begin with a short history of helplines and then give a brief overview of the functioning and the significance of suicide prevention helplines or crisis hotlines, the world over. We then lay our emphasis on the discussion about various suicide prevention helplines in India and their role. Subsequently, we discuss various aspects of setting up of a new suicide prevention helpline.

■ HISTORY

Suicide prevention helplines can be considered as an element similar in construct to "telehealth" or "telemedicine," which is delivery of healthcare over telephone when distance or time is an issue.[1,2] History of telehealth dates to the time as early as late 19th century when telephone was invented. Alexander Graham Bell invented telephone in 1876 and Lancet spoke about telehealth in 1879.[2] Radio consultations, which are still happening, in fact began in 1920s.[3]

However, it took a while for people to realize that telephones can be used for counseling people who are contemplating death by suicide. It was in 1953, when "The Samaritans," a charity organization, began the first telephone helpline for providing emotional support to people at risk of suicide in the United Kingdom. The Samaritans then also established their services in the United States in 1974.[4] The United States, however, had its first suicide prevention center in 1958.[5]

In India, "Befrienders Worldwide/Samaritans," a public charity registered in Mumbai, was the first to start helpline services in 1960. Other nongovernmental organizations such as the SNEHA, Sumaitri, and the Befrienders India began their suicide prevention helplines since 1986, 1988, and 1992, respectively. While the United Kingdom and the United States have national helplines from a long time, "Kiran," the first national mental health helpline that also deals with suicidal callers was launched in 2020. Today, there are >50 helplines that focus on suicide prevention from India in different states.[6] Several state governments have initiated regional suicide prevention helpline services.

SUICIDE PREVENTION HELPLINES FOR INDIA

Attitudes to death and suicide vary from one culture to another and within a culture they change from time to time too.[7] Indian culture is different from that of the western and in fact the spectrum of cultural variations within India is quite wide. Moreover, the risk factors, motives and modes of suicide also seem to be distinct for India compared to the west.[8] This implies that India needs a distinct and custom-made suicide prevention policy and strategies. While the United States got its *National Strategy for Suicide Prevention* in 2001,[5] India is still due for one. Since the time American strategy came into force, the need for a national strategy to reduce suicides for India has been raised.[9] Very recently, again an urgent call for materializing India's national suicide prevention strategy has been made in a health policy paper in the *Lancet Psychiatry*.[10] Suicide prevention helpline services are an inherent part of such strategy. In fact, helplines form one of the best practice elements for suicide prevention along with means of restriction and gatekeeper training,[11] and have emerged as one of the major effective strategies for preventing suicides.[12]

However, recently it has been understood that there is lack of awareness among Indians, especially youth, toward suicide support services.[13]

Are suicide prevention helplines effective?
While the overall empirical evidence in terms of effectiveness of suicide prevention helpline services is sparse,[12] the evidence from India is almost nonexisting except for a couple of anecdotal papers. These papers have mostly assessed helplines for improving contact with health services and reducing the treatment delay.[14,15]

A recent systematic review of effectiveness of crisis lines shows that most available studies (none from India) in this regard have assessed user and provider reports and suggest that helplines to be effectiveness in suicide prevention indeed. However, they also report that high quality data in this regard is still lacking.[16]

Is there a need for more suicide helplines?
While suicide prevention helplines or crisis hotlines exist for a long time, their need in recent times has increased. In the times of coronavirus disease 2019 (COVID-19) pandemic, several online news media reported increase in the number of suicides from India.[17] The importance of these helplines might be twofold because of the ensuing restrictions to physical consultations and rise in awareness of teleconsultations. When we tracked the interest over time for "suicide helpline" using the "Google trends" for the last 10 years, we found that it was web-searched the most during the COVID-19 pandemic in India (**Figs. 1A and B**).

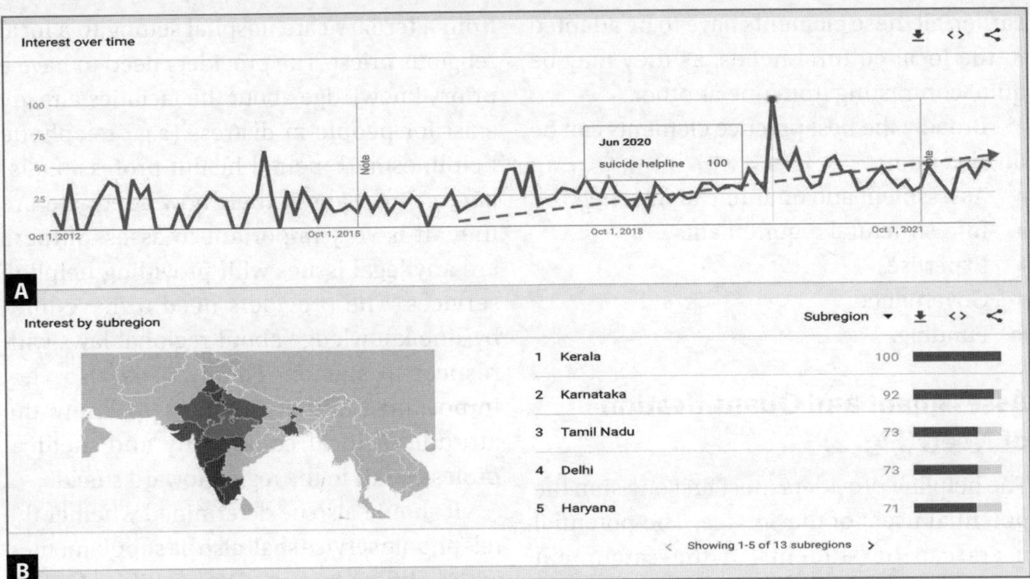

Figs. 1A and B: Google trends for "suicide helpline" in India in the last 10 years. (A) (Interest by time): X-axis represents time – 9/25/12 to 10/25/22; Y-axis represents "interest over time" – A value of 100 is the peak popularity for the term. A value of 50 means that the term is half as popular. A score of 0 means there was not enough data for this term. The most popular point was June 2020. The gray-dotted arrow indicates progressively increasing trend for the interest in the last 6–7 years; (B) (Interest by subregion): Interest over time across various states.

Figures 1A and B also shows that there is a progressively increasing trend for the interest in the search of "suicide helpline" in the last 6–7 years. The South Indian states of Kerala, Karnataka, and Tamil Nadu have the highest "interest over time." Therefore, we deem that revamping the suicide helplines is mandated.

There are several reported concerns regarding the confidence, training, and competence among the providers and follow-up care of the callers.[16,18] Barring a few,[19,20] there are no reported quality assessments or internal audits for suicide helplines, too. Moreover, several media reports from India have reported that many suicide helpline calls go unanswered and questions have been raised on the training of providers.[21-24] This implies that rather than increasing the number of suicide helpline services, the existing services need to be refined in terms of quality of the service they provide.

BEST PRACTICE ELEMENTS FOR SUICIDE PREVENTION HELPLINES

The World Health Organization (WHO) has laid down a comprehensive resource material for establishing a crisis line.[25] Perhaps, this resource contains the best practice elements not only for establishing a helpline but also for ensuring viable maintenance of the services. Complying to these guidelines ensures that all the best practice elements are followed. Additionally, one may also look up resource documents by the "Befrienders Worldwide" on "checklist of considerations for setting up a helpline," "planning framework for the establishment of a new service" and "guiding policies and practice."[26] Below in this section we sum up some crucial best practice elements for suicide prevention helplines. As mentioned earlier, all these elements have to be adapted to the local cultural needs, as they may be quite contrasting from one another.

Broadly the best practice elements can be divided into:

- Assessment and quantification of need
- Infrastructural requirements
- Expertise
- Governance
- Funding.

Assessment and Quantification of Need (Fig. 2)

The helpline providers must first envision the potential users of the service. The potential users can be students, if the catchment contains a lot of educational institutes, it can be elderly if the region is an aging one, it can be persons with mental illnesses, if there are no available mental health centers in the catchment. It is also important to have an accurate estimate about the suicide rate, the common modes of suicide in the catchment. It should also be noted that there can be many reasons for not reporting suicides in the given area. The reasons and the number not reported may again vary quite significantly from region to region. Next, it is important to have an idea about which other agencies or services the potential callers would have contact with. These services may range from a tertiary care hospital setting to a local religious priest. The providers need to have a priory knowledge about the facilities already exist for people in distress (e.g., telephone helplines and mental health professionals) and an idea about their how adequate are they. It is very important to assess if there are any legal issues with providing helpline services. The providers need to have line-by-line knowledge about regional laws with respect to suicide. Finally, it is also very important for the providers to know the attitude of local community and medical professionals in the region toward suicide.

It should also be determined whether the telephonic service shall also be supplemented with helpline by text (SMS or WhatsApp). It is also very relevant to have an idea about telephone network facilities in the catchment. It is also important to envisage if 24-hours services are required or if not then then the best-suited time slot for helpline operations must be determined. Suicide helpline service providers may also like to combine these services with community outreach programs too.

Infrastructure

Infrastructural needs for a suicide prevention helpline will be:

- Identify, design, and furnish premises

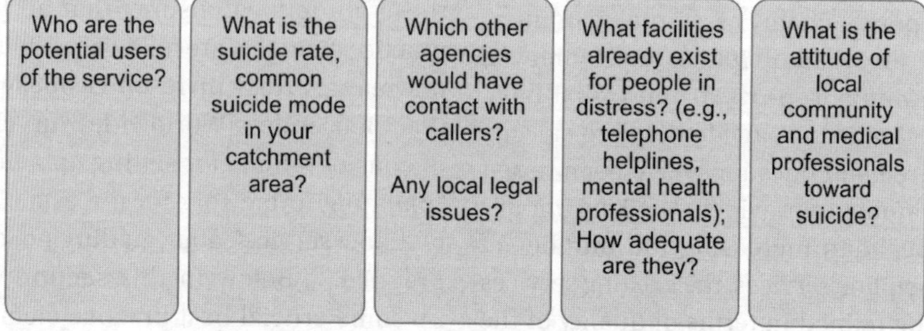

Fig. 2: Assessment of need and quantification of it.

- Maintenance of essentials
  - Electricity
  - Internet
  - Furniture
  - Water
  - Refreshments
- Equipment
  - Telephone system
  - Computer system
  - Stationary.

The need for physical space (a nodal call center) or the premises of the suicide prevention helpline may vary depending upon the extent of usage of online material and access to online storage. If physical space is deemed to be necessary then other essentials such as electricity, internet services, furniture, water and refreshments also have to be taken care of. Irrespective of the kind of space that is determined the telephone system (landline or a mobile service, number of lines, etc.) and a computer system has to be ascertained. Need for a vanity number (specific number which is easy to remember, for example, 9000090000) may also be decided based on local needs and preferences. Call forwarding services are now available as mobile applications and many are free of charge. It is, however, important to determine if the application follow privacy regulations. There are various tele-forwarding and call-log maintenance software that are available, which charges depend upon the extent of ease in services they provide. If the helpline service operate from a physical space and the access to many online resources is less, then some stationary (for physical records) becomes necessary.

Expertise

Expertise at several levels will be required for operating suicide prevention helpline services.

- Administrative and organizational
- First response
- Escalation
- Technical assistance
- Collaborations for referral.

The administrative and organizational responsibilities have to be taken care of by personnel who are preferably not involved in call responding. Their responsibilities will be in arranging funds and finances, maintaining the infrastructural requirements and also selecting and training of call responders (this aspect will be covered separately in the subsequent sections). The call responders will be at least at two levels: first response (first responders) and call escalation. The first responders will be to attend the call and will deliver the suicide first response or also called as suicide first aid. The call may be escalated (in other words transferred) to a specialist, who can be a clinical psychologist, psychiatric nurse, a psychiatrist, etc.), if the first responders determine that there is a need for an intervention beyond the suicide first response or if the caller is not responding well to the suicide first response. The number of first responders and experts for call escalation also has to be determined. Expertise from technical assistance teams such as telecommunications or an information and technology (IT) is very important while setting up the services and also for troubleshooting technical glitches. The callers, in most instance, will have to be referred for various other services, such as medical, police, fire service, women organizations, local government bodies, schools/colleges, transport services, etc., and even to other available suicide helpline services. Apart from having a close collaboration with these services, it is important to ascertain adequate level of expertise is available with such resources.

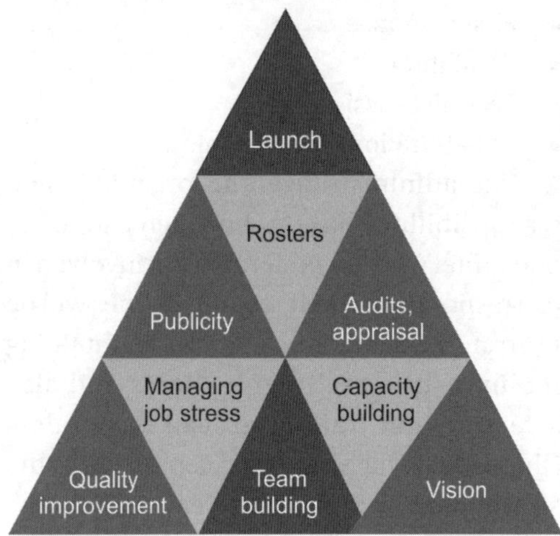

Fig. 3: Governance.

Governance (Fig. 3)

Governance is not only the responsibility of the administration and the personnel involved in organizational activities but also by the other technical people involved with the suicide prevention helpline service. While the launch, publicity, and preparing rosters for call response may be taken up by the administration, they all should be aided by the first responders and experts available for call escalation. Call allocation algorithms must be prepared before-hand. While regular audits and appraisals are part of quality improvement, feedback from callers will also help in improving the quality of services provided (these aspects will be covered separately in the subsequent sections). The task of responding to suicidal callers is not an easy one, it comes with a lot of stress. One has to keep improving the communication skills as each caller is very different from one other and this adds to the stress. Therefore, regular team building and capacity building exercises will help to reduce or manage the stress levels. The team including all the various stakeholders need to have a clear vision for the helpline services and need to re-evaluate that vision periodically.

Funding

With all the envisioned needs—infrastructural, expert level or technical and governance, a realistic estimate of the finances has to be determined. Once the budget, one time and recurring, is estimated, possible funding resources have to be identified. These funding resources may be governmental or nongovernmental or private/commercial. It is important to note that once a suicide helpline service is started, withholding it or stopping it may implicate sudden seize of an extremely important life-saving tool to someone. Therefore, realistic budgeting and funding is very important. In fact, even waitlisted funding resources may be determined if need arises. The major burden of funding is in the recruitment of first responders and personnel for escalation and their salaries or renumerations. Based on the availability of funding resources, these services may be undertaken by volunteers. Voluntary services, though, bring along other challenges such as availability and continuity in service.

QUALITY IMPROVEMENT: AUDITING AND APPRAISAL

Based on the WHO's resource material for establishing a crisis line,[25] a questionnaire to appraise the practice, perceived feasibility, and perceived effectiveness of suicide helpline providers has been prepared **(Table 1)**. This 50-item questionnaire is an exhaustive one. The items have been divided into those tapping practice (items 13–16, 19–45, etc.); perceived feasibility (items 5, 11, 12, 23, etc.); and perceived effectiveness (items 7, 17, 47–50). The responses, if honest, will help the providers to understand the

TABLE 1: Questionnaire to audit/appraisal of suicide prevention helpline services.		
1	Name of the suicide helpline:	
2	When was your "Suicide Helpline" established? (Year)	
3	Since when is it fully operational? (Year)	
4	Briefly describe how was the idea of your suicide helpline conceived?	Open
5	How was the strategic planning to start the suicide helpline services based or guided?	Open
6	When your suicide helpline services began, were you aware of any guidelines for setting up such services?	
	If yes, please mention the ones that were considered?	
7	Do you feel your suicide prevention helpline has any unique proposition that makes it successful or distinctive?	
	If yes, please describe?	
8	Is your suicide helpline service profit-oriented or non-profit?	
9	Is it part of any organization/society?	
	If yes, is the organization/society government funded or nongovernmental or commercial?	
10	Were there any breaks in service?	
	If yes, when?	
	If yes, what were the reasons for each break?	
11	How difficult or easy is it to receive funds for this service on regular basis?	Very difficult 1–10 very easy
12	Do you believe that you have enough infrastructures to run the suicide helpline service?	
	If no, what are the infrastructural lacunae?	
13	What are the service timings for your suicide helpline?	
14	What are the service days for your suicide helpline?	
15	What is the average number of calls received per day?	
16	What is the average number of calls received per week?	
17	What is the percentage number of calls that are deemed genuinely related to suicidality?	
18	What is the ratio of "calls received: calls made" during the service hours?	
	If the ratio is <1, what are the possible reasons?	

Contd...

Contd...

19	Do you keep track of number of calls made during the nonservice hours or days?	
	If yes, what is the average number of such calls received per day?	
20	What is the mechanism to maintain the confidentiality of the callers' identity details in your service?	
21	How many call responders work in your suicide helpline service?	
22	Do you use any selection criteria for recruiting them?	
	If yes, please describe.	Open
23	Are the call responders' volunteers or are they paid?	
	If voluntary, how difficult or easy is it to access volunteers on continuous basis?	Very difficult 1–10 very easy
	If paid, is it prepaid or contingent payment?	
	If paid, how difficult or easy is it to receive funds for their service on regular basis?	Very difficult 1–10 very easy
24	Are the call responders' adequately qualified?	
25	What is the qualification of the call responders in your suicide helpline service? (Choose as many as relevant)	• ANM/GNM • BSc (Psychology/Sociology Honours) • BSc Nursing • MSc (Psychology/Social Work/ Sociology) • MSc Nursing • MPhil (Psychology/Social Work/ Sociology) • PhD (Psychology/Social Work/ Sociology) • BA/BCom Bachelors with certificate course in counseling • MBBS doctors • MD Psychiatry/CFM specialists
26	Are the call responders trained specifically in suicide prevention strategies?	
27	Are the call responders trained specifically in helpline management?	
28	Are the call responders trained specifically in ethical standards and guidelines related to suicide prevention helplines?	
29	Do you arrange for induction training programs in suicide prevention counseling for call responders?	
	If yes, please briefly describe the modules used.	Open
	If no, what are the barriers?	Open

Contd...

Contd…

30	What is the average experience of each of the call responders in attending suicide helpline calls?	
31	Is there a mechanism to supervise/monitor the call responders?	
	If yes, please briefly describe the mechanism.	Open
	If no, what are the barriers?	Open
32	How confident are you that your call responders are comfortable with standard principles of suicide prevention strategies?	• Not at all confident 1–10 • Very much confident
33	How confident are you that the quality of counseling and support is uniform across all the call responders?	• Not at all confident 1–10 • Very much confident
	If not much confident, how do you intend to improve that?	
34	Is there a mechanism to receive call responders' feedback and assess their satisfaction?	
	If yes, please briefly describe the mechanism.	Open
	If no, what are the barriers?	Open
35	Are phone queues or automated call routing operational?	
36	What are the resources used for referral? (Choose as many as relevant)	• Police • Fire service • Ambulance hospitals • Mental health services • General practitioners and other health and social workers • Private medical clinics • Domestic violence services • Rape crisis services • Services for LGBTQ persons • Women's organizations • Youth organizations • Organizations working to help people with HIV/AIDS • Emergency accommodation services • City, town, and village leaders, and municipal and local governments • Religious bodies • Schools/colleges • Transport services (e.g., railway)
37	What are the three most commonly sought referral resources? (In descending order, the most common first)	• A • B • C

Contd…

Contd...

38	Are there formal agreements with these resources for referrals? Please indicate those with an agreement?	Same response options as above
39	Is there a mechanism to assess caller compliance to call responder's referrals?	
	If yes, what are the compliance rates, i.e., what percentage of callers complies by contacting the referring resource?	
	If no, what are the barriers?	Open
	If no, what is the likelihood the client will be complaint to the suggested referrals?	Highly unlikely 1—Highly likely
	What do you believe are the likely barriers for compliance to referrals?	Open
40	Is follow-up contact of callers operational in your helpline service?	
	If yes, what is the average number of callers who accept contact calls?	
	If no, what are the barriers?	Open
41	Are there any supplementary contact services such as email, online chats, text messages or social media platforms?	
	If yes, what is the average percentage of callers who avail these supplementary services?	
	If no, what are the barriers?	Open
42	Is there a mechanism to assess reutilization of your helpline service by the clients?	
	If yes, what is the reutilization rate?	
	If no, what are the barriers?	Open
43	Are there any internal audits on the functioning of the helpline service?	
	If yes, please describe in brief the procedure followed.	Open
	If no, what are the barriers?	Open
44	Do you periodically conduct quality assurance checks?	
	If yes, how often?	
	If yes, how do you assure quality of services provided?	Open
	If no, what are the barriers?	Open
45	Did you try to scientifically assess the effectiveness and client/caller satisfaction?	
	If yes, how?	Open
	If yes, please briefly describe the findings.	Open
	If no, what are the barriers?	Open

Contd...

Contd...

46	Has COVID-19 posed any problems in the operational functioning of your suicide helpline?	
	If yes, please describe what are these problems based on the questions you responded above.	Open
	If yes, please describe how have you planned to resolve these problems?	Open
47	"Overall I believe that our suicide helpline service is effective in helping clients with suicidality". I can say this with:	• Very low confidence 1–10 • Very high confidence
48	Overall in terms of feasibility I believe that running a suicide helpline service is:	• Very difficult 1–10 • Very easy
49	Things that are important to improve the overall functioning of our suicide helpline are:	Open
50	What are the three most important challenges you face in running our suicide helpline service? (In descending order, the most important one first)	

current practice of their suicide helpline and help them to appraise various factors with regard to smooth operation of the suicide helpline service. It will also help them to understand what are the areas that need a revamp.

■ TRAINING

All the first responders as well as experts for call escalation must be trained in suicide first response. Typically, the first part of training is generally a basic orientation regarding specific ethical standards for first responders on induction. These ethical standards include confidentiality and honesty. The next level training, which is also called as suicide first response training, includes the following elements.

- Understanding of values and attitudes of the first responders toward suicide
- Suicide education
- The core guiding elements during the call:
  - Recognize
  - Ask
  - Listen
  - Explore
    - Support
    - Safety plan
  - Where to refer?
  - When to escalate?

While it is important to understand the individual values and attitudes toward suicide as it determines the way we would listen and understand the caller, it is also important to provide the actual scenario regarding suicides the world over and regionally. The suicide education not only includes definition, various terminology (specifically the preferred terms and the terms to be avoided), epidemiology, and the common modes and reasons for suicide, but also includes education regarding the hidden numbers, the kind of impact suicide has on the kin and the society at large, the suicide continuum (death wish > suicidal ideas > suicidal plan > attempt to die by suicide), etc.

The core guiding principles will then be explained. First important step is to recognize suicidality in the callers' initial talk, and then if not specified, asking about it. Once the caller mentions about suicide, it is important to let the caller speak more about it. At this phase, the responders only try to facilitate caller to speak more about it and the responders only listen (active listening). When the caller is exhausted after his description of suicidality and circumstances surrounding it, and stops for a moment, the moment is considered to be best for achieving "pause." Responder tries to suggest the caller if it is possible for taking a pause from thinking about suicide and tries to explore various risk factors for suicide and various protective factors. Then the responder tries to engage the caller in selecting the most feasible support and make the "safety plan." Safety plan is to remove all the sources that can be modes of suicide or even triggers for suicidal thoughts, at both immediate and future. Next the training involves selection of suitable referral source. The first responders are also trained to determine the need for an intervention beyond the suicide first response or if the caller is not responding well to the suicide first response. They may then escalate the call to the person available for call escalation. Training in first response must also involve a predetermined set of mocks. There can be one induction and periodic refresher training for the call responders. Mock calls should also be conducted more periodically, if possible every fortnight.

The certification training in suicide first response is being provided by many agencies such as the "suicide first aid,"[27] "safe talk,"[28] etc.

SUICIDE PREVENTION HELPLINES/CRISES HOTLINES: WORLDWIDE SCENARIO

Suicide rates vary 10-fold and range from 5 per one lakh population to 20 per one lakh population globally (GBD 2019).[29] Hence, worldwide suicide remains a pressing concern. Youth helplines (mostly from the US and Australia) have been shown to benefit myriad psychosocial concerns with suicidality being one of them.[30] Expectedly, worldwide prevention helplines are established so that helpers aim to reduce the crisis states, psychological distress, and risk of suicide. These helpline services do tend to lend help via calls, chat, or text. The countries providing crisis helplines are the US, the United Kingdom (UK), Australia, Israel, Canada, Amsterdam, Spain, China, Hungary, and Belgium to name a few. Hoffberg and colleagues[16] recently published a systematic review of 33 studies of crisis line services (including two RCTs, four cohort studies, and rest a mix of observational and quasi-experimental design). They did determine whether helpline calls do have any significant impact on immediate proximal and distal outcomes.

For immediate proximal evidence, single-time measurement or single-group before-after (pre- post-crises intervention) study design was employed. Proximal outcome measures included helper responses/approaches used during the call, client mood/satisfaction change from the beginning to the end of the call, the provision of referrals, etc. Outcome measurement was done via silent monitors or call/chat log ratings and some studies used validated assessment tools. However, some studies relied upon administrative and clinical records such as routine call sheets (to be filled by responders).[16] In the most robust proximal evidence of effectiveness, Gould et al.[31] evaluated silent monitoring of >1,500 calls to the US National Suicide Prevention Lifeline (NSPL) network of crisis hotline centers. They found that helpers with Applied Suicide Intervention Skills Training (ASIST) were significantly more likely to impact caller behavioral and affect changes during the call, including callers feeling less depressed (OR: 1.31; 95%

CI: 1.01–1.71; $p < 0.05$) and less suicidal (OR: 1.74; 95% CI: 1.39–2.18; $p < 0.001$), compared with those without ASIST. As per the most recent Spanish suicide prevention helpline study, almost three-fourths (72.37%) of calls resulted in an emergency rescue evacuation to the emergency department, 4.61% were referred to a professional, and 1.96% denied to be attended.[32]

Distal evidence of the effectiveness of suicide prevention helplines ranged from a follow-up about 1 week up to 4 years.[16] Distal outcomes included mood/satisfaction, helper responses/approaches, the provision of referrals, as well as self-directed violence. Outcome measurement was similar to those utilized for immediate proximal evidence. Almost two-thirds callers expressed satisfaction post 1-week crises service with female callers responding better than males.[33] In the only RCT measuring distal effects of four suicide prevention program arms for crisis line callers. The study participants were the family and friends of high-risk suicidal men. Participation in any of the crisis line programs have shown to reduce suicidal ideation/ attempts at 2 and 6 months, respectively.[34] But, this RCT had high risk of bias and problems with the design. One retrospective study comparing suicide among users versus nonusers of helplines reported far higher suicide rates among helpline users [Males: 86.3 vs. 32.6 per 100,000; Females: 42.8 vs. 16.7 per 100,000; both incident rate ratio (IRR) = 2.6]. Factors associated with suicide were male, old age, isolation, and mental illness.[35]

Volunteers versus Paid Responders

Overall, helpers with 140+ hours of call training had better outcomes than those with less experience like less likelihood of high suicide risk from beginning to the end of the call, better response in suicide emergency, and more likelihood for the safety agreement to be respected.[33] But, when comparing the individual outcomes of volunteers and paid responders, there have been mixed findings reported. Gould and colleagues[36] reported that paid responders are more likely to engage in more collaborative active rescue interactions with callers than volunteers. But as per Mishara and colleagues,[33] there were no significant differences between volunteers and paid employees in outcomes.

Frequent Callers versus Infrequent Callers

Worldwide frequent callers comprise very less proportion of callers (<5%) but they buy majority of calls (>60%) inflicting emotional drain on the helpers.[37] Frequent callers when compared to infrequent callers are more of old age, unmarried, living in isolation and having physical illness and anxiety. Frequent callers were more likely to visit the psychiatrists in last 1 month. Some authors have termed these "typical callers" as "dominant, hostile, and exhibitionistic." There have been *recommendations* made to address this issue of frequent callers:[37]

- Encouraging frequent callers to severely limit use of the helpline. This is recommended because of belief that crises intervention (for acute events) is different from psychotherapy (for more long-term relationship).

- Limiting the number of calls and duration of calls accompanied by continued suicide risk assessment (help is ensured when needed).

- Assigning a precise helper to respond to all calls from each frequent caller. This brings continuity and consistency in care and saves time for re-evaluation.

- Initiating regular contact rather than waiting for the callers to re-initiate the contact.
- Individualized case management plans are created for each caller.
- Involving family and friends in the interventions.

Studies have documented the preferable cost-effectiveness of the national suicide prevention helpline (Belgium) and its modest effect on quality-adjusted life years (QALYS).[38]

Android Apps and Suicide Prevention Helpline

In a recent review of 43 suicide prevention mobile apps, 85% of the apps provide national suicide helpline numbers. Around 76% of apps provide connectivity to the suicide helpline within the app. Interestingly, 15 of these apps provide helpline numbers listed on each page of the app. Only one quarter of the apps would include motivational elements (beyond one liners) to break barriers in help seeking. These app would include the brief descriptions of common mental issues and situations when to seek help. These apps also displayed motivational quotes and some quoted positive experiences of past callers.[39]

Suicide Prevention Helpline Notices

Studies have found that search engine helpline notices are not associated with harm, i.e., escalation of suicidal tendencies. And if any positive change in search behavior was found to be small. Pages with higher rank (being neutral to suicide) and those showing more antisuicide pages were more likely to be clicked on. Having more antisuicide webpages displayed has been shown to be the only factor associated with further searches for suicide prevention information.[40]

CONCLUSION

Suicide helpline services are life-saving and perhaps be considered as emergency services. Therefore, policies guiding setting up of and maintaining suicide helpline services must be in place. In fact, formation of India's national suicide prevention strategy might well be a much-needed milestone in policies and regulations pertaining to suicide helplines in India. Although there are several suicide helpline services in India, there is no regulatory body guiding and monitoring them. Our chapter implies that although suicide prevention helplines are needed, there need to be more research into their effectiveness and more so on audit/appraisal aspects of them. By providing an overview of how such appraisals can be conducted, our chapter also provides best practice elements for setting up and operating suicide prevention helpline services and also the best practice elements for training the call responders.

REFERENCES

1. Cipolat C, Geiges M. The History of Telemedicine. In: Burg G (Ed). Telemedicine and Teledermatology. Current Problems in Dermatology. Basel: Karger; 2003. pp. 6–11.
2. Nesbitt TS. The Evolution of Telehealth: Where Have We Been and Where Are We Going? In: Board on Health Care Services, Institute of Medicine (Eds). The Role of Telehealth in an Evolving Health Care Environment: Workshop Summary. Washington DC: National Academies Press; 2012.
3. Ryu S. History of Telemedicine: Evolution, Context, and Transformation. Healthc Inform Res. 2010;16:65-6.
4. Evans R. Samaritans Radar app. Nurs Stand. 2014;29:33.
5. Brief History of Suicide Prevention in the United States. In: Office of the Surgeon General (US); National Action Alliance for Suicide Prevention (US). 2012 National

Strategy for Suicide Prevention: Goals and Objectives for Action: A Report of the U.S. Surgeon General and of the National Action Alliance for Suicide Prevention. Washington DC: US Department of Health and Human Services; 2012.

6. AASRA. (2019). Suicide Prevention Helpline Directory (India). [online] Available from: http://www.aasra.info/helpline.html [Last accessed Jan., 2023].

7. Carstairs GM. Attitudes to Death and Suicide in an Indian Cultural Setting. Int J Soc Psychiatr. 1955;1:33-41.

8. Radhakrishnan R, Andrade C. Suicide: An Indian perspective. Indian J Psychiatry. 2012;54:304-19.

9. Manorantjtham S, Abraham S, Jacob KS. Towards a national strategy to reduce suicide in India. Natl Med J India. 2005;18:118-22.

10. Vijayakumar L, Chandra PS, Kumar MS, Pathare S, Banerjee D, Goswami T, et al. The national suicide prevention strategy in India: context and considerations for urgent action. Lancet Psychiatry. 2022;9:160-8.

11. Menon V, Subramanian K, Selvakumar N, Kattimani S. Suicide prevention strategies: An overview of current evidence and best practice elements. Int J Adv Med Health Res. 2018;5:43-51.

12. Zalsman G, Hawton K, Wasserman D, van Heeringen K, Arensman E, Sarchiapone M, et al. Suicide prevention strategies revisited: 10-year systematic review. Lancet Psychiatry. 2016;3:646-59.

13. Cherian AV, Menon V, Rathinam B, Aiman A, Shrinivasa Bhat U, Arahantabailu P, et al. Awareness and preferences about suicide crisis support service options among college students in India: A cross sectional study. Asian J Psychiatr. 2022;74:103172.

14. Chavan BS, Garg R, Bhargava R. Role of 24 hour telephonic helpline in delivery of mental health services. Indian J Med Sci. 2012;66:116-25.

15. Shrivastava AK, Johnston ME, Stitt L, Thakar M, Sakel G, Iyer S, et al. Reducing treatment delay for early intervention: evaluation of a community based crisis helpline. Ann Gen Psychiatry. 2012;11:20.

16. Hoffberg AS, Stearns-Yoder KA, Brenner LA. The Effectiveness of Crisis Line Services: A Systematic Review. Front Public Health. 2020;7:399.

17. Pathare S, Vijayakumar L, Fernandes TN, Shastri M, Kapoor A, Pandit D, et al. Analysis of news media reports of suicides and attempted suicides during the COVID-19 lockdown in India. Int J Ment Health Syst. 2020;14:88.

18. Wakai S, Schilling EA, Aseltine RH Jr, Blair EW, Bourbeau J, Duarte A, et al. Suicide prevention skills, confidence and training: Results from the Zero Suicide Workforce Survey of behavioral health care professionals. SAGE Open Med. 2020; 8:2050312120933152.

19. Department of Children and Families. (2012). The effectiveness and sufficiency of services provided by the New Jersey-based suicide prevention hotlines. [online] Available from: https://www.state.nj.us/humanservices/news/reports/NJ%20HOTLINE%20SURVEY%20REPORT%2011%2028%2012.pdf [Last accessed Jan., 2023].

20. Gould MS, Lake AM, Galfalvy H, Kleinman M, Munfakh JL, Wright J, et al. Follow-up with Callers to the National Suicide Prevention Lifeline: Evaluation of Callers' Perceptions of Care. Suicide Life Threat Behav. 2018;48(1):75-86.

21. Homegrown. (2021). 40 Unanswered Calls Show Us The Grim Reality Of Suicide Helplines In India. [online] Available from: https://homegrown.co.in/article/802586/40-unanswered-calls-show-us-the-grim-reality-of-suicide-helplines-in-india [Last accessed Jan., 2023].

22. https://theprint.in/opinion/pov/suicide-helplines-go-unanswered-in-india-or-you-get-untrained-volunteers/499565/

23. The Print. Most suicide helplines are of little help as they don't work when people need them. [online] Available from: https://theprint.in/health/most-suicide-helplines-are-of-little-help-as-they-dont-work-when-people-need-them/442287/ [Last accessed Jan., 2023].

24. Fact Checker. (2022). Govt's Mental Health Helpline Offers Little Help, Other Suicide Prevention Hotlines too Face Challenges. [online] Available from: https://www.factchecker.in/context-check/govts-mental-health-helpline-offers-little-help-other-suicide-prevention-hotlines-too-face-challenges-834837 [Last accessed Jan., 2023].

25. World Health Organization. (2018). Preventing suicide: a resource for establishing a crisis line. Geneva: World Health Organization; 2018 (WHO/MSD/MER/18.4). Licence: CC BY-NC-SA 3.0 IGO. [online] Available from: https://apps.who.int/iris/bitstream/handle/10665/311295/WHO-MSD-MER-18.4-eng.pdf?ua=1 [Last accessed Jan., 2023].

26. Befrienders Worldwide. (2022). Setting up an Emotional Support Service. [online] Available from: https://www.befrienders.org/setting-up-a-helpline [Last accessed Jan., 2023].

27. https://suicidefirstaid.org.au

28. LivingWorks. (2022). LivingWorks safeTALK: Learn and practice powerful, life-saving skills in just four hours. [online] Available from: https://www.livingworks.net/safetalk [Last accessed Jan., 2023].

29. GBD 2019 Diseases and Injuries Collaborators. Global burden of 369 diseases and injuries in 204 countries and territories, 1990-2019: a systematic analysis for the Global Burden of Disease Study 2019. Lancet. 2020;396(10258):1204-22. Erratum in: Lancet. 2020;396(10262):1562.

30. Mathieu SL, Uddin R, Brady M, Batchelor S, Ross V, Spence SH, et al. Systematic Review: The State of Research Into Youth Helplines. J Am Acad Child Adolesc Psychiatry. 2021;60(10):1190-233.

31. Gould MS, Cross W, Pisani AR, Munfakh JL, Kleinman M. Impact of Applied Suicide Intervention Skills Training on the National Suicide Prevention Lifeline. Suicide Life Threat Behav. 2013;43(6):676-91. Erratum in: Suicide Life Threat Behav. 2015;45(2):260.

32. Mokkenstorm JK, Eikelenboom M, Huisman A, Wiebenga J, Gilissen R, Kerkhof AJFM, et al. Evaluation of the 113 Online Suicide Prevention Crisis Chat Service: Outcomes, Helper Behaviors and Comparison to Telephone Hotlines. Suicide Life Threat Behav. 2017;47(3):282-96.

33. Mishara BL, Daigle M, Bardon C, Chagnon F, Balan B, Raymond S, et al. Comparison of the Effects of Telephone Suicide Prevention Help by Volunteers and Professional Paid Staff: Results from Studies in the USA and Quebec, Canada. Suicide Life Threat Behav. 2016;46(5):577-87.

34. Mishara BL, Houle J, Lavoie B. Comparison of the effects of four suicide prevention programs for family and friends of high-risk suicidal men who do not seek help themselves. Suicide Life Threat Behav. 2005;35(3):329-42.

35. Chan CH, Wong HK, Yip PS. Exploring the use of telephone helpline pertaining to older adult suicide prevention: A Hong Kong experience. J Affect Disord. 2018;236:75-79.

36. Gould MS, Lake AM, Munfakh JL, Galfalvy H, Kleinman M, Williams C, et al. Helping Callers to the National Suicide Prevention Lifeline Who Are at Imminent Risk of Suicide: Evaluation of Caller Risk Profiles and Interventions Implemented. Suicide Life Threat Behav. 2016;46(2):172-90.

37. Mishara BL, Côté LP, Dargis L. Systematic Review of Research and Interventions With Frequent Callers to Suicide Prevention Helplines and Crisis Centers. Crisis. 2022. Erratum in: Crisis. 2022.

38. Pil L, Pauwels K, Muijzers E, Portzky G, Annemans L. Cost-effectiveness of a helpline for suicide prevention. J Telemed Telecare. 2013;19(5):273-81.

39. Sudarshan S, Mehrotra S. Suicide Prevention Mobile Apps for Indian Users: An Overview. Cureus. 2021;13(7):e16770.

40. Cheng Q, Yom-Tov E. Do Search Engine Helpline Notices Aid in Preventing Suicide? Analysis of Archival Data. J Med Internet Res. 2019;21(3):e12235.

18

Assessment of Suicide Risk

Sujit Sarkhel

ABSTRACT

The chapter highlights the need to assess risk in all cases exhibiting suicidal behavior. The role of risk factors, warning signs, protective factors and suicide enquiry leading to a proper estimation of risk hierarchy into mild, moderate and severe has been explained. Finally, the basic outlines of management following risk stratification have been mentioned.

Keywords: Risk assessment; Suicide risk.

INTRODUCTION

Suicide depends on a multitude of factors and it is not possible to predict suicide based on a single encounter in the emergency room or in the clinic. Suicide is a low base-rate phenomenon (the number of suicides in expressed per lakh population, e.g., current rate of suicide in India is 12 per lakh population). Hence, any instrument which attempts to predict the risk of suicide is bound to have low predictive value. Another important drawback is that we depend a lot on the patient's subjective account when we assess suicidal behavior in terms of frequency, intensity, plans, intent, and lethality. Thus, a person with a strong intent to die may easily mislead the clinician by concealing his real intent. The best clinical practice should include a thorough assessment of suicidal risk covering all possible domains through a well-conducted clinical interview, gathering additional information whenever possible from multiple sources like friends, family members, blogs, diaries, personal notes and treatment records, and coming to a conclusion after giving due weightage to all the factors. The available guidelines only provide a broad outline based on which the clinician may proceed.

THE BASIC STEPS IN RISK ASSESSMENT

Although there is no rigid format for risk assessment it is better to keep the core areas and broad headings in mind so that the important aspects are not missed. A typical risk assessment interview progresses through the following stages which may not always follow the same order:[1]

- Engagement
- Thorough psychiatric assessment
- Presence of recent stressful event
- Assessment of risk factors
- Assessment of warning signs
- Presence of hopelessness, anxiety, depression, and sleep disturbances
- Assessment of impulsivity/self-control

- Assessment of protective factors
- Suicide enquiry proper.

Engagement

This is the step of establishing rapport with the patient. Suicidal thoughts are extremely private to the patient and he is unlikely to open up to a clinician unless adequate trust and rapport is established. If the first encounter occurs in a busy emergency setup which lacks privacy, it is desirable to wait for some time till the patient has been stabilized medically and privacy is ensured. It is better to get a screen in the emergency to talk to the patient in case it is not possible to arrange a separate room. Apart from being calm, assuring, and nonjudgmental in approach, certain cognitive techniques have been found helpful in putting the patient at ease and promoting engagement. In normalization, the clinician says that there are cases where people have thought of suicide when they have been put into similar situations. In shame attenuation, the clinician says that if he were to face as much ordeal as the patient, he might have also had suicidal thoughts.[2] Establishing rapport with family members is of paramount importance not only to gather corroborative information but also to ensure their support and collaboration while planning management. Once the engagement phase has been adequately negotiated, the interview can gently flow through various phases of proper assessment.

Thorough Psychiatric Assessment

This is a significant initial step where a proper psychiatric interview and mental status examination must be done to establish the presence of psychiatric diagnosis if any. Psychiatric conditions which are commonly associated with suicidal behavior include major depressive disorder (depressive, mixed, and manic phases), bipolar disorder, substance use disorder (especially alcohol), schizophrenia, borderline personality disorder, anxiety disorders, and post-traumatic stress disorder. Comorbid alcohol use disorder with another Axis I diagnosis significantly elevates the risk of suicide. Additional information should always be sought from family members whenever deemed necessary.

Presence of a Recent Stressful Event

The presence of any recent loss or stressor should be specifically probed. This includes financial loss, stressor in interpersonal relationship, recent loss of near and dear one, chronic or sudden disabling physical illness, or loss of reputation or professional identity. *Stressful events like failures in love affairs and examination failures have been documented as risk factors in Indian data.*

Assessment of Risk Factors

Risk factors are those factors which have been shown to correlate with suicidality irrespective of the time frame. Although a multitude of risk factors have been described in literature, only the most important ones have been mentioned here **(Box 1)**.[3] It is always better to divide the risk factors into modifiable and nonmodifiable ones so that

---

BOX 1: Risk factors for suicide.[3]

Modifiable:
- Alcohol and abuse of other substances
- Recent stressful life events (especially financial/relational loss)
- Access to lethal means
- Hopelessness/despair
- Anhedonia
- Impulsivity

Nonmodifiable:
- Past suicide attempt
- Current or lifetime psychiatric disorders
- Family history of suicide
- Chronic medical illness
- History of physical/sexual abuse
- Recent discharge from a psychiatric facility
- Poor support system

special emphasis could be laid on the former while planning management.

Assessment of Warning Signs

Unlike risk factors which do not always denote immediately elevated risk, warning signs of suicide were specifically conceived to denote those signs and symptoms which denote an elevated risk of suicide in the very near future—hours, days to weeks.[4] Another important feature of warning signs is that these can be easily recognized and reported by the family members or close associates in addition to patient's self-report. **Box 2** mentions a list of important warning signs which must be looked for at the time of risk assessment.

Presence of Hopelessness, Anxiety, Depression, and Sleep Disturbances

During the risk assessment interview, it is always better to ask separately about certain domains, which have been found to be closely associated with suicidality. The assessment should be done in a scale of 1–10 and the scores should be compared on subsequent assessments. Feeling of hopelessness should be specifically asked. Anxiety and depressive symptoms should be separately asked and rated based on subjective report. This should be done in addition to any Axis I diagnosis of anxiety or depressive disorder. Finally, sleep disturbances should be separately probed and recorded.

Assessment of Impulsivity and Self-control

Impulsivity and self-control should be assessed subjectively in a scale of 1–10 as per the patient's own version of his self-control. It should be supplemented by information from family members and treatment records regarding objective evidence of impulsivity in

BOX 2: Warning signs of suicide.[4]

- Active suicidal thinking
- Preparation and rehearsal behavior
- Hopelessness
- Anger
- Recklessness, impulsivity, dramatic mood changes
- Anxiety and agitation
- Feeling trapped
- No reasons for living, no purpose in life
- Increased alcohol or substance abuse

terms of impulsive aggression and substance abuse. Assessment of impulsivity is of paramount importance in the Indian context. Unlike the data available in the West which reports underlying psychiatric disorders in more than 90% cases of suicidal deaths, Indian data reveal around 50% and have underlying psychiatric disorders and the remaining are unplanned, impulsive acts.

Assessment of Protective Factors

This is an important area which has an important role not only in risk stratification but also in planning management. If the patient is not kept in an inpatient facility, it is always necessary to assess available support system which can be utilized effectively while planning management on an outpatient basis. The common protective factors which need to be assessed are enumerated in **Box 3**.

Suicide Enquiry Proper

This is the most pivotal step in the entire assessment interview. The areas to be covered in suicide enquiry are: (1) Suicidal idea, (2) Suicide plan, (3) Suicide intent—subjective and objective, (4) Lethality of attempt/plan, and (5) Past suicide attempts.

- *Suicidal idea:* To elicit suicidal idea, it is better to ask the patient directly. Questions like, "Have you thought of killing yourself?" or "Are you having suicidal thoughts of

BOX 3: Protective factors for suicide.[1,3]

- Presence of social support. Support needs to be both present and accessible
- Children at home
- Sense of responsibility to family
- Pregnancy/motherhood
- Religiosity/spiritualty
- Life satisfaction
- Intact reality testing ability
- Positive coping skills
- Positive problem-solving skills
- Positive therapeutic relationships
- Easy access to support for help seeking
- Fear of social disapproval

late?." Suicidal ideas should be clearly distinguished from morbid ruminations in which the patient wishes that he were dead but does not actively think of killing himself. Once the presence of suicidal ideas is established, a series of questions are asked to establish the frequency, intensity, and duration of suicidal thoughts in the last 48 hours. Some questions that can be of use are—"How often do the thoughts come to you?," "How long do the thoughts last?," and "How intense are the thoughts (in a scale of 1–10)?."

- *Suicidal plan:* This should include detailed assessment of plan if any. Questions should be directed to elicit whether the patient has a definite plan, how, when, and where does he intend to carry it out, whether he has access to means, whether there are any preparatory acts involved and how lethal is the plan as per the patient's knowledge and perception.
- *Suicidal intent:* Intent to carry out the plan should be assessed both subjectively and objectively. For subjective intent, the patient can be directly asked, "Do you have any intention to act on your thoughts?," "Can you express your intent in a scale of 1–10?." Objective measures

of intent include preparation behavior and rehearsal behavior. In the former, the patient engages in behaviors to set things in order prior to his death like writing a will or giving away his belongings or making preparations to find out the various means of killing himself. In rehearsal behavior, patient actually practices his planned method before carrying it out. Presence of such behaviors denotes strong intent on the part of the patient.

- *Lethality:* This term denotes objective danger to life associated with a method of suicide. The measure of lethality should be objectively assessed by the clinician and may not coincide with the patient's perception of lethality. A common example in our country involves sudden, impulsive ingestion of pesticide by young individuals in villages, sometimes following trivial quarrel or disputes. The act is often accompanied by subjective perception of low lethality but would be rated as a means of high lethality on objective assessment.
- *Past suicide attempts:* A selective but detailed enquiry of past suicide attempts can provide valuable information which may help in determining risk of suicide for the current state. A detailed history of all suicide attempts taking place in the last 2 months should be recorded. Beyond this period, one need not assess each and every attempt in detail. In such cases, especially if the patient has history of multiple attempts spanning several years, only the "first" attempt and the "worst" or the most severe suicidal attempt as per the patient needs to be assessed and noted down.[2] The contextual factors of the past attempts may be assessed under the following headings (conveniently remembered by the acronym "PMOR")—Precipitant,

Motivation for the attempt, Outcome, and Reaction. Precipitant deals with the triggering factor, Motivation assesses how strong was the intent to die, Outcome probes the events following the attempt and what steps were taken to get medical attention and finally, and Reaction assesses how the person felt after surviving the attempt.[1] Probing the past suicidal attempts should always be done after the initial questions about current suicidal ideation. Once the past attempts are assessed and recorded, the clinician should proceed to ask about the current suicidal ideation.

Box 4 summarizes the points to be covered in suicide risk assessment. This may serve as a useful checklist for carrying out risk assessment in a busy clinic.

■ RISK STRATIFICATION

This is to be done after thorough assessment and evaluation of all the facets discussed above. **Table 1** shows basic outlines of risk stratification.[5,6]

BOX 4: Checklist for suicide risk assessment.

1. *Engagement:* Ensure privacy, establish rapport by communicating in a gentle, nonjudgmental manner; use normalization and shame attenuation if necessary. Communicate effectively with family members and gain their confidence
2. *Thorough psychiatric assessment:* Brief history and mental status examination to establish psychiatric diagnosis if any
3. *Presence of recent stressful event:* Financial, interpersonal or any other stressor
4. *Assessment of risk factors:* Lay special emphasis on modifiable risk factors
5. *Assessment of warning signs:* Assess imminence based on warning signs
6. *Presence of hopelessness, anxiety, depression, and sleep disturbances:* Ask directly and rate patient's subjective account
7. *Assessment of impulsivity/self-control:* Use both subjective and objective measures
8. *Assessment of protective factors:* Take special note of available support system
9. *Suicide enquiry proper:* Probe for current suicidal idea, then probe for past suicidal events, and finally assess the current suicidal idea further including plan, intent, and lethality

TABLE 1: Risk stratification and outlines of management.[5,6]

Risk level	Risk/protective factor	Suicidality	Possible interventions
High	Psychiatric diagnoses with severe symptoms or acute precipitating event; protective factors not relevant; substance abuse/dependence; severe depression, command hallucinations; poor support system	Potentially lethal suicide attempt or persistent ideation with strong intent or suicide rehearsal	Admission generally indicated unless a significant change reduces risk. Suicide precautions
Moderate	Multiple risk factors, few protective factors; moderate depression; support system inconsistent	Suicidal ideation with plan, but no intent or behavior. Preparatory acts are usually absent	Admission may be necessary depending on risk factors. Develop crisis plan including safety planning. Give emergency/crisis numbers. Frequent reevaluation of suicide risk
Low	Modifiable risk factors, strong protective factors; good support system	Thoughts of death, no plan, intent, or behavior	Outpatient referral, symptom reduction. Give emergency/crisis numbers

Chronic Risk

Those who make two or more serious suicide attempts (strong intent and/or lethality) are known as multiple suicide attempters. Such individuals usually have comorbid Axis I diagnosis and usually have chronically elevated risk of suicide. The elevated risk of subsequent attempt is usually within 1 year of the last attempt. Such individuals are said to be having chronic risk of suicide.[7] A potentially serious situation occurs when an individual with chronic risk develops acute exacerbation following a sudden precipitating event or crisis.

■ CONCLUSION

Suicide is one of the most intriguing medical emergencies across the world. India is no exception. Suicide rates in the country are rising steadily over the last few years. It is essential that all emergency medical facilities in the country, whether government or a private setup, must be equipped to handle a person presenting with suicidal crisis. It should be clear at the outset that the aim of risk assessment is not to predict suicidality with accuracy. Rather the purpose is to identify a state of heightened risk for suicide and manage it properly. This chapter tries to formulate the essential features of a comprehensive assessment of suicide risk and would be useful to all categories of healthcare professionals who have to deal with suicidal crisis.

■ REFERENCES

1. Rudd MD. Core competencies, warning signs, and a framework for suicide risk assessment in clinical practice. In: Nock MK (Ed). The Oxford Handbook of Suicide and Self-Injury: Oxford Library of Psychology. Oxford University Press; 2014.
2. Shea SC. The Chronological Assessment of Suicide Events: A Practical Interviewing Strategy for the Elicitation of Suicidal Ideation. J Clin Psychiatry. 1998; 59:58-72.
3. Jacobs DG, Baldessarini RS, Conwell Y, Fawcett JA, Horton L, Meltzer H, et al. Practice Guideline for the Assessment and Treatment of Patients with Suicidal Behaviors. Am J Psychiatry. 2003;160(11 Suppl):1-60.
4. Rudd MD, Berman AL, Joiner TE Jr, Nock MK, Silverman MM, Mandrusiak M, et al. Warning signs for suicide: Theory, research, and clinical applications. Suicide Life Threat Behav. 2006;36:255-62.
5. Substance Abuse and Mental Health Services Administration. Suicide Assessment Five-step Evaluation and Triage for clinicians (SAFE-T). [online] Available from: https://store.samhsa.gov/product/SAFE-T-Pocket-Card-Suicide-Assessment-Five-Step-Evaluation-and-Triage-for-Clinicians/sma09-4432 [Last accessed January, 2023].
6. Bryan CJ, Rudd MD. Advances in the Assessment of Suicide Risk. J Clin Psychol. 2006;62(2):185-200.
7. Rudd MD, Joiner TE, Rajab MH. The relationships between suicide ideators, attempters, and multiple attempters in a young adults sample. J Abnorm Psychol. 1996;105(4):541-50.

19

Ethical and Legal Aspects of Suicide in India

Guru S Gowda, Ravindra Neelakanthappa Munoli, Bevinahalli Nanjegowda Raveesh

ABSTRACT

"Ethical and Legal Aspects of Suicide" is a topic of debate in the fields of medicine and law. On one side, both advocate for individual autonomy, while on the other, the sanctity of life. In light of these considerations, ethical considerations have a significant impact on the legal standpoint on suicide. This continuous realm led to various positions on suicide, assisted suicide, and euthanasia in different parts of the world. This chapter provides an in-depth look at the socio-cultural and religious context, cultural and moral perspectives, and current legal status of suicide and attempted suicide in India. It also briefly discusses India's current medico-legal and ethical position on "Assisted Suicide" and "Do Not Resuscitate". The final part discusses the virtual world, the internet, and social networks in community suicide. The role of the World Health Organization (WHO), Mental Health Care Act-2017 (MHCA-2017), and Press Council of India (PCI) in suicide prevention.

Keywords: Suicide and law; Mental healthcare act.

COMMUNITY AND RELIGIOUS ATTITUDES TOWARD SUICIDE

Life is a gift; however, there are instances when people intentionally end their lives through unnatural means (suicide). Suicide is not merely an event related to an individual. Significant social dynamics and attitudes determine the probability of suicide. Individual integration with society and the degree of solidarity or cohesiveness play a vital role in suicidal behavior. The majority of people who attempt suicide are conflicted about their decision; the attempt is often a cry for help. Suicide psychological autopsy studies (among people who were prevented from committing suicide by outside intervention) show that people who have suicidal thoughts do not have a permanent desire to die or are ambivalent about their decision. One study in Seattle, Washington, for example, found that 75 of the 96 suicide attempters were quite uncertain about their intentions to die. Subsequent studies also noted that individuals desire to accomplish something by the attempt rather than the desire to die.[1] Stigma and punitive attitudes impede suicide prevention. These attitudes are eager to punish suicidal behavior and frequently blame living people for suicidal deaths. They foster an environment in which suicidal behavior is hidden, and people who are suicidal are afraid to speak up. Punitive attitudes remained when suicide was considered a crime and an unforgivable sin, and those who committed suicide were denied Christian burial (Vetting 1997).[2]

There are social and cultural impediments in place, in addition to the formal restraints on passing a suicide verdict. A person who commits suicide has traditionally been considered a mortal sin by Christian churches, particularly the Roman Catholic Church. In the Chinese culture, Confucianism emphasizes the importance of family ties and stresses not to harm one's own body because it was given to them by their parents. In addition, it emphasizes that individuals are must learn to cope with suffering from human life.[3] On the other hand, attempting suicide is implicitly forbidden, except in cases where it promotes family loyalty.

Various religious and philosophical writings in Indian Hindu culture have expressed opinions on suicide. Some religious groups permitted suicide (the best sacrifice being man's own life), while others forbade it. For example, "sati", a widow's self-immolation (by self-destruction on her husband's funeral pyre, the widow would atone for her husband's sins, and also have the belief that it frees husband from punishment, and opens the gates to heaven for him), was sanctioned by religious belief. There was a compassionate attitude toward suicide in Hinduism. Death, after all, eventually leads to rebirth in a new body[3-5] (Rao, 1975). However, there are saintly sayings that the soul of a suicide victim descends into lower forms of life, such as a dog or a cow.

In terms of Islam, the Quran does not contain any explicit prohibitions against suicide. Suicide is still considered a violation of a divine command found in Islam's holy books. Suicide may be allowed by social and cultural structures, which may even suggest it as an appropriate or honorable course of action in certain circumstances. Many Japanese people, for example, believe that death brings forgiveness for any sins committed during one's lifetime. As a result, suicide may be considered as a means of resolving one's problems. It could be a dignified death committed to upholding a family's, state's, or nation's hierarchy (Ong and Leng, 1992).[5] Committing suicide or individual involvement in another's suicide is considered a crime also in some societies. It is punishable in many countries as it is a crime, and it is based on societal, cultural, and religious values. As a result, suicide laws differed from country to country (Ong and Leng, 1992).[6]

■ INDIAN LAWS ON SUICIDE: PAST

According to the Indian legal system, an individual's life is valuable to himself and the state. In that mindset, "Right to life" is a natural/fundamental right embodied in Article 21 of the Constitution of India. Fundamental rights of many democratic countries express that suicide is an unnatural way to end one's life that is incompatible with the concept of a right to life (Pandey 1998).[7] According to Section 309 of the Indian Penal Code (IPC), "Whoever attempts to commit suicide or acts toward the commission of such offense shall be punished with simple imprisonment for a term which may extend to 1 year or a fine or both. In addition, Sections IPC 306 and 304b add to the strength of IPC Section 309.

There are numerous gaps and conflicting views in the law of the land (India) regarding suicide. For example, (a) The Indian law is unclear when it comes to declaring a fast unto death and self-immolation [Ram Sunder vs. State, 1961 ALLLJ 550, 1962 AIR (All) 262]; (b) If the person took an overdose of poison by accident or is intoxicated, attempted suicide is not punishable (Emperor vs. Dwaraka Poonja, BOMLR 146;1912: Queen Emperor vs. Ramakka, 1884 ILR 8 Mad 5); (c) Even though attempting suicide is punishable under Section 309 of the IPC,[8] different High Courts and Supreme Court in India have provided conflicting judgments. It may be because the legal system bases its decision on the individual's desire to end his life after gathering adequate information than just passing judgment by looking at the nature of the suicidal act.

Few Court laws provide more insight in this area, *"Maharashtra vs Maruthy Sripati Dubal (1987)"*[9] held that Article 21 of the constitution guarantees the right to life, including the right to die. As a result, the court ruled that Section 309 of the IPC is unconstitutional since it punishes someone who attempts suicide. The court concluded that their wish to die is distinct rather than unnatural. Court also listed the possible reasons why people might want to end their lives; these include (a) illness, (b) cruel or unbearable living conditions, and (c) feelings of shame or disenchantment with life. Further, Judges also advocated for the right to life, saying that they believe everyone should choose how and when to end their lives. In this case, a depressed policeman was denied permission to start a shop and earn a living. Out of frustration, he tried to light himself in the office of Bombay Corporation. Contrary to previous judgment, In 1988, the *Chenna Jagadeeswar v. State of Andhra Pradesh* (1988) case,[10] the court held Section 309 of the IPC was declared constitutional and rejected the argument that Section 309 violated Article 14 (Right to Equality), even though attempting suicide is an unspecified and unsupervised act. Further, the court explained its decision by saying, "To humanize our penal laws, Section 309 IPC should be revoked. It said that the harsh and illogical provision of IPC 309 may result in a person being punished twice: (a) due to his failure to commit suicide, who has suffered agony, and (b) facing indignity as a result of his failure to commit suicide".

In P Rathinam *vs* Union of India (1994),[11] the petitioners challenged Section 309. The plaintiff contended that it violated the Constitution's Articles 14 and 21. A Supreme Court division bench, agreeing with Maharashtra V. Maruthy Sripati Dubal (1987) viewpoint, stated that a person has the "right to die". It noted that Section 309 of the Indian Penal Code, which defines "attempt to commit suicide" as a criminal offense, is unconstitutional. Furthermore, the divisional branch determined that Article 21 of the Constitution's "right to live" also encompasses the "right not to live", or the right to die or end one's life. The Supreme Court overruled the prior judgment of "P Rathinam *vs* Union of India"[12] after 2 years in the "Gian Kaur *vs* the State of Punjab (1996)" case. It was upheld that the "right to die" is not included in Article 21 of the Constitution.

To conclude all these judgments together, retaining Section 309 will not protect the morality principle and value. But, human beings' most basic instinct is to protect themselves and live. So, the desire to attempt suicide goes against the instincts of most people in society. In addition, attempting suicide is against the accepted norm and could happen to few individuals in the community. In addition, individual autonomy can never be granted to the point of allowing the individual to take his own life, which is against the accepted social norm. Finally, the attempt to suicide considered is unnatural and goes against the moral values of ordinary people who make up society. On the whole, the different viewpoints, judgments, and opinions show that a law relating to the attempt to suicide in India is unclear, inconsistent, and confounding with the decisions given in different cases by the high and supreme courts.

INDIAN LAWS ON SUICIDE: PRESENT

"If any person dies by suicide, whoever abets the commission of such suicide will be punished with imprisonment of either description for a term which may extend to 10 years, and shall also be liable to fine," according to Section 306, IPC.[8] Further, Section 108 IPC explains that "the abetment of an offense being an offense, the abetment of such an abetment is also an offense."

Whoever abets any offense shall, if the act abetted is committed in consequence of the abetment, and this Code makes no express provision for the punishment of such abetment, be punished with the penalty provided for the offense, according to Section 109 of IPC (Mrs K Kamala *vs* State of Karnataka, Crl.P.No. 2759 of 2007).[8] Further, whoever abets a crime punishable with imprisonment shall, if that offense is not committed in consequence of the abetment, be punished with imprisonment of any description provided for that offense for a term which may extend to one-fourth part of the most extended term provided for that offense; or with such fine as is provided for the crime, or with both, according to Section 116 IPC [Satvir Singh *vs* State of Punjab (2001) 8 SCC 633].

The perspectives of psychiatrists, psychologists, and sociologists on suicide have provided the legal community with newer insights into this area. This contemporary perspective on an attempt at suicide yielded the decriminalization of Article 309 in the MHCA, 2017.[13] However, It is worth noting that a similar attempt was made in the past, and the law commission recommended repealing IPC Section 309 in 1971. The Indian Government accepted the recommendation, but the bill was not passed in the Lok Sabha in 1979 because the elected body had been dissolved, and the bill had lapsed (Trivedi, 1997).[14]

An attempt to commit suicide was a punishable offense under IPC Section 309.[8] Under the MHCA, 2017, the application of this section is limited by the premise that people who completed or attempted suicide may have mental illness and be under severe stress.[9] It does not decriminalize the IPC 309, but it enforces the appropriate Government to (a) provide care, treatment, and rehabilitation to a person, having severe stress and who attempted to commit suicide; (b) to plan for reducing the risk of recurrence of attempt to commit suicide. Even though MHCA, 2017, changed the status of "attempts to suicide" from legal to medical, the IPC 309 provisions have not been repealed in their entirety. So, there is a possibility of misuse of existing IPC 309 laws that cannot be ruled out.[15]

Every new law generates a debate about what is right and what is wrong. It is the same with the decriminalization of Article 309 in the MHCA, 2017 has been widely panned by the general public and by legal professionals.[9] However, there are a few compelling arguments that attempt suicide should be regulated and make a punishable offense. Therefore perspective form stakeholders includes: (a) Suicide has a harmful effect and causes significant loss to the community; (b) It is the government's responsibility to look after the health of the people and to address the problems leading to the life-ending tendency; (c) There is the proper inquiry of suicide attempter can be made by the concerned authorities, only when there is a law against suicide.

There are a few compelling arguments that attempting suicide should not be regulated or make a punishable offense. These arguments are (a) The right to privacy is the most potent argument against punishment and regulatory oversight on suicide attempts; (b) As everybody knows, the court and legal investigation negatively affect the already depressed suicide attempter and his family; (c) In addition, there may be unwarranted harassment of close friends or family; (d) If the suicide attempter is punished, the family will be financially burdened even more after all the costs of rescuing the individuals from the self-physical damage on the body; and (e) Can it be justified to harm those still alive for an act committed by a family member if the person dies in the attempt?.

A few processes have been outlined in **Table 1** to manage a person who has attempted suicide to ensure the provision of Part 2 of Section 115(2) of the MHCA

TABLE 1: Medico-legal approach to managing an attempted suicide person in a hospital setting.

Step 1	Assess and triage: Rapid assessment and triaging in the emergency room
Step 2	Stabilize: Initiate necessary medical or surgical treatment to stabilize the patient
Step 3	Medico-legal case (MLC): Medico-legal case registration, and depending on the severity, admission if required
Step 4	Psychiatry referral: Mandatory psychiatric referral for required assessment (making a diagnosis and assessing the severity of stress and suicidal intent) and treatment
Step 5	Inform: Inform the patient regarding Section 115 of MHCA 2017
Step 6	Inquiry by the health team and police regarding Sections 108, 109, and 116 IPC
Step 7	Discharge planning and follow-up care with medical, surgical, and psychiatric teams as per guidelines

2017. According to that, "individuals who have attempted suicide and are enduring significant stress should be provided with care, treatment, and rehabilitation to limit the likelihood of recurrence of a suicide attempt".[9]

To summarize, the MHCA, 2017, changed the legal status of "attempts to suicide" to biopsychosocial issue and obligated the government to provide "care, treatment, and rehabilitation to a person who is experiencing severe stress and has attempted to die by suicide, to reduce the risk of a suicide and also recurrence of suicide."

ETHICAL AND LEGAL ASPECTS OF ASSISTED SUICIDE AND DO NOT RESUSCITATE

Assisted suicide is legally and factually distinct from euthanasia and suicide. In assisted suicide, a third party intentionally assists a person in committing suicide by providing drugs for self-administration at the request of that person, who is willing and competent and does not per se terminate the life. Whereas in euthanasia, life is ended by the intervention of a third party through omission or action.[16] Assisted suicide is a legally punishable offense in India. **Table 2** distinguishes between suicide, assisted suicide, do not resuscitate (DNR), and euthanasia.

Suicide, assisted suicide, DNR, and euthanasia are all prohibited and punishable offenses in India, according to the IPC and Article 21 of the Indian Constitution.[8] Suicide, assisted suicide, DNR, and euthanasia are illegal and punishable crimes in India as per IPC and against Article 21 of the Indian Constitution.[8] The various perspectives, judgments, and opinions received on Article 21 on the right to die. Nonetheless, on March 7, 2011, the Indian Supreme Court issued a ruling on involuntary passive euthanasia in Ms Aruna Shanbaug, resulting in a paradigm

TABLE 2: Distinguishes between suicide, assisted suicide, "do not resuscitate", and euthanasia.

	Suicide	*Assisted suicide*	*Do not resuscitate*	*Passive euthanasia*	*Active euthanasia*
Person's intent to end their life	Present	Present	Not applicable	Not applicable	Present
Assist in the death of others	Absent	Present	Not applicable	Present	Present
External interventions by others in ending a life	Absent	Absent	Absent	Present	Present
Lethal medication administration	It could be one of the forms	It could be one of the forms, and the third party intentionally assists a person	Not applicable	Not present	Present
The physician withdraws the life-support system	Not applicable	Not applicable	Not applicable	Present	Not Applicable
Withholding cardiopulmonary resuscitation	Not applicable	Not applicable	Present	Not applicable	Not Applicable
Current legal status in India	IPC 305, 306, 309	IPC 306	No legal sanctity	The Euthanasia (Regulation) Bill, 2019	The Euthanasia (Regulation) Bill, 2019

shift.[17] The Supreme Court ordered the Government to develop a euthanasia law. Consequently, the Law Commission of India proposed a bill that allows passive euthanasia. In 2016, the Ministry of Health and Family Welfare (MoHFW), Government of India, issued a draft bill on the "euthanasia regulation bill" for public comment and to make an informed decision and take a general perspective. Currently, The Euthanasia (Regulation) Bill, 2019 now introduced in Lok Sabha.[18] One such law is passed, passive euthanasia may have a considerable impact on India's cultural, religious, political, public, and medical sectors soon.

Furthermore, it may impact the Hippocratic Oath, which prohibits medical professionals from practicing euthanasia. So, the Hippocratic Oath, particularly on this phrase—"I will neither give a deadly drug to anybody who asked for nor will I make a suggestion to this effect—needs to be changed or omitted in India, when medical graduates take the oath.[19]

"Do not resuscitate" is an option in the patient's best interest, where cardiopulmonary resuscitation (CPR) would be inappropriate. It will be done and exercised by treating physician(s) with their best judgment, where CPR would be likely to prolong the suffering of the patient.[20] DNR is distinct from passive euthanasia, which involves withdrawing or withholding other ongoing life-supporting treatments for patients.

In India, recent Indian Council of Medical Research, bioethics unit consensus guidelines, and court order say that DNR is to be made collaboratively with parents or the spouse or other close relatives. Few situations where, absence of any of the parents or the spouse or other close relatives, the decision about DNR can be taken by a person or a body of persons acting as a next friend. In extraordinary circumstances, it can be taken by the doctors attending to the patient. However, the decision about DNR should be taken bona fide in the patient's best interest.[20] In addition, approval of the High Court is required when the decision about DNR is accepted by the near relatives or doctors or the next friend. The acceptance of the High Court is kept to prevent misuse and vested interest of the third party.

ROLE OF VIRTUAL WORLD: INTERNET AND SOCIAL NETWORKS IN COMMUNITY SUICIDE

The growing use of the internet and smartphones by an ordinary person in India has resulted in easily accessible online resources, markets, and virtual worlds. The online media platforms/virtual world (Facebook, WhatsApp, Telegram, and Twitter) have enabled near-instantaneous dissemination of information to the general public and community. The "Werther" effect has been linked to a rapid spike in suicides in the community, with media coverage sensationalizing celebrity/prominent personality suicides, including a detailed account of the incident or speculations on the reasons for the same.[21,22] Furthermore, the "Papageno Effect" has been linked to lower rates of suicide in the community by considerate reporting of suicide, highlighting the provision of hope, and offering alternative ways to cope with stress, who has a suicidal idea or thoughts.[21]

According to studies conducted in India and other Southeast Asian countries, the overall responsibility and quality of suicide reporting was low and not at an optimal level. They also observed differences between reports published in vernacular newspapers and those published in English newspapers. For example, it was discovered that vernacular newspapers avoided reporting on potentially harmful characteristics, whereas their English counterparts included protective elements in their reports.[23,24] A recent Indian study noted a significant increase in online search interest for suicide-related keywords, associated with poor adherence to quality reporting guidelines, linked with celebrity suicide.[25] Furthermore, while covering the incident, it also noted that there was less emphasis on creating awareness and educating the public about suicide and its prevention at the community level.[26]

ETHICAL AND LEGAL ROLES OF MEDIA (PRINT AND AUDIO-VISUAL) IN SUICIDE COVERAGE AND SUICIDE PREVENTION

Through the broadcast of information, the media plays a vital role in bridging the gap between communities and the world. How suicide is presented in the media has a significant impact on public knowledge, comprehension, acceptance, help-seeking, and societal attitudes toward suicide. So, the responsible media reporting of suicides has been considered an essential population-based suicide prevention strategy worldwide. To improve the responsible reporting of suicides by media, the World Health Organization (WHO) and the International Association for Suicide Prevention (IASP) launched SUPRE (SUicide PREvention). The SUPRE is a suicide prevention initiative.[27] Through this initiative, resources materials

TABLE 3: Press Council of India guidelines on reporting of suicide by media professionals.[27]

Dos while reporting suicide by media professionals	Don'ts while reporting suicide by media professionals
Provide accurate information about where to seek help and how to get help for suicidal thoughts or ideas	Place stories about suicide prominently and unduly repeat such stories
Educate the public about the facts of suicide and suicide prevention without spreading myths	Use language which sensationalizes or normalizes suicide or presents it as a constructive solution to problems
Report stories of how to cope with life stressors or suicidal thoughts	Explicitly describe the suicide method used
Apply particular caution when reporting celebrity suicides	Provide details about the site/location
Apply caution when interviewing bereaved family or friends	Use sensational headlines
Recognize that media professionals themselves may be affected by stories about suicide	Use photographs, video footage, or a social media link

were developed to help journalists. These resources are to guide media professionals on how to report such deaths to raise public awareness about the issue of suicide and avoid the risk of imitation.[28,29] Media portrayal of suicides has an important influence on suicidal behaviors in society. Recently Press Council of India (PCI) adapted the WHO guidelines, and **Table 3** shows the PCI guidelines on reporting suicide by media professionals.[28,29]

▎ FUTURE DIRECTION AND CONCLUSION

"Suicide, assisted suicide, do not resuscitate, and euthanasia" are all prohibited and punishable offenses in India. The viewpoints, judgments, and opinions on "Attempt to Suicide" in India show that it is still unclear, inconsistent, and confounding with the decisions given in different cases by the High Court and the Supreme Court. However, the Mental Health Care Act of 2017 changed the legal status of "attempts to suicide" as maybe a biopsychosocial problem. It obligated the government to provide "care, treatment, and rehabilitation to a person who is experiencing severe stress and has attempted to die by suicide, to reduce the risk of suicide, and also recurrence of suicide. All the sections of the society, viz., police, judiciary, media personals, and journalists need to be sensitized about the legal nuances of IPC Sections 108, 109, 116, 306, and 309 in the background of Section 115 of the Mental Health Care Act and Press Council of India guideline on suicide reporting. In addition, concerning bodies should develop and implement protocols, policies, and procedures to manage a person who attempted suicide and emphasize suicide prevention in the community. Concerned bodies can be made mandatory to maintain an online register to document all suicides/suicide attempts in hospitals and submit it periodically to review boards. This will help in policy-making decisions. It also helps to make national and region-specific suicide prevention strategies.

■ REFERENCES

1. Daly M, Conway M, Kelleher MJ. Social determinants of self-poisoning. Br J Psychiatry. 1986;148:406-13.
2. Vetting (1997).
3. Hassan R. Suicide in Singapore. Eur J Sociol. 1980;21(2):183-219.
4. Balodhi JP. Indian Mythological Views on Suicide. NIMHANS J. 1992;10:101-5.
5. (Rao, 1975).
6. (Ong and Leng, 1992).
7. Pandey JN. The Constitutional law of India. Allahabad: Central Law Agency; 1998.
8. The Indian Penal Code. (1860). Sections 40, 108, 109, 116, 306, 309, 511. [online] available from: https://indiacode.nic.in/bitstream/123456789/2263/3/A1860-45.pdf. [Last accessed July, 2022].
9. Patil BK, Sawant P. (1987). The Bombay High Court in Maharashtra vs. Maruthy Sripati Dubal (1987). [online] Available from: https://indiankanoon.org/doc/490515/ [Last accessed July, 2022].
10. Chenna Jagadeeswar vs. State of AP (1988).
11. P. Rathinam vs. Union of India (1994).
12. Smt. Gian Kaur vs. The State Of Punjab 1996 AIR 946, 1996 SCC (2) 648.
13. The Mental Healthcare Act - 2017, Ministry of Law and Justice; Gazette of India; 2017. [online] Available from: http://www.egazette.nic.in/WriteReadData/2017/175248.pdf. [Last accessed July, 2022].
14. Trivedi JK. Punishing attempted suicide: Anachronism of the twentieth century. Editorial, Indian J Psychiatry. 1997;39:87-9.
15. Vadlamani LN, Gowda M. Practical implications of Mental Healthcare Act 2017: Suicide and suicide attempt. Indian J Psychiatry. 2019;61:S750-5.
16. Medical News Today. (2022). What are euthanasia and assisted suicide? [online] Available from: https://www.medicalnewstoday.com/articles/182951 [Last accessed July, 2022].
17. Supreme Court of India. (2011). Bench: Markandey Katju, Gyan Sudha Misra. Aruna Ramchandra Shanbaug vs Union of India and Ors on 7 March, 2011. [online] Available from: https://indiankanoon.org/doc/235821/ [Last accessed July, 2022].
18. Lok Sabha. (2019). The Euthanasia (Regulation) Bill, 2019. [online] Available from: http://164.100.47.4/billstexts/lsbilltexts/asintroduced/916ls%20as%20int..%20euthanasia%20as%20introduced..pdf [Last accessed July, 2022].
19. National Library of Medicine. (2002). The Hippocratic Oath. [online] available from: https://www.nlm.nih.gov/hmd/greek/greek_oath.html [Last accessed July, 2022].
20. Mathur R. ICMR Consensus Guidelines on 'Do Not Attempt Resuscitation. Indian J Med Res. 2020;151(4):303-10.
21. Niederkrotenthaler T, Voracek M, Herberth A, Till B, Strauss M, Etzersdorfer E, et al. role of media reports in completed and prevented suicide: Werther v. Papageno effects. Br J Psychiatry. 2010;197(3):234-43.
22. Hittner JB. How robust is the Werther effect? A re-examination of the suggestion-imitation model of suicide. Mortality. 2005;10(3):193-200.
23. Chandra PS, Doraiswamy P, Padmanabh A, Philip M. Do newspaper reports of suicides comply with standard suicide reporting guidelines? A study from Bangalore, India. Int J Soc Psychiatry. 2014;60(7):687-94.
24. Armstrong G, Vijayakumar L, Niederkrotenthaler T, Jayaseelan M, Kannan R, Pirkis J, et al. Assessing the quality of media reporting of suicide news in India against World Health Organization guidelines: A content analysis study of nine major newspapers in Tamil Nadu. Aust N Z J Psychiatry. 2018;52(9):856-63.
25. Ganesh R, Singh S, Mishra R, Sagar R. The quality of online media reporting of celebrity suicide in India and its association with subsequent online suicide-related search behaviour among general population: An

infodemiology study. Asian J Psychiatr. 2020;53:102380.

26. Menon V, Kar SK, Varadharajan N, Kaliamoorthy C, Pattnaik JI, Sharma G, et al. Quality of media reporting following a celebrity suicide in India. 2022;44(1):e133-40.

27. WHO. (2017). Preventing suicide: a resource for media professionals—update 2017. [online] Available from: https://www.who.int/mental_health/suicide-prevention/resource_booklet_2017/en/ [Last accessed July, 2022].

28. WHO. (2020). Responsible and deglamorized media reporting. [online] Available from: https://www.who.int/mental_health/mhgap/evidence/suicide/q9/en/ [Last accessed July, 2022].

29. Vijayakumar L. Media Matters in suicide-Indian guidelines on suicide reporting. Indian J Psychiatry. 2019;61(6):549-51.

Suicide Prevention in India

Lakshmi Vijayakumar

ABSTRACT

The chapter takes a public health approach to suicide prevention. It discusses various suicide prevention strategies adopted by the World Health Organization. Then it goes through the steps taken by the government of India so far. Finally, a National Action Plan for suicide prevention in India is proposed.

Keywords: Suicide Prevention; Suicide Prevention Strategies.

◼ INTRODUCTION

The World Health Organization estimated that 173,347 people died by suicide in India in 2019 and that it was the highest in the world.[1] Suicide has been identified as the leading cause of death among the 15–39 years age group[2,3] with 52.6% of all suicide deaths among females and 47.4% among males belonging to this age group.[3] India, in 1990, had contributed 27.3% of global suicide deaths among females and 16.7% among males and this has increased to 36.5% and 20.9%, respectively in 2019.

It is estimated that in 2019 about 85,900 females and 109,470 males died by suicide in India accounting for 2.1% of the 9.4 million deaths that occurred in the country during the year according to Global Burden of Disease estimates.[3,4] India's age-standardized suicide death rate (ASDR) for 2019 is estimated at 13.8/100,000 population with suicide mortality rate among Indian females being 2.1 times higher than the global rate.[2,5]

It has been assessed that for every death by suicide in India, there are 15 suicide attempts and >200 people who are suicidal.[4] Reports estimate that 5·1% of the Indian population over the age of 18 years had some level of nonfatal suicidal thoughts and behavior with 68.5% reporting suicidal ideation.[5]

Suicide death rates vary in India by region, religion, and by caste.[6] A 15-fold variation for females and sevenfold variation for males in ASDR has been reported at the state level.[2] The male-to-female ratio of ASDR for the country was 1.28 in 2019 and ranged from 0.78 to 4.62 between the states.

India is unlikely to reach its goal of one-third reduction in suicide rates as part of its commitment to the sustainable development goal (SDG) 2030.[3] The World Health Organization (WHO) has in its report indicated suicide as a major public health concern in India and has advocated a comprehensive suicide prevention strategy taking into account the country's socio-cultural, economic, and health conditions.[7] At present the Indian Government is in the process of developing a national suicide prevention strategy.

A PUBLIC HEALTH APPROACH TO SUICIDE PREVENTION

Suicide has traditionally been viewed as a mental health issue that is addressed primarily through clinical intervention, especially through the treatment of depression. However, it has been suggested that the role of mental disorders within suicide is not as significant in countries like India compared to the West.[8,9]

It is now clearly established that suicide is a public health issue, and as such it should be addressed by social and public health programs rather than as part of mental health programs, especially in a country like India where the association between mental disorders and suicide is comparatively less.

Other factors for arguing for a public health approach in India include the fact that social reasons for suicide are more readily acceptable than emotional reasons. Apart from this on a practical note, there is the extremely limited availability of mental health professionals[8] (India as such has around 9,000 psychiatrists for a population of 1.3 billion people). Suicide is also accorded low priority in the competition for meagre resources,[10] and this can be gauged from the fact that the whole mental health component comprises only 2% of the national health budget.[11] Given the resource constraints (manpower and finance) it would be a major challenge to roll out an expensive healthcare system driven model for suicide prevention. It is therefore logical that a low resource country like India has primarily depended on low-cost interventions that are often delivered by lay volunteers.[8] This situation has led to the emergence of nongovernmental organizations (NGOs) in the field of suicide prevention.[10]

ROLE OF NONGOVERNMENTAL ORGANIZATIONS

As mentioned, the government has limited resources to address the issue of suicide and NGOs have stepped in to fill the gap. SNEHA (Society for Nutrition, Education, and Health Action), a volunteer driven nongovernmental organization based in Chennai, pioneered suicide prevention helplines in India as early as 1986[9] and since then several other NGOs have followed suit. Most of them operate crisis centers or hotlines and offer free service and as such play a crucial role.

The primary goal of these prevention centers is to provide emotional support to those who are suicidal in the population through befriending and counseling in person or by telephone. They are the premier NGOs in suicide prevention, and they are instrumental in increasing the awareness about suicide and its prevention in their respective populations. The crisis centers have adapted to local needs and do not follow the approach as practiced in the West. For instance, crisis centers are often the entry point for people with psychological problems into clinical services. The volunteers are trained in the identification of mental disorders, and they make appropriate referrals. Furthermore, they undertake education of gatekeepers, raise awareness in the public as well as media. Although many innovative programs for raising awareness and increasing help-seeking behavior have been developed to prevent suicide, majority of them have not been evaluated.[9]

SUICIDE PREVENTION STRATEGIES IMPLEMENTED IN INDIA

Interventions need to be locally devised. A direct transfer of the strategies employed in the West are unlikely to work in India as the interventions are derived from theoretical models based upon data from the West. The significant differences in terms of gender ratio, age structure, and methods employed for suicide in the West from India mean that interventions must be suitably adapted to factor in local requirements and be consistent with the local social and cultural practices.[8]

When devising suicide prevention strategies, it is also essential to take into account the risk and protective factors that are relevant at the national, regional, state and also at the local community level. These are likely to vary across the various parts of the country. However, some risk factors that apply to the whole country have been identified; these include the contribution of social and cultural factors across the life course of an individual such as family problems, financial setbacks, grief over the death of a loved one, academic failure, breakup of a marriage, poverty, poor physical health and abuse,[11,12] in addition to globally known risk factors such as depression and alcohol use. Not much data on protective factors for suicide is available from India. Higher education and religiosity[13-15] along with social support and having children have been identified as protective factors from suicide.[14,16]

As indicated previously due to resource constraints most suicide prevention activities and programs have been delivered by NGOs using lay health workers and in collaboration with other community stake holders. Interventions which are evidence-based and those that have been evaluated are presented in this chapter.

The prevention efforts have been classified into three levels:

1. *Universal prevention*: Universal interventions target the general population with coverage of the population as a whole.
2. *Selective prevention*: Selective interventions focus on subpopulations that have an elevated risk and can be employed on the basis of sociodemographic characteristics, geographical distribution, or prevalence of mental and substance use disorders.
3. *Indicated prevention*: Indicated interventions are aimed at persons who are already known to be vulnerable to suicide or who have attempted suicide.[16]

Universal Prevention Strategies

India has not had a national suicide prevention strategy and it is only currently a policy paper is being considered. However, despite its absence the government has taken actions over the years across the health and social domains that facilitate suicide prevention. These include the introduction of several new laws and policies.[17,18]

National Mental Health Policy

The National Mental Health Policy of India launched in 2014 aimed to reduce suicide deaths and suicide attempts using suicide prevention programs, restricting access to the means of suicide (primarily pesticides), framing guidelines for responsible media reporting, community gatekeeper training, improving data on suicide and addressing alcohol abuse, and depression as key risk factors.

The District Mental Health Program (DMHP, which is currently operational in 500 of the 725 districts in the country currently with a psychiatrist as part of a multidisciplinary team) was identified as a key stakeholder in the delivery of the service. Along with the nearly 5,000 primary care doctors across the country who have been trained under the DMHP in mental health assessment and treatment.[18]

In the proposed reorganization of primary healthcare through Health and Wellness Centers, mental healthcare is one of six identified noncommunicable diseases that they are tasked with, but suicide prevention is not explicitly mentioned.[18]

Decriminalization of Suicide

Suicide attempt was a criminal offense in India until it was in a roundabout fashion decriminalized under the Mental Healthcare Act of 2017, which stated that any person who attempts to commit suicide shall not be tried and punished.[19-22] As per the Act, the government has the duty to provide care, treatment and rehabilitation to the person who attempts suicide to reduce the risk of recurrence. However, the conflict with Section 309 of the Indian Penal Code, under which suicide attempt is punishable, is yet to be addressed in practice.[23]

Policy Changes (Education)

India sees an increase in adolescent suicides in the months of June to July each year when examination results are announced. The enormous competition to get into colleges, the media hype associated with the announcement of the top rankers, and the shame associated with failure pushes distressed students to suicide.[24] Some states and local governments offer suicide prevention helplines during these months; however, their effectiveness is not known as there has been no systematic evaluation of these helplines. SNEHA an NGO working in suicide prevention started a campaign and the state government of Tamil Nadu was responsive and introduced a system of supplementary board examinations in 2004 allowing those who have failed the board examination to take another examination immediately in the same month as results were declared. A study showed that after this was introduced, there was almost 50% reduction in related suicides over a decade.[25] The states of Andhra Pradesh, Karnataka, and Maharashtra have also initiated similar laws, but these have yet to be implemented nationally.

Restricting Access to Lethal Means of Suicide (Pesticides)

Restricting access to means of suicide is one of the effective strategies to prevent and reduce death by suicide and suicide attempts. In India, the most common means used for suicide is consumption of pesticides. To manage this, the registration, production, distribution, and sale of 18 toxic pesticides were banned in 2018, and there is a proposal to expand this ban to an additional 27 highly lethal pesticides.[26] There is evidence to show from the state of Kerala that suicide rates have fallen after pesticides were banned.[27]

Establishing a Good Monitoring and Reporting System

While India has a system to record and report suicides, it is acknowledged that the quality of the data is variable and that there is vast underreporting and as such the available data is not reliable. This hinders the formulation of appropriate strategies. A comprehensive surveillance system is required which to bridge this gap.[28]

An attempt to setup a comprehensive surveillance system in rural Gujarat by adding a community-based component has been reported where the data was gathered through key informants such as village heads, teachers, priests, shopkeepers, private physicians, private hospitals, and community healthworkers and was compared with data from hospital and police records. Information was collected for a period of 12 months from 116 villages. The community surveillance system identified 67 cases of suicide compared with 30 cases by hospital and police records and 70 attempted suicides compared with 51 from the hospital and police records.[28] This study clearly indicated the potential of this system of combining community surveillance and official data from hospital and police records to address the problem of underreporting of suicide and suicide attempts in India.[28]

Guidelines for the Media

The Press Council of India, in 2019, released a set of guidelines on reporting on suicides, based on the recommendations of the World Health Organization and the International Association for Suicide Prevention guidelines.[29] The Indian guidelines state that news agencies while reporting the cases of suicide must *not* (a) Place stories about suicide prominently and unduly repeat such stories, (b) Use language which sensationalizes or normalizes suicide or presents it as a constructive solution to problems, (c) Explicitly describe the method used, (d) Provide details about the site/location, (e) Use sensational headlines, and (f) Use photographs, video footage, or social media links.[30]

Effective implementation of the Press Council's guidelines requires active collaboration between media personnel and mental health professionals. Apart from that a monitoring mechanism has to be initiated to ensure that the guidelines are followed, which should fall within the broader national strategy of suicide prevention.[30]

Selective Prevention Strategies

Contact and Use of Safety Planning Cards among Refugees

Refugees have been identified as a vulnerable group with increased suicide risk because of forced migration, traumatic events and resettlement in unfamiliar environments. An intervention of regular contact and use of safety planning cards by community volunteers to reduce suicidal behavior among Sri Lankan refugees residing in camps in Tamil Nadu, South India was carried out among consenting adults in two refugee camps (one intervention and one control). High-risk individuals (those scoring >16 on Centre for Epidemiological Studies Depression or >30 on Post-traumatic Stress Disorder (PTSD) or with active/passive suicidal ideation or a history of previous suicidal attempts) were targeted for intervention by the trained community volunteers.[31]

The study reported that of the 288 high-risk refugees in intervention camp, 139 completed the intervention. In the control camp, 187 were categorized as high risk. Prevalence of suicide attempts was 6.1%. Following intervention, differences between sites in changes in combined suicide (attempted suicides and suicides) rates per 100,000 per year were 519 (95% confidence interval (CI): 136–902; p < .01) indicating that contact and use of safety planning (CASP) cards as an intervention was feasible and effective in reducing suicidal behavior.[31]

Central Storage Facility to Reduce Pesticide Suicides

Using a central storage facility to delay and reduce access to pesticide and thereby reducing suicides was a strategy that was examined in a trial that assessed the feasibility and acceptability of a centralized pesticide storage facility as a preventive strategy. In the trial conducted in rural south India two villages were randomized to be intervention sites and two were designated as control site. Two centralized storage facilities with lockable storage boxes were constructed. Farmers could access their pesticide storage boxes with the key to their own locker, and a duplicate key was kept with the manager of the central storage facility.[32] The results of the study revealed that most participants found the storage facility to be both useful and acceptable. In addition to protecting against wastage, they felt that it had also helped to prevent pesticide suicides as the pesticides stored here were not as easily and readily accessible. The study also reported that at baseline at the intervention site there were 13 suicides and attempted suicides which reduced to 6 postintervention, whereas there was no change in the control site. Further analysis of the data showed that reported changes in completed and attempted suicide rates per 100,000 person-years were 295 for pesticide suicide and 339 for suicide by all methods. The study demonstrated that reducing access to pesticides through safe central storage is simple, culturally acceptable, and potentially sustainable.[32]

Promoting Nonpesticide Management

In a study conducted in four villages in Andhra Pradesh that had stopped using chemical pesticides in favor of nonpesticide management (NPM) the authors reported that the number of suicides had come down from 14 to 3 after introduction of NPM. They concluded that restriction of pesticide availability and accessibility by NPM has the potential to reduce pesticide suicides when combined with psychosocial and health interventions.[33]

Helplines and Guidelines

During coronavirus disease 2019 (COVID-19), the Government of India launched some preventive activities that indirectly addressed suicide prevention.[34] Two toll-free helplines for psychosocial support and one for domestic violence were established. Written and audio-visual guidelines were also released regarding mental health issues for various groups, including people living with mental disorders and also for healthcare providers to enable management of mental health issues.[35] However, the impact of these measures has not been assessed.

Indicated Prevention Strategies

Brief Intervention and Contact

Brief intervention and contact (BIC) was evaluated to assess its potential as a preventive strategy for suicide in a randomized control trial, the Suicide Prevention Multisite Intervention Study (SUPRE-MISS). Individuals above the age of 12 years ($N = 680$) who had attempted suicide and were admitted in intensive care unit of a general hospital in the city of Chennai were randomly allotted to treatment as usual (control arm) and to BIC (intervention arm). The BIC process involved a standard 1-hour individual session with the participant at the time of discharge and subsequent periodic follow-up contacts. This session addressed risk and protective factors, social, and psychological distress underlying the suicidal behavior, alternative and healthier coping strategies, referral options, and relapse prevention. Review visits were done at 1st, 2nd, 4th, 7th, and 11th week as well as 4th, 6th, 12th, and 18th month after discharge. Suicide deaths and suicide attempts were significantly lower in the BIC group in comparison to the treatment as usual group. This low-cost intervention is effective and can easily be scaled up in healthcare settings in India.[36]

Healthy Activity Program

The Healthy Activity Program (HAP), an intervention for individuals with moderate to severe depression in primary care, was assessed through a randomized control trial wherein the intervention was provided by lay counselors in the intervention arm and enhanced usual care was provided in the comparative arm and was found to be acceptable and cost-effective, and it reduced suicidal thoughts and attempts [adjusted mean difference: 0·61 (0.45–0.83); p = 0.001).[37]

A NATIONAL ACTION PLAN FOR SUICIDE PREVENTION IN INDIA

It is essential that India has a national suicide prevention policy and action plan. Typically, national strategies comprise a range of prevention strategies, such as means restriction, media guidelines, and training for health workers. It would also cover resource allocation for achieving the short-to-medium and long-term objectives identified. It would also in addition lay out the plans and strategies that would be implemented effectively and lay the framework for regular evaluation and feeding back the findings to fine-tune and re-strategize ongoing programs and inform future planning and in the designing of future programs.

India should develop and strengthen surveillance, resulting in better quality and availability of both suicide and suicide attempt data, and to provide and disseminate data that are necessary to inform action.[38]

A national suicide prevention strategy needs to be multisectoral, involving not only the health sector but also sectors such as education, labor, social welfare, agriculture, business, justice, law, defense, politics, and the media.[16]

A national action plan for suicide prevention for India with four primary objectives is proposed. They are: (1) Policy changes to be implemented to reduce and prevent suicide, (2) Enhancing the capacity of health services to provide suicide prevention services, (3) Promoting community resilience and societal support for suicide prevention, and (4) Strengthening surveillance of self-harm and suicide. The activities that can be undertaken to reach each of the above-mentioned objectives are presented below **(Fig. 1)**.

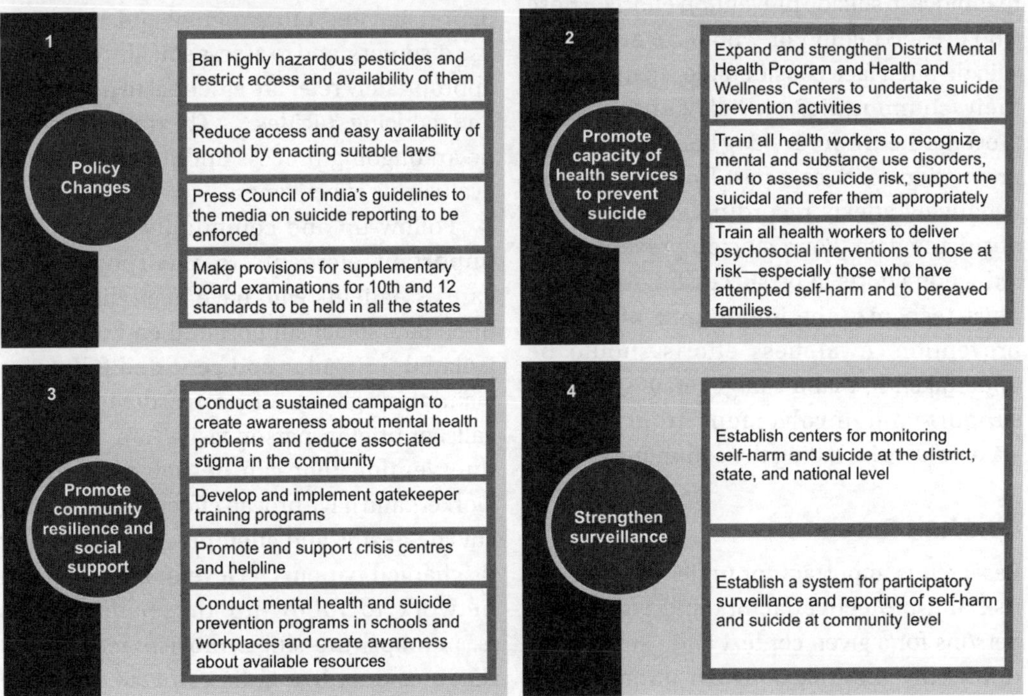

Fig. 1: Action plan for suicide prevention in India.

■ FUTURE DIRECTIONS

The following need to be undertaken to ensure the success and sustainability of a national strategy and it is essential that these gaps should be addressed going forward.

Improving Case Registration

As suicide often remains misclassified, unreported, or underreported, and improved surveillance systems are needed to enhance the quality of the available data. Capturing suicide attempt data, a more challenging endeavor, is equally important as a prior suicide attempt is the strongest predictor of subsequent suicide in the general population. A systematic approach for gathering data in a sustained manner is essential.[16]

Increase Awareness and Reduce Stigma

Stigma related to suicide is a significant roadblock to suicide prevention efforts. Those who are left behind or who have attempted suicide often face considerable stigma within their communities, which subsequently prevents them from seeking help from suicide prevention services. Apart from that stigma negatively affects recording and reporting of suicide data. For a suicide prevention or reduction efforts to be successful, the public must recognize the importance of suicide prevention. Awareness efforts should be undertaken so that it can generate sustained support and involvement from all the stakeholders including the community.[16]

Conduct Research

Research is important for understanding the risk and protective factors and vulnerable persons for a given context and can be used to identify the link between intermediate outcomes of a strategy's action plan. India currently does not have sufficient evidence-based intervention strategies for suicide prevention or reduction that are based on the various risk and protective factors identified locally.[16]

Strengthening Health Services

The health sector should incorporate suicide prevention as a core component of its service as this will ensure early detection and intervention. Protocols for clinical decision-making and management have been developed through WHO Mental Health Gap Action Program (mhGAP) Intervention Guide in nonspecialized health settings[39] for use in low resource settings.

A key element of this is training of healthworkers especially those in primary care services (who are often the first contacts) on the protocols to ensure that psychosocial support is provided to those in need.[40] Training healthcare workers to recognize depression and other mental and substance use disorders, and to assess suicide risk and to appropriately refer are essential to preventing and reducing suicides.[41,42] The training should be an ongoing process and it is essential to evaluate its effectiveness.

Follow-up and community support are important elements to incorporate into care as patients who have been discharged often lack social support and end up feeling isolated.[39] Regular and repeated follow-up visits through use of postcards, telephone calls, or brief in-person visits[43] are a low cost intervention that can be delivered by lay workers and have proved effective in reducing suicide deaths and attempts among recently discharged patients.[44] Developing a support network to follow-up these individuals is, perhaps, the single most practical step that a country like India can take to reduce suicides.[45]

Support for Survivors of Suicide

Suicide causes great suffering to survivors such as spouses, parents, children, family, friends, coworkers, and peers who are left behind. The impact on them is both immediate and in the long-term. Reaching out to this vulnerable group is crucial, as they can be prone to depression and suicidal behaviors.[46] It is therefore essential to provide support to the survivor and this can be achieved by establishing self-help groups for survivors.[16]

Conduct Monitoring and Evaluation

A comprehensive monitoring and evaluation framework needs to be evolved that would investigate the various aspects of the suicide reduction and prevention strategies. Evaluations are important for indicating whether changes need to be made and where it must be made. Intermediate and primary outcomes (reducing suicides and suicide attempts) should be clearly defined with time-linked targets. Monitoring and evaluation is critical as it provides continuous feedback that facilitates redesigning and fine-tuning of strategies on an ongoing basis.[16]

Apart from these, efforts must be made to identify the various stakeholders involved, assess the manpower and financial resources available through a situation analysis and identify the extent of the problem, region and statewise, along with identifying the barriers. It is essential to obtain political commitment, otherwise strategies are likely to remain only on paper or only partially implemented, if implemented at all.[16]

■ CONCLUSION

Suicide is a major public health problem in India. The enormity of suicide deaths in the country calls for immediate action. The magnitude of the problem and the paucity of resources necessitates collaboration and cooperation across a variety of stakeholders to implement strategies that are culturally relevant and cost-effective. There is an immediate need for implementation of a comprehensive surveillance system for recording suicides and attempted suicides which is a necessary first-step in quantifying the scale of the problem and subsequently offering guidance for intervention and policy provision. More research with a focus on adapting interventions to the cultural context taking into considering the local risk and protective factors are needed. A bottom-up approach based on local or regional suicide prevention activities can provide a basis for the development of a national suicide prevention strategy. Efforts to destigmatize suicide and encourage help seeking are of paramount importance and awareness creation is essential at the individual, social, and community level. There is a strong requirement for political will to ensure prioritization and implementation of suicide prevention strategies, failing which India is unlikely to meet its commitment on the SDG 2030.

■ REFERENCES

1. World Health Organization. (2021). Suicide worldwide in 2019: global health estimates. [online] Available from: https://www.scribd.com/document/519919274/9789240026643-eng [Last accessed July, 2021].
2. Institute for Health Metrics and Evaluation. (2021). Global Health Data Exchange. [online] Available from: http://ghdx.healthdata.org/gbd-results-tool [Last accessed July, 2021].
3. India State-Level Disease Burden Initiative Suicide Collaborators. Gender differentials and state variations in suicide deaths in India: the Global Burden of Disease Study 1990-2016. Lancet Public Health. 2018;3(10):e478-89

4. Indian Council for Medical Research, Public Health Foundation of India, Institute for Health Metrics and Evaluation. (2021). GBD India Compare Viz Hub. [online] Available from: https://vizhub.healthdata.org/gbd-compare/india [Last accessed July, 2021].

5. Amudhan S, Gururaj G, Varghese M, Benegal V, Rao GN, Sheehan DV, et al. A population-based analysis of suicidality and its correlates: Findings from the National Mental Health Survey of India, 2015-16. Lancet Psychiatry. 2020;7(1):41-51.

6. Arya V, Page A, Dandona R, Vijayakumar L, Mayer P, Armstrong G. The geographic heterogeneity of suicide rates in India by religion, caste, tribe, and other backward classes. Crisis. 2019;40(5):370-4.

7. World Health Organization. (2021). Suicide. [online] Available from: https://www.who.int/india/health-topics/suicide [Last accessed July, 2021].

8. Vijayakumar L, Phillips M. Suicide Prevention in Low- and Middle-Income Countries. In: O'Connor RC, Pirkis J (eds). The International Handbook of Suicide Prevention. United States: John Wiley & Sons, Ltd.; 2016.

9. Vijayakumar L, Armson. Volunteer Perspective on Suicides. In: Hawton K (Ed). Prevention and Treatment of Suicidal Behaviour. Oxford: Oxford University Press; 2005. pp. 335-50.

10. Vijayakumar L, Daly C, Arafat Y, Arensman E. Suicide prevention in the Southeast Asia region. Crisis: J Crisis Interven Suicide Prevent., 2020;41(Suppl 1):S21-29.

11. Jacob K, Sharan P, Mirza I, Garrido-Cumbrera M, Seedat S, Mari J, et al. Mental health systems in countries: Where are we now? Lancet. 2007;370:1061-77.

12. Vijayakumar L, Nagaraj K, John S. Suicide and Suicide Prevention in Developing Countries. Disease Control Priorities Project Working Paper No 27; 2004.

13. Gururaj G, Isaac MK, Subbakrishna DK, Ranjani R. Risk factors for completed suicides: A case-control study from Bangalore, India. Inj Control Saf Promot. 2004;11(3):183-91.

14. Kumar PN, George B. Life events, social support, coping strategies, and quality of life in attempted suicide: A case-control study. Indian J Psychiatry. 2013;55(1):46-51.

15. Arya V, Page A, River J, Armstrong G, Mayer P. Trends and socio-economic determinants of suicide in India: 2001-2013. Soc Psychiatry Psychiatr Epidemiol. 2018;53(3):269-78.

16. Vijayakumar L. Suicide in women. Indian J Psychiatry. 2015;57(Suppl 2):S233-8.

17. World Health Organization. (2018). National suicide prevention strategies: progress, examples and indicators. [online] Available from: https://www.who.int/publications/i/item/national-suicide-prevention-strategies-progress-examples-and-indicators. [Last accessed July, 2021].

18. Vijayakumar L, Chandra PS, Kumar MS, Pathare S, Banerjee D, Goswami T, et al. National suicide prevention strategy in India: Context and considerations for urgent action. The Lancet Psychiatry. 2022;9(2):160-8.

19. Patel V, Ramasundarahettige C, Vijayakumar L, Thakur JS, Gajalakshmi V, Gururaj G, et al. Suicide mortality in India: A nationally representative survey. Lancet. 2012;379(9834):2343-51.

20. Dandona R, Bertozzi-Villa A, Kumar GA, Dandona L. Lessons from a decade of suicide surveillance in India: Who, why and how? Int J Epidemiol. 2017;46(3):983-93.

21. Vijaykumar L. Suicide and its prevention: The urgent need in India. Indian J Psychiatry. 2007;49(2):81-4.

22. Behere PB, Sathyanarayana Rao TS, Mulmule AN. Decriminalization of attempted suicide law: Journey of fifteen decades. Indian J Psychiatry. 2015;57(2):122-4.

23. Mahapatra D. (2020). Attempt to suicide punishable or survivor requires rehabilitation, asks SC. Times of India. [online] Available from: https://timesofindia.indiatimes.com/india/should-suicide-bid-be-punished-or-survivor-treated-with-care-sc/articleshow/78069068.cms. [Last accessed July, 2022].

24. Vijayakumar L, Pirkis J, Whiteford H. Suicide in developing countries (3) prevention efforts. Crisis. 2005;26(3):120-4.

25. National Crimes Record Bureau. Accidental deaths and suicides in India—2019. New Delhi: Government of India; 2020.

26. The Gazette of India. (2020). [online] Available from: http://egazette.nic.in/

WriteReadData/2020/219423.pdf [Last accessed July, 2022].

27. Bonvoisin T, Utyasheva L, Knipe D, Gunnell D, Eddleston M. Suicide by pesticide poisoning in India: A review of pesticide regulations and their impact on suicide trends. BMC Public Health. 2020;20:251.

28. Vijayakumar L, Pathare S, Jain N, Nardodkar R, Pandit D, Krishnamoorthy S, et al. Implementation of a comprehensive surveillance system for recording suicides and attempted suicides in rural India. BMJ Open. 2020;10:e038636.

29. World Health Organization. Preventing Suicide: A Resource for Media Professionals Update 2017. Reference No WHO/MSD/MER/17.5. Geneva, Switzerland: World Health Organization; 2017.

30. Vijayakumar L. Media matters in suicide—Indian guidelines on suicide reporting. Indian J Psychiatry. 2019;61:549-51.

31. Vijayakumar L, Mohanraj R, Kumar S, Jeyaseelan V, Sriram S, Shanmugam M. CASP—An intervention by community volunteers to reduce suicidal behaviour among refugees. Int J Soc Psychiatry. 2017;63(7):589-97.

32. Vijayakumar L, Jeyaseelan L, Kumar S, Mohanraj R, Devika S, Manikandan S. A central storage facility to reduce pesticide suicides—a feasibility study from India. BMC Public Health. 2013;13:850.

33. Vijayakumar L, Satheesh–Babu R. Does 'No Pesticide' reduce suicides? Int J Soc Psych. 2008;55(5):401-6.

34. Dandona R, Sagar R. COVID-638 19 offers an opportunity to reform mental health in India. Lancet Psychiatry. 2021;8(1):9-11.

35. Ministry of Health and Family Welfare, Government of India. (2020). Caring for Health Care Warriors—Mental Health Support During COVID-19. [online] Available from https://www.mohfw.gov.in/pdf/HCWMentalHealthSupportGuidanceJuly20201.pdf. [Last accessed July, 2022].

36. Vijayakumar L, Umamaheswari C, Ali ZS, Devaraj P, Kesavan K. Intervention for suicide attempters: A randomized controlled study. Indian J Psychiatry. 2011;53(3):244-8.

37. Patel V, Weobong B, Weiss HA, Anand A, Bhat B, Katti B, et al. The Healthy Activity Program (HAP), a lay counsellor-delivered brief psychological treatment for severe depression, in primary care in India: A randomised controlled trial. Lancet. 2017;389(10065):176-85.

38. World Health Organization. Preventing Suicide: A Global Imperative: WHO Report on Suicide. Geneva, Switzerland: World Health Organization; 2014.

39. World Health Organization. mhGAP Intervention Guide for Mental, Neurological and Substance use Disorders in Non-specialized Health Settings: Mental Health Gap Action Programme (mhGAP). Geneva: World Health Organization; 2016.

40. World Health Organization. (2014). Preventing suicide: A resource for nonfatal suicidal behavior case registration. [online] Available from: https://apps.who.int/iris/bitstream/10665/112852/1/9789241506717_eng.pdf [Last accessed July, 2022].

41. Wasserman D, Rihmer Z, Rujescu D, Sarchiapone M, Sokolowski M, Titelman D, et al. The European Psychiatric Association (EPA) guidance on suicide treatment and prevention. Eur Psychiatry. 2012;27:129-41.

42. Kapur N, Steeg S, Webb R, Haigh M, Bergen H, Hawton K, et al. Does clinical management improve outcomes following self-harm? Results from the multicentre study of self-harm in England. PLoS One. 2013;8:e70434.

43. Fleischmann A, Bertolote JM, Wasserman D, De Leo D, Bolhari J, Botega NJ, et al. Effectiveness of brief intervention and contact for suicide attempters: A randomized controlled trial in five countries', randomized controlled trial in five countries. Bull World Health Organ. 2008;86:703-9.

44. Luxton DD, June JD, Comtois KA. Can post discharge follow-up contacts prevent suicide and suicidal behaviour? A review of the evidence. Crisis. 2013;34:32-41.

45. Vijayakumar L, Silverman M. Suicide and the prevention of suicidal behaviours (chapter 38). in: Bhugra D, Bhui K, Wong SYS, Gilman SE (Eds). Textbook of Public Mental Health. Oxford: Oxford University Press; 2018.

46. World Health Organization. (2012). Public health action for the prevention of suicide: A framework. Geneva: World Health Organization.

Index